ATLAS OF
Ultrasound-Guided Musculoskeletal Injections

ATLAS OF
Ultrasound-Guided Musculoskeletal Injections

Gerard A. Malanga, MD

Clinical Professor
Department of Physical Medicine and Rehabilitation
UMDNJ—New Jersey Medical School
Newark, New Jersey
Founding Partner
New Jersey Sports Medicine, LLC
Summit, New Jersey

Kenneth R. Mautner, MD

Assistant Professor
Department of Orthopaedics
Physical Medicine and Rehabilitation
Emory Healthcare
Atlanta, Georgia

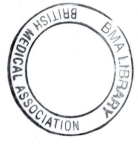

McGraw Hill Education | Medical

New York   Chicago   San Francisco   Athens   London   Madrid
Mexico City   Milan   New Delhi   Singapore   Sydney   Toronto

Atlas of Ultrasound-Guided Musculoskeletal Injections

1 2 3 4 5 6 7 8 9 0   CTP/CTP   19 18 17 16 15 14

ISBN 978-0-07-176967-9
MHID 0-07-176967-6

This book was set in Times by Thomson Digital.
The editors were Brian Belval and Christina M. Thomas.
The production supervisor was Catherine Saggese.
Project management was provided by Ritu Joon, Thomson Digital.
The text designer was Janice Bielawa.
The cover designer was Thomas De Pierro.
China Translation & Printing Services, Ltd. was printer and binder.

Library of Congress Cataloging-in-Publication Data

Atlas of ultrasound-guided musculoskeletal injections / [edited by] Gerard Malanga, Kenneth R. Mautner.
  p. ; cm.
Includes bibliographical references and index.
ISBN-13: 978-0-07-176967-9 (print book : alk. paper)
ISBN-10: 0-07-176967-6 (print book : alk. paper)
ISBN-13: 978-0-07-177204-4 (ebook)
I. Malanga, Gerard A. II. Mautner, Kenneth R.
[DNLM: 1. Musculoskeletal Diseases—ultrasonography—Atlases. 2. Injections—methods—Atlases. 3. Nerve Block—methods—Atlases. 4. Orthopedic Procedures—methods—Atlases. 5. Ultrasonography, Interventional—methods—Atlases. WE 17]
RC925.7
616.7'07543—dc23

                                                                      2013014104

McGraw-Hill Education books are available at special quantity discounts to use as premiums and sales promotions, or for use in corporate training programs. To contact a representative, please visit the Contact Us pages at www.mhprofessional.com.

CONTENTS

SECTION V Pelvis   183

SECTION VIII Special Procedures   419

CONTRIBUTORS

Joseph J. Albano, MD

Private Practice of Regenerative and Sports Medicine
Team Physician for US Speedskating, Real Salt Lake Soccer,
  US Military Cycling
Westminster College
Salt Lake City, Utah

Danielle Aufiero, MD

Clinical Assistant Professor
Department of Physical Medicine and Rehabilitation
Western University of Health Sciences
Pomona, California

Matthew Axtman, DO

Sports Medicine Fellow
Department of Orthopaedics
Emory University
Atlanta, Georgia

Luis Baerga-Varela, MD

Assistant Professor
Department of Physical Medicine, Rehabilitation and Sports Medicine
University of Puerto Rico
San Juan, Puerto Rico

Darryl Eugene Barnes, MD

Consultant
Department of Orthopedics
Mayo Clinic Health System
Austin, Minnesota

Marko Bodor, MD

Assistant Professor
Department of Neurological Surgery
University of California San Francisco
San Francisco, California

Jay E. Bowen, DO

Assistant Professor
Department of Physical Medicine and Rehabilitation
University of Medicine and Dentistry of New Jersey
Newark, New Jersey

Alberto Capa-Grasa, MD, PhD

Attending Physician
Physical Medicine and Rehabilitation
University Hospital La Paz
Attending Physician
Sports Medicine and Physical Education
University Hospital La Paz
Madrid, Spain

Gary P. Chimes, MD, PhD

Assistant Professor
Department of Physical Medicine and Rehabilitation
University of Pittsburgh Medical Center
Fellowship Director, Musculoskeletal Sports & Spine Fellowship
Division Chief of Physical Medicine and Rehabilitation, UPMC-East
Pittsburgh, Pennsylvania

John C. Cianca, MD

Clinical Associate Professor
Baylor College of Medicine
Department of Physical Medicine and Rehabilitation
Private Practice
Baylor College of Medicine
Houston, Texas

Jackson Cohen, MD

Resident
Department of Rehabilitation Medicine
University of Miami School of Medicine
Miami, Florida

Sean Colio, MD

Sports Medicine Physiatrist
Swedish Spine, Sports, and Musculoskeletal Medicine
Swedish Medical Group
Seattle, Washington

Paul A. Cook, MD

Physician
Hand and Microsurgery Associates, Inc.
Columbus, Ohio

Megan Helen Cortazzo, MD

Assistant Professor
Vice Chair of Outpatient Services
Department of Physical Medicine and Rehabilitation
University of Pittsburgh School of Medicine
University of Pittsburgh Medical Center
Pittsburgh, Pennsylvania

Jerod A. Cottrill, DO

Private Practice
Department of Physical Medicine and Rehabilitation
Rebound Orthopedics
Portland, Oregon

B. Elizabeth Delasobera, MD

Sports Medicine Fellow
Department of Family Medicine
Fairfax Family Practice - VCU
Fairfax, Virginia
Attending Physician
Department of Emergency Medicine
Georgetown University Hospital
Washington, District of Columbia

Rahul Naren Desai, MD

Sports and Pain Interventionalist
Musculoskeletal Radiology
EPIC Imaging
Portland, Oregon

Kevin deWeber, MD, FAAFP, FACSM

Assistant Professor
Department of Family Medicine
Uniformed Services University of the Health Sciences
Bethesda, Maryland
Director, Military Sports Medicine Fellowship
Department of Family Medicine
Ft. Belvoir Community Hospital
Ft. Belvoir, Virginia

Kevin B. Dunn, MD, MS

New Jersey Sports Medicine, LLC
Cedar Knolls, New Jersey

John FitzGerald, MD

Associate Clinical Professor
David Geffen School of Medicine
Department of Medicine and Rheumatology
University of California Los Angeles
Los Angeles, California

Michael Fredericson, MD

Professor and Attending Physician
Department of Orthopaedic Surgery
Stanford University, Hospital and Clinics
Stanford, California

Bradley D. Fullerton, MD

Medical Director
Private Practice Physiatrist
Department of Physical Medicine and Rehabilitation
Specialty Care Center Pediatric Spasticity Clinic
Dell Children's Medical Center of Central Texas
Austin, Texas

Charles E. Garten II, MD

Private Practice
Sports Medicine
Myers Sports Medicine and Orthopaedic Center
Atlanta, Georgia

Ched Garten, MD

Myers Sports Medicine and Orthopaedic Center
Atlanta, Georgia

Alfred C. Gellhorn, MD

Clinical Assistant Professor
Department of Rehabilitation Medicine
University of Washington
Seattle, Washington

Michael Goldin, MD

Fellow
Department of Physical Medicine and Rehabilitation
University of Medicine and Dentistry of New Jersey
Newark, New Jersey

Bradly S. Goodman, MD

Associate Professor
Department of Physical Medicine and Rehabilitation
University of Alabama at Birmingham
Birmingham, Alabama
Associate Professor
Department of Physical Medicine and Rehabilitation
University of Missouri at Columbia
Columbia, Missouri

Joshua G. Hackel, MD, FAAFP

Associate Professor
Florida State School of Medicine
Tallahassee, Florida
Team Physician
Department of Athletics
University of West Florida
Pensacola, Florida

Nelson A. Hager, MS, MD

Associate Clinical Professor
Department of Physical Medicine and Rehabilitation
University of Washington School of Medicine
Medical Director
Bone and Joint, Sports and Spine Center
University of Washington Medical Center
Seattle, Washington

Mederic M. Hall, MD

Assistant Professor
Department of Orthopaedics and Rehabilitation
University of Iowa Sports Medicine Center
Iowa City, Iowa

Jonathan S. Halperin, MD

Clinical Associate
Division of Physiatry
Sharp Rees Stealy Medical Group
San Diego, California

Ronald W. Hanson Jr, MD, CAQSM

Fellowship Director, Interventional Orthopedics
Center for Regenerative Medicine
The Centeno-Schultz Clinic
Broomfield, Colorado

Keith Hardy, MD

Clinical Instructor
Department of Rehabilitation Medicine
University of Washington
Seattle, Washington

Kimberly G. Harmon, MD

Clinical Professor
Family Medicine and Orthopaedics and Sports Medicine
University of Washington
Team Physician
University of Washington
Seattle, Washington

Eric Robert Helm, MD

Resident
Department of Physical Medicine and Rehabilitation
University of Pittsburgh School of Medicine
Pittsburgh, Pennsylvania

Troy Henning, DO

Assistant Professor and Attending Physician
Department of Physical Medicine and Rehabilitation
University of Michigan
Ann Arbor, Michigan

John C. Hill, DO, FACSM, FAAFP

Professor
Director of Primary Care Sports Medicine Fellowship
Department of Family Medicine
University of Colorado School of Medicine
Denver, Colorado

Garry Wai Keung Ho, MD, CAQSM

Assistant Program Director
Sports Medicine
VCU-Fairfax Family Practice and Sports Medicine
Fairfax, Virginia
Assistant Professor
Family Medicine
Virginia Commonwealth University School of Medicine
Richmond, Virginia

Anne Z. Hoch, DO

Professor
Department of Orthopaedic Surgery
Medical College of Wisconsin
Milwaukee, Wisconsin

Thomas M. Howard, MD, FACSM

Assistant Clinical Professor
Department of Family Medicine
VCU School of Medicine
Richmond, Virginia

Mandy Huggins, MD

Staff Physician
Department of Orthopaedics
Broward Health Physician Group
Ft. Lauderdale, Florida

Mark-Friedrich Berthold Hurdle, MD

Assistant Professor
Department of Physical Medicine and Rehabilitation
Mayo Clinic College of Medicine
Jacksonville, Florida

Garrett S. Hyman, MD, MPH

Clinical Assistant Professor
Department of Rehabilitation Medicine
University of Washington
Seattle, Washington
Consulting Physician
Northwest Spine and Sports Physicians, PC
Kirkland, Washington

Victor Ibrahim, MD

Assistant Professor
Department of Rehabilitation Medicine
Georgetown University School of Medicine
Director, Ultrasound and Regenerative Medicine
National Rehabilitation Hospital
Washington, District of Columbia

Jon A. Jacobson, MD

Professor
Director, Division of Musculoskeletal Radiology
Department of Radiology
University of Michigan
Ann Arbor, Michigan

Prathap Jayaram, MD

Resident
Department of Physical Medicine and Rehabilitation
Baylor College of Medicine/University of Houston Alliance
Houston, Texas

Mark Edward Lavallee, MD, CSCS, FACSM

Associate Clinical Professor
Department of Family Medicine
Indiana University School of Medicine
Co-Director
South Bend-Notre Dame Sports Medicine Fellowship Program
Memorial Hospital
South Bend, Indiana

Matthew Leiszler, MD

Fellow
Primary Care Sports Medicine
University of Colorado
Denver, Colorado

Paul H. Lento, MD

Associate Professor
Department of Physical Medicine and Rehabilitation
Temple University School of Medicine
Attending Physician
Department of Physical Medicine and Rehabilitation
Temple University Hospital
Philadelphia, Pennsylvania

John M. Lesher, MD, MPH

Adjunct Assistant Professor
Department of Physical Medicine and Rehabilitation
University of North Carolina
Chapel Hill, North Carolina
Attending Physician
Department of Physical Medicine and Rehabilitation
Carolina Neurosurgery and Spine Associates
Charlotte, North Carolina

John L. Lin, MD

Assistant Professor
Department of Rehabilitation
Emory University
Director of Post Acute Spinal Cord Services
Shepherd Center
Atlanta, Georgia

Arthur Jason De Luigi, DO, FAAPMR, DAPM

Assistant Professor
Department of Rehabilitation Medicine
Georgetown University School of Medicine
Director, Sports Medicine
Department of Rehabilitation Medicine
National Rehabilitation Hospital/Georgetown University Hospital
Washington, District of Columbia

Gerard A. Malanga, MD

Clinical Professor
Department of Physical Medicine and Rehabilitation
UMDNJ—New Jersey Medical School
Newark, New Jersey
Founding Partner
New Jersey Sports Medicine, LLC
Summit, New Jersey

Jennifer K. Malcolm, DO

Sports Medicine Fellow
Sports Medicine Institute
Saint Joseph Regional Medical Center
Mishawaka, Indiana
Mark Lavallee, Maryland
Department of Sports Medicine
Memorial Hospital
South Bend, Indiana

Srinivas Mallempati, MD

Attending Physician
Department of Physical Medicine and Rehabilitation
St. Vincents East
Attending Physician
Department of Physical Medicine and Rehabilitation
Trinity Medical Center
Birmingham, Alabama

Sean N. Martin, DO

Faculty
Family Medicine Residency
HQ Air Armament Center
Eglin Air Force Base, Florida
Sports Medicine Physician

Javier Vaquero Martín, MD, PhD

Professor
Department of Orthopaedic Surgery
University of Gregorio Marañón
Madrid, Spain

R. Amadeus Mason, MD

Assistant Professor
Department of Orthopaedics
Emory University School of Medicine
Atlanta, Georgia

Kenneth R. Mautner, MD

Assistant Professor
Department of Orthopaedics
Physical Medicine and Rehabilitation
Emory Healthcare
Atlanta, Georgia

Matthew D. Maxwell, MD

Department of Physical Medicine and Rehabilitation
University of Pittsburgh Medical Center
Pittsburgh, Pennsylvania

John M. McShane, MD

McShane Sports Medicine
Villanova, Pennsylvania

Brandon J. Messerli, DO

Evergreen Sport and Spine Center
Department of Physiatry
Evergreen Health
Kirkland, Washington

Johan Michaud, MD, FRCPC

Associate Professor of Physiatry
Centre Hospitalier de l'Université de Montréal
Ultrasound Consultant
Institut De Physiatrie du Québec
Montreal, Québec
Canada

Megan Groh Miller, MD

Department of Primary Care Sports Medicine
UMDNJ-Robert Wood Johnson
New Brunswick, New Jersey

Robert Monaco, MD

Director of Sports Medicine
Department of Athletics
Rutgers University
Piscataway, New Jersey
Clinical Assistant Professor
Department of Family Medicine
UMDNJ-Robert Wood Johnson Medical School
New Brunswick, New Jersey

Sean W. Mulvaney, MD

Assistant Professor
Department of Emergency and Military Medicine
Uniformed Services University
Bethesda, Maryland

Rebecca Ann Myers, MD

Sports Medicine Fellow
Sports Medicine
University of Notre Dame
South Bend, Indiana

Megan L. Noon, MD

Assistant Professor
Department of Orthopaedic Surgery, Physical Medicine
  and Rehabilitation
Medical College of Wisconsin
Milwaukee, Wisconsin

Kambiz Nooryani, MD

Department of Physical Medicine and Rehabilitation
New Jersey Medical School
Newark, New Jersey

Prasanth Nuthakki, MD

Fellow
Interventional Physiatry
Alabama Orthopedic Spine and Sports Medicine Associates
Birmingham, Alabama

Jeffrey M. Payne, MD

Mayo Clinic Health System
Faribault, Minnesota

Evan Peck, MD

Associate Staff
Section of Sports Medicine
Department of Orthopaedic Surgery
Cleveland Clinic, Florida
West Palm Beach and Weston, Florida
Affiliate Assistant Professor
Charles E. Schmidt College of Medicine, Florida Atlantic University
Boca Raton, Florida

Scott Jeffery Primack, DO, FAAPMR, FACOPMR

Senior Clinical Instructor
Department of Physical Medicine and Rehabilitation
School of Public Health, University of Colorado School of Health
Aurora, Colorado

Guillermo Emilio Rodríguez-Maruri, MD

Resident
Department of Physical Medicine and Rehabilitation
Gregorio Marañón Hospital
Madrid, Spain

Eugene Yousik Roh, MD

Clinical Assistant Professor
Department of Orthopedics, Physical Medicine and Rehabilitation
Stanford University Medical Center
Redwood City, California

Jose Manuel Rojo Manaute, MD, PhD

Dr. Prof. Javier Vaquero Martín
Department of Orthopaedic Surgery
University Hospital Gregorio Marañón
Madrid, Spain

Joseph J. Ruane, DO

Associate Clinical Professor
Sports Medicine
Ohio University College of Osteopathic Medicine
Athens, Ohio
Medical Director
Spine, Sport & Joint Center
Riverside Methodist Hospital
Columbus, Ohio

Gregory R. Saboeiro, MD

Associate Professor
Department of Radiology
Weill Cornell Medical Center
Attending Physician
Department of Radiology
Hospital for Special Surgery
New York, New York

Steven Sampson, DO

Clinical Instructor
Medicine
David Geffen School of Medicine at UCLA
Los Angeles, California
Clinical Assistant Professor
Department of Physical Medicine and Rehabilitation
Western University of Health Sciences
Pomona, California

Jacob L. Sellon, MD

Sports Medicine Fellow
Sports Medicine Center
Department of Physical Medicine and Rehabilitation
Mayo Clinic
Rochester, Minnesota

Asal Sepassi, MD

Extern
Department of Physical Medicine and Rehabilitation
University of Medicine and Dentistry
Newark, New Jersey

Brian J. Shiple, DO

Assistant Clinical Professor
Department of Family Medicine
Temple University School of Medicine
Philadelphia, Pennsylvania

Jevon Simerly

RestorePDX
Portland, Oregon

Jay Smith, MD

Professor
Department of Physical Medicine and Rehabilitation
Mayo Clinic
Consultant
Departments of Physical Medicine and Rehabilitation and Radiology
Mayo Clinic
Rochester, Minnesota

Matthew Thomas Smith, MD
Spine Health Institute
Altamonte, Florida

Joanne Borg Stein, MD
Associate Professor
Department of Physical Medicine and Rehabilitation
Harvard Medical School
Boston, Massachusetts

Henry A. Stiene, MD, FACSM
Team Physician
Department of Family Medicine
Beacon Orthopaedics and Sports Medicine Xavier University
Cincinnati, Ohio

Todd P. Stitik, MD
Professor
Department of Physical Medicine and Rehabilitation
New Jersey Medical School
Director, Occupational/Musculoskeletal Medicine
Physical Medicine and Rehabilitation
New Jersey Medical School
Newark, New Jersey

Jeffrey A. Strakowski, MD
Clinical Associate Professor
Department of Physical Medicine and Rehabilitation
The Ohio State University School of Medicine
Associate Director of Medical Education
Department of Physical Medicine and Rehabilitation
Riverside Methodist Hospital
Columbus, Ohio

Kate E. Temme, MD
Clinical Instructor
Department of Orthopaedic Surgery
Medical College of Wisconsin
Milwaukee, Wisconsin

Jose A. Ramirez-Del Toro, MD
Clinical Instructor
Department of Physical Medicine and Rehabilitation
University of Pittsburgh Medical Center (UPMC)
Director of Sports Medicine
California University of Pennsylvania
Director of Sports Medicine and Spine Care
The Orthopedic Group, PC
Pittsburgh, Pennsylvania

Paul D. Tortland, DO, FAOASM
Medical Director
Valley Sports Physicians and Orthopedic Medicine
Avon, Connecticut
Assistant Clinical Professor
Department of Medicine
University of Connecticut School of Medicine
Farmington, Connecticut

Ricardo J. Vasquez-Duarte, MD
Assistant Professor
Department of Physical Medicine and Rehabilitation
University of Miami Miller School of Medicine
Miami, Florida

Christopher J. Visco, MD
Assistant Professor
Department of Rehabilitation and Regenerative Medicine
Columbia University College of Physicians and Surgeons
Assistant Attending Physician
Department of Rehabilitation and Regenerative Medicine
New York Presbyterian Hospital
New York, New York

Brandee L. Waite, MD
Assistant Professor
Associate Director Sports Medicine Fellowship
Department of Physical Medicine and Rehabilitation
University of California Davis School of Medicine
Sacramento, California

Nicholas H. Weber, DO
Resident Physician
Department of Physical Medicine and Rehabilitation
University of Pittsburgh Medical Center
Pittsburgh, Pennsylvania

Adam D. Weglein, DO, DABMA
Assistant Clinical Professor
Department of Family Medicine
University of Texas Houston Medical School
Houston, Texas

Beth M. Weinman, DO
Resident Physician
Department of Orthopaedics
Medical College of Wisconsin
Milwaukee, Wisconsin

Steve J. Wisniewski, MD
Assistant Professor
Department of Physical Medicine and Rehabilitation
Mayo Clinic
Rochester, Minnesota

Amy X. Yin, MD
Resident Physician
Department of Physical Medicine and Rehabilitation
Harvard Medical School/Spaulding Rehabilitation Hospital
Boston, Massachusetts

This book is long overdue. Since I started using ultrasound to inject hip joints in our sports medicine center in October 2003, the use of ultrasound to perform diagnostic and therapeutic interventional procedures has increased dramatically. In 2003, ultrasound-guided musculoskeletal interventions were primarily performed by radiologists, dedicated musculoskeletal ultrasound (MSK US) courses emphasizing interventional procedures were sparse, and the peer-reviewed literature contained perhaps a few dozen articles focusing on interventional MSK US. Nearly a decade later, US-guided musculoskeletal interventions are regularly performed by not only radiologists but also physiatrists, family practitioners, rheumatologists, anesthesiologists, orthopedic surgeons, podiatrists, neurologists, and multiple other groups. Interventional MSK US training has been integrated into many residency and fellowship training programs. Dedicated MSK US courses are relatively easy to find, and many include specific interventional training on cadavers. Finally, depending on the journals you read (and my friends and colleagues know that my list is long), there are one or more articles pertaining to interventional MSK US published every month. Admittedly, it is becoming increasingly difficult to keep up with the field.

Although I, like many others, have reflected upon these past 10 years with both astonishment and a sense of accomplishment, I could not help but recognize that one important task had not yet been completed. Every well-established field has a reference text…a foundation…a "go to" resource. Yet, no such text existed in the field of interventional MSK US. Beginners in the field had no textbook from which to learn the basics of interventional MSK US. More experienced practitioners had no easily accessible reference to review less frequently performed procedures or efficiently familiarize themselves with new procedures. And finally, those who might be considered "experts" in the field of interventional MSK US by many had no place to share the wisdom they had gained through years of experience (and many mishaps). Consequently, I am extremely pleased that Drs. Gerry Malanga and Kenneth Mautner decided to produce this multi-authored textbook in which the "state of the art" of interventional MSK US is presented.

Atlas of Ultrasound-guided Musculoskeletal Injections provides a comprehensive overview of interventional MSK US presented in a logical and user-friendly format. Whereas the initial chapters cover the fundamentals of interventional MSK US, the main body of the text dedicates one chapter to each US-guided procedure. The format of each chapter has been standardized for learning efficiency and includes sections on key points, pertinent anatomy, common pathology, US imaging, indications, and technique. Perhaps most impressive is the vast spectrum of procedures covered in the text, which ranges from basic US-guided joint injections to perineural injections, tenotomies, and surgical procedures such as percutaneous A1 pulley release. Consequently, this text will appeal to practitioners from diverse backgrounds and skill levels.

Of particular importance to me is that this text is authored by experienced practitioners from multiple disciplines. In my opinion the dramatic advances of the past decade have been a direct result of the collaboration between enthusiastic practitioners from multiple disciplines who shared a common goal of improving patient care. Thus, *Atlas of Ultrasound-guided Musculoskeletal Injections* appropriately provides a written record of the field of interventional MSK US as told by many of those who actively participated in its development. Thanks to Gerry, Ken, and the multidisciplinary group of authors who have dedicated their expertise, time, and effort to fill an important gap in the field of interventional MSK US. In many ways, the publication of this textbook was necessary to provide a foundation from which we can move into the future and explore new methods to utilize US-guided interventions to improve patient care. As I said, this textbook is long overdue.

Jay Smith, MD
Mayo Clinic
Rochester, Minnesota

The use of diagnostic and interventional musculoskeletal ultrasound has greatly enhanced our abilities in the diagnosis and treatment of a variety of musculoskeletal conditions. Through our years of performing and teaching ultrasound-guided injections, it became apparent that there was no textbook to assist clinicians on how to properly perform various ultrasound-guided injections. The medical literature has increasingly demonstrated the superiority in accuracy of ultrasound-guided injections when compared to palpation-guided ("blind") injections. Many clinicians have experienced increased treatment options that can now be offered to patients through the use of ultrasound-guided injections.

As we write this book, the field of orthopedic medicine and the way we practice are facing a paradigm shift. For years, physicians of various specialties have used corticosteroid injections as a mainstay of treatment for issues from tendinitis to arthritis. We have done this with limited proof of their efficacy and significant evidence of the negative effects of corticosteroids on tendons and chondral cartilage that may result from this treatment. Over the past 5 years, orthobiologics treatments (i.e., the use of endogenous substances such as platelet-rich plasma and bone marrow stem cells) have been increasingly used and studied in treating soft tissue and cartilage disorders. The evidence for these treatments continues to evolve. In the next 10 years, it is likely that the old paradigm of treating supposed inflammation with steroid injections will continue to be replaced by using agents that will promote tissue repair and modulation (inhibition) of degenerative inflammatory mediators. Many minimally invasive techniques are being developed to deliver these orthobiologics, and ultrasound guidance is the predominate modality for delivering these injections to the target tissue.

The focus of this textbook is to describe the techniques for performing ultrasound-guided procedures without an emphasis on what is to be injected. Our goal is that each chapter could be read independently describing the equipment for the procedure, setup of the US machine, and approach to the target area for each specific procedure. As an atlas, we hope to cover almost every injection: joint, tendon, ligament, and major nerves of the body that one may encounter in clinical practice. We have also included some cutting-edge procedures, such as ultrasound-guided carpal tunnel release, which will likely expand in the years to come.

This book was a major collaborative effort among clinicians of various specialties who are considered to be leaders in the field of musculoskeletal ultrasound. We selected chapter authors based on current practice experience, as many of these injections have never been described in the literature and hence there are no studies to compare techniques. For these chapters we have tried to provide the most efficient way to reach the target tissue. We hope that this book will challenge the readers, should they not agree with us, to set up comparative studies that may further evaluate the effectiveness of these procedures. Such studies are already being carried out in various centers around the world. We hope that the readers of this Atlas find it helpful in optimizing the treatments that they offer to their patients providing a state-of-the-art approach to the use of ultrasound guidance. We look forward to your feedback to enhance this Atlas in the future.

We would like to thank the multiple chapter authors for their diligence in producing high-quality chapters. Special thanks to Brian Belval who initially approached us regarding the concept of this textbook. Many, many thanks to Sarah M. Granlund, the Project Manager of this textbook. It is only through her efforts in working with us as well as all the chapter authors that this textbook has become a reality.

Sincerely,

Gerard A. Malanga, MD
Kenneth R. Mautner, MD

We would like to thank all the authors who contributed to this book and all those who have advanced the field of Musculoskeletal Ultrasound over the past decade. We especially want to acknowledge Keith Hardy, a friend and contributor to this textbook, who recently passed away. Most importantly, none of this could be possible without the loving support of our wives and children.

Gerard A. Malanga, MD
Kenneth R. Mautner, MD

SECTION I

Introduction

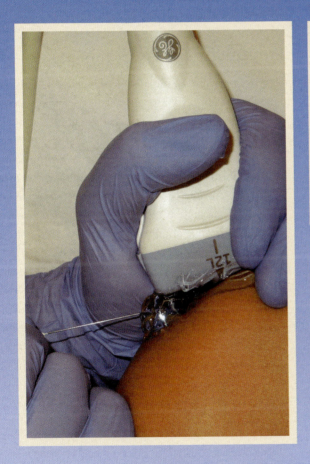
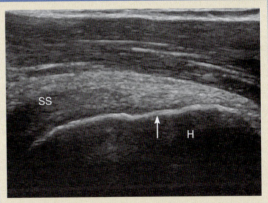
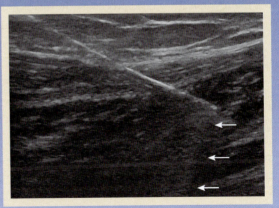

Christopher J. Visco, MD

General Considerations

Ultrasound guidance (USG) allows the physician to identify target structures for aspiration or injection with improved accuracy compared to nonguided procedures.[1] This improved accuracy is conferred because the needle shaft, tip, and target structure are constantly visualized in real time. The addition of USG requires a high level of anatomic knowledge, focus, manual skill, and substantial practice. Each soft tissue or boney structure has a different ideal technique, method of visualization, and needle choice; these details are more fully developed in each chapter in this text. Ultrasound has no absolute contraindication and is generally considered safe, but is subject to the limitations and skill of the user.

Indications

The indication for utilization of USG for any particular procedure should be considered, discussed during the informed consent, and documented. Indications are evolving in the literature and may be practice specific. Common indications could include lack of surface anatomic landmarks because of body habitus, proximity to neurovascular structures, a bleeding diathesis, aberrant anatomy, deeper structures, or a need to avoid radiation exposure in someone who would otherwise undergo a fluoroscopically guided procedure. In some cases, the failure of a nonguided procedure, or a need to be extremely accurate for a diagnostic injection may drive the utilization of ultrasound guidance.

Ultrasound Machine, Knobology, and Physics

A prerequisite to performing USG procedures includes a familiarity with the machine and image optimization. Choose the type of transducer that best accommodates the injection. A linear array transducer is often best for most procedures where the structure is superficial and the needle angle is shallow. A curvilinear array is best for the deep structures such as the hip, or where body habitus necessitates. Visualize structures in both orthogonal planes (long axis and short axis). Adjust the depth, frequency, and focus with each new target structure to best optimize the image. Then adjust gain, and then time-gain compensation as needed. Use color or power Doppler

to evaluate for vascular structures. Anisotropy, a property of certain tissues that causes them to appear differently as waves hit them in varying directions (eg, ultrasound waves that hit tendon in a nonperpendicular direction cause reflection at an angle too great to return the signal to the transducer), can cause dense ligamentous or tendon structures to appear artificially dark. When structures are darker relative to other structures in the field of view, the ultrasound waves pass through, are absorbed, or reflected, and this is described as *hypoechoic*. Hyperechoic is a term used when structures are brighter relative to others (waves return to transducer). *Isoechoic* describes equal echogenicity to other structures in the field of view, and an *anechoic* image is devoid of signal (black).

Preparation and Pre-Scanning

Routinely perform an initial scan prior to each injection. This is done to obtain key information about the target structure and plan for the procedure. Adjust the patient height, ultrasound screen, and machine location for the best ergonomic setup. The best transducer type, needle length, and trajectory can be determined at this time. Anticipate obliquity by assessing depth; if a structure is deep, a longer needle may be needed; if a very steep angle is taken, it will be difficult to visualize the needle because of anisotropy. The preferred trajectory is in plane, but certain procedures are performed out of plane for anatomic reasons. The pre-scan is also helpful for identifying adjacent structures to avoid, such as neurovascular structures, anomalous anatomy, or unintended masses and pathology.[2] Optimize the image during the pre-scan by adjusting the depth, frequency, and focus. Consider adding multiple focal zones to best visualize both the target structure and the needle.

Performing the Procedure

Before performing an USG procedure, an appropriate time out should be taken.[3] Aseptic technique should be maintained and is discussed more in Chapter 3. Prepare the injectate and procedure materials in close proximity to the machine and patient. Use the same trajectory that was determined during the pre-scan; often a skin mark is helpful to return to the same position. The freehand technique allows physicians to stabilize the transducer with the nondominant hand, anchoring it to the patient's skin with their fingers or heel of the hand and inject with the dominant

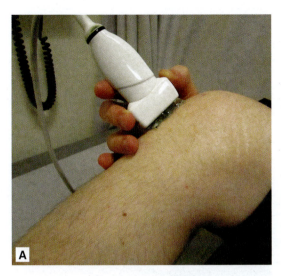 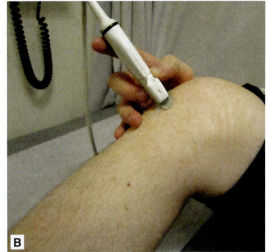

FIGURE 1-1 ■ Long axis (**A**) and short axis (**B**).

hand. Advance slowly moving only the needle or the transducer at once, not both simultaneously. Avoid advancing the needle without visualizing the tip. Techniques to help with identifying a needle in the field of view include rotating the bevel, using a small amount of jiggle, and manipulating the stylet.

Documentation

Store any relevant images of key structures for future reference. An image of the needle in place at the target structure should routinely be saved. When relevant, include pre- and postinjection images, particularly any measurements (tendon tear, cyst, or effusion size), and annotate accordingly. Document the procedure in the medical record and include ultrasound findings from the pre-scan. Include a brief discussion of the indications for using ultrasound in each documented procedure.

Definitions

1. Transducer relative to target (Figure 1-1)
   (1) Long axis (longitudinal): The transducer is parallel to the normal anatomic alignment of the target structure (eg, the tendon fibers are running across the screen).
   (2) Short axis (transverse): The transducer is perpendicular to the target structure.
2. Needle relative to transducer (Figure 1-2)
   (1) In plane: Generally, this is the preferred technique. The entire needle shaft and tip as well as the target structure are visualized constantly.
   (2) Out of plane: The transducer is oriented perpendicular to the needle shaft, so only a point of hyperechoic needle is seen when in the field of view. The main disadvantage is the inability to ascertain if the needle

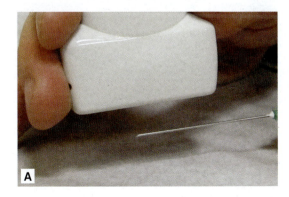 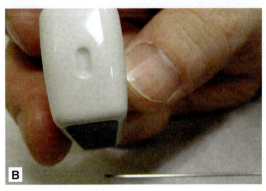

FIGURE 1-2 ■ In plane (**A**) and out of plane (**B**).

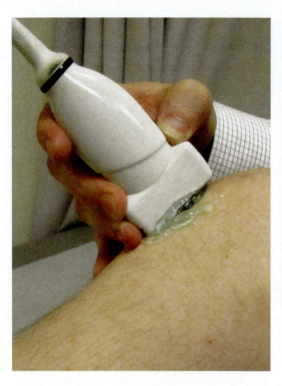 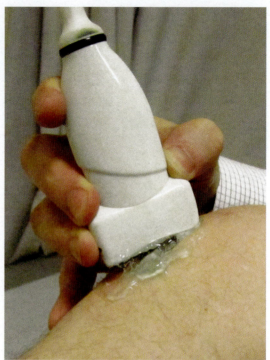

FIGURE 1-3 ■ Heel-Toe of transducer in the long axis.

has passed the plane of the transducer. Used sparingly for superficial joints. Use the walk-down technique to ensure visualization of the needle tip.

3. Transducer positioning for USG procedures
   (1) Translation: The transducer is moved in one orthogonal direction (long axis or short axis) in reference to the target structure.
   (2) Rotation: The transducer is spun.
   (3) Heel-Toe: The transducer is angled in the long axis (Figure 1-3).
   (4) Tilt/Wag: The transducer is angled in the short axis (Figure 1-4).
   (5) Compression: Increasing or decreasing the direct physical pressure with the transducer.
   (6) Stand-off oblique: Build up the gel under one end of the transducer. This oblique technique allows the needle

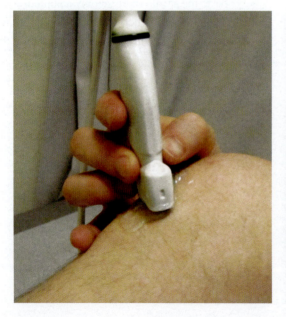 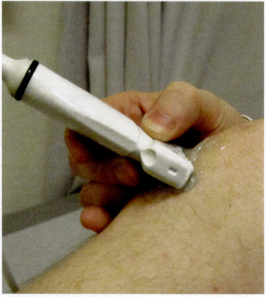

FIGURE 1-4 ■ Tilt/Wag of transducer in the short axis.

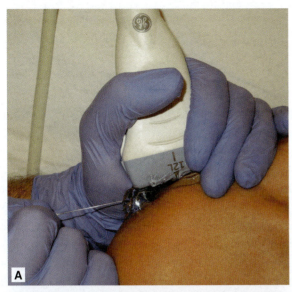

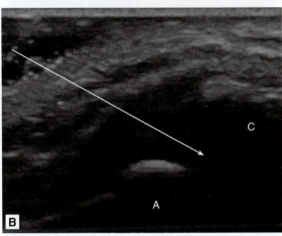

FIGURE 1-5 ■ **A.** Setup demonstrating stand-off oblique technique to superficial injection (acromioclavicular joint in this example). **B.** Accompanying ultrasound view. *Arrow* represents needle path. Top left corner is stand-off gel to reduce angle of entry. A, acromion; C, clavicle.

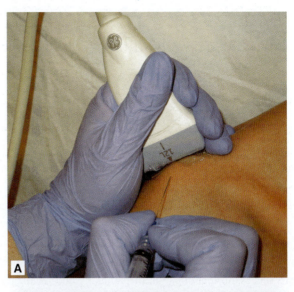

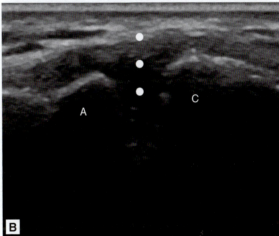

FIGURE 1-6 ■ **A.** Setup demonstrating walk-down technique to superficial joint injection (acromioclavicular joint in this example). **B.** Accompanying ultrasound view. *Dots* represent needle path toward joint. A, acromion; C, clavicle.

to pass through the gel and decreases needle anisotropy (similar to the Heel-Toe effect) (Figure 1-5).

(7) Walk Down: A technique used during an out-of-plane injection to prevent inserting the needle too deeply or beyond the plane of transducer (Figure 1-6).

- Insert the needle relatively superficially until the tip can be seen.
- Withdraw and angle more steeply until the tip of the needle again meets the plane of transducer.
- Continue to withdraw and approach more deeply until the needle tip meets the target structure.

References

1. Daley EL, Bajaj S, Bisson LJ, Cole BJ. Improving injection accuracy of the elbow, knee, and shoulder: does injection site and imaging make a difference? A systematic review. *Am J Sports Med*. 2011;39(3):656–662.
2. Smith J, Finnoff JT. Diagnostic and interventional musculoskeletal ultrasound: part 1. fundamentals. *PM&R*. 2009;1(1):64–75.
3. Standards and Guidelines for the Accreditation of Ultrasound Practices. American Institute of Ultrasound in Medicine. www.aium.org. 2011.

CHAPTER 2 Ultrasound Physics for Interventional Procedures

Matthew D. Maxwell, MD / Nicholas H. Weber, DO / Gary P. Chimes, MD, PhD

Ultrasound Physics

Ultrasound (US) imaging is unique in that it uses sound waves to create high-resolution images in real time, allowing for dynamic imaging with minimal ionizing radiation. However, US waves can be physically altered, obscuring the clarity of the images and hindering its use for diagnostic and therapeutic purposes. Therefore, it is important to understand the basic physics of US imaging and the technical difficulties that may arise from it. Proper understanding will allow the clinician more successful identification of pathology and localization of clinically relevant structures during intervention.

Basic Principles

Although there are many types of transducers available, all share a fundamental component that makes US imaging possible: the piezoelectric crystal. A piezoelectric crystal allows for the conversion of physical energy (in this case, in the form of sounds waves) into electrical energy. Arrays of these crystals both project and receive sound waves, converting them into functional images. Various transducers have different array designs; however, all perform this basic function. Piezoelectric crystals have variable physical characteristics beyond the scope of this chapter; however, it is important to note that crystals selected for medical imaging are able to transmit and receive a wide range of frequencies while minimizing signal interference that may degrade image quality.

When voltage potential is applied to the array of crystals, they emit sound waves into the adjacent tissues. As the waves encounter tissues of different densities, a portion of them are bounced back to the transducer as a series of echoes; these echoes provide the necessary data to create a two-dimensional image of the underlying tissue. The resulting image is comprised of a number of pixels, each of which represents three inherent properties of each reflected echo. The first property is the intensity of the echo; the more of the sound that is reflected, the brighter the image. The second property is the depth at which the echo is reflected, corresponding to the vertical position of the image provided. This is a function of the echo's "time of flight" or the time elapsed between sound wave emission and its echo's return; the deeper the structure, the longer the time of flight. The third property is the horizontal position of each pixel, which is simply a function of the crystal's position on the transducer.

Several physical factors interfere with beam transmission, making a functional image difficult to produce—a principle known as *attenuation*. First, a portion of the energy is absorbed as frictional forces convert wave energy into heat. Second, as the beam encounters different tissue interfaces, reflection causes a portion of the wave to travel in different directions; the principles governing reflection are discussed further below. Last, as the US beam encounters irregular surfaces, the beam is essentially "reflected" into many different directions, known as *scattering*. These factors combine to attenuate the intensity of the returning echo, with energy decreasing exponentially with greater tissue depth. For this reason, *time-gain compensation* (TGC) is used to amplify echoes with longer time of flight. Thus, the amplitude of the returning wave is amplified exponentially to provide image brightness that is comparable to superficial tissues. Although TGC provides a functional image despite this exponential beam attenuation, it may produce artifact as noted below. These factors combine to make image interpretation more tenuous at greater tissue depths.

Frequency

Ultrasound frequencies used in medical imaging typically range from 2–18 megahertz (MHz), depending on the structure being evaluated. Lower frequencies (~2–5 MHz) are typically used to evaluate deeper structures such as the hip; low frequencies allow for less attenuation and deeper beam penetration. Mid-range frequencies (~8–12 MHz) are typically used to evaluate structures such as the knee or deeper structures of the shoulder. Higher frequencies (10–18 MHz) are used for evaluation of superficial structures such as the wrist, foot, and ankle, which allows for greater resolution in cases where tissue depth is not a concern.

Frequency selection and structure of interest are both critical to selection of the appropriate US transducer. Lower frequencies are typically produced by a curvilinear array probe. Middle- and higher-range frequencies can be produced by linear array transducers of varying size. In most cases, a classic linear array is appropriate. However, in situations where bony prominences may interfere with transducer-to-skin contact, a small-footprint linear array (ie, a "hockey stick" transducer) may produce better-quality images.

With few exceptions, the sound frequency selected remains unchanged as it travels through the human body. It is important to note that frequency selection can markedly affect the quality of images and information obtained during your examination. As noted above, attenuation obscures images at greater tissue depths. Of the many factors that affect wave energy absorption, frequency is the only one that can be controlled by the examiner; others include tissue viscosity, relaxation time, and temperature. Absorption increases proportionally with frequency: As frequency doubles, energy absorption doubles. Thus, one uses lower frequencies for deep tissue imaging to reduce energy absorption. Notably, frequency is also directly related to spatial image resolution, that is, higher frequencies provide greater resolution in the axis of the transducer beam. Thus, when selecting beam frequency, there is a trade-off; higher frequencies provide greater resolution, and lower frequencies allow for greater depth of penetration. As a practical matter, using the highest frequency possible that allows for sufficient depth penetration is recommended.

Velocity

Although the frequency of a given sound wave remains constant in human tissues, its velocity can vary significantly. The velocity of sound increases with tissue density; for example, sound travels faster underwater. This is because less compressible tissues transmit sound at a greater velocity. As another example, sound travels more than twice as fast through cortical bone than through muscle or fat. This variation in velocity, along with tissue density, determines tissue impedance. Specifically, impedance (Z) is the product of velocity (V) and density (p): $I = pV$. Tissue differences in velocity, density, and impedance, thus, determine how sound waves are reflected back to the transducer or distorted by refraction.

Reflection

Sound wave reflection—and refraction—occurs where one tissue type transitions to another, that is, from fat to muscle, muscle to tendon, tendon to bone. Each tissue type has a characteristic density and velocity at which sound will travel, determining that tissue's impedance. The magnitude of difference in impedance determines how much sound will be reflected.

This principle explains the need for ample transmission gel when applying the transducer to the skin. The impedance of air is immensely different from those of all human tissue types; thus, any interface between air and tissues will reflect essentially all sound waves, without providing further tissue penetration for imaging purposes. Similarly, the impedance of cortical bone is much greater than those of other tissues; thus, when transmitted waves encounter bone, essentially all of the beam is reflected and cannot provide images of deeper structures.

The angle of incidence (AOI) and its effects on image quality and interpretation are crucial to understand during any diagnostic or interventional procedure. Most importantly, AOI predicts how the sound beam is reflected from the tissue interface. As AOI approaches zero—and the sound beam approaches perpendicular—a greater proportion of the reflected beam returns to the transducer to produce a functional image. As a correlate, when AOI increases, the sound beam is reflected away from the transducer (Figure 2-1A). The AOI determines the angle at which sound is reflected. During interventional procedures, this principle governs how well the needle tip is visualized within human tissues. When the needle is oriented more obliquely relative to the US beam, it is more difficult to visualize because the beam is reflected away from the transducer (Figure 2-1B). It also dramatically affects image quality when visualizing curved surfaces, for example, the femoral condyle. When imaging a curved interface, the wave beam must travel in line with its radial vector or, in other words, perpendicular to its tangent, in order to reflect toward the transducer (Figure 2-1C). This principle must be carefully observed when planning any intervention along a curvilinear structure.

Refraction

Just as the velocity and AOI influence sound wave reflection, they also determine the degree of wave refraction. Refraction is crucial when interpreting US imaging, particularly when used for needle guidance; it is best thought of as the curving of sound waves occurring at tissue interfaces. Just as transitions between air and water can distort underwater images—think of the underwater window at the aquarium—so can transitions between tissue types distort the sound waves transmitted through the body.

The extent of refraction is determined by the velocity and the AOI of the wave beam. As noted above, the velocity of the transmitted wave beam changes as it travels into different tissue types; as this occurs, the wavelength of the beam must also change because the frequency remains constant—recall *velocity = frequency × wavelength*. As the wavelength travels through the interface of two tissues—each with their characteristic density, velocity, and impedance—the direction of the wave may be refracted. The magnitude of refraction is directly proportional to the difference in velocity between the two tissue types and to the AOI, as determined by Snell's law:

$$\frac{\sin \theta_i}{V_i} = \frac{\sin \theta_r}{V_r}$$

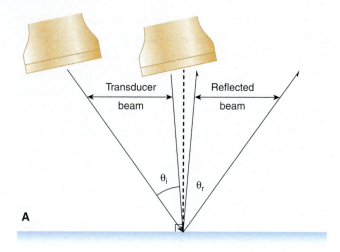

A

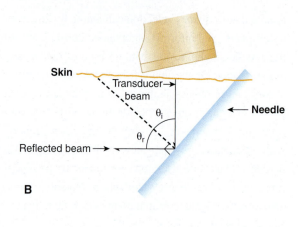

B

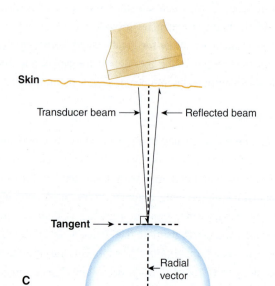

C

FIGURE 2-1 ■ **A.** Reflection. As the angle of incidence (AOI) approaches 0°, a greater portion of the beam returns to the transducer. **B.** Needle identification. As the needle's angle becomes more oblique, the beam is reflected away from the transducer, making need identification difficult. **C.** Curved surfaces. Directing the beam along the radial vector of curved structures maximizes reflection back to the transducer.

where θ_i is the AOI, θ_r is the angle of refraction, and V_i and V_r are the long-axis velocities of the wave beam in the respective tissues.

Therefore, as the sound wave approaches perpendicular to the tissue interface—and sin θ_i therefore approaches zero—the degree of refraction approaches zero. For this reason, it is *vital* to maintain the wave beam as close to perpendicular whenever possible to minimize the amount of image distortion caused by refraction. It is also important to note that the magnitude of the angle of refraction—whether it is more acute or oblique than the AOI—is not easily predicted, as it will vary according to the relative tissue velocities at the tissue interface (Figure 2-2).

Doppler Flow Imaging

When sound is reflected from a moving object, one observes a change in that sound's frequency. This is known as the

Doppler effect and is used in US to detect moving tissues beneath the skin. When tissues move with respect to the sound beam emitted from the transducer, there is a change in the frequency of the sound reflected from that tissue, for example, blood within an artery. This change in frequency is directly proportional to the velocity of the moving interface relative to the transducer. The use of Doppler flow imaging allows for improved assessment of tissues findings such as hyperemia, which may indicate an inflammatory process, granulation tissue in areas of healing, and other alterations in tissue vascularity. It is important to note that Doppler is most sensitive when the direction of movement is in the same direction as the US beam and is least sensitive when the direction is oriented perpendicularly. Thus, Doppler imaging can be very useful to identify vascular structures during interventional procedures, but it is important to recognize its limitations.

FIGURE 2-2 ■ Refraction. The extent of refraction is dependent on the angle of incidence (AOI) and relative long-axis velocities on each side of the tissue interface, dictated by Snell's law. θ_i, AOI; θ_r, angle of refraction. Note that θ_r may be more acute or oblique compared to θ_i, depending on the relative long-axis velocities of sound within each tissue along the interface.

Image Optimization

Modes of Scanning

B-mode scanning, or "brightness" mode, is essentially the only US mode used in musculoskeletal imaging. Each US beam pulse from the transducer reflects from different tissues within the body according to their physical properties; the amplitude of the returning echo is represented as "brightness" in a designated pixel on the screen. As noted above, the vertical position, or depth, of the pixel is determined by "time of flight" and the horizontal position, or width, is determined by the crystal receiving the echo. Thus, sequential echoes are transmitted from and reflected back to the transducer to produce real-time, two-dimensional imaging. Two additional modes of scanning include *A-mode* ("amplitude" mode) and *M-mode* ("motion" mode), neither of which is particularly relevant to musculoskeletal imaging and will therefore not be described in detail.

Gain

As noted above, the sound beam is attenuated by many interfering factors as sound travels through the body; the gain function compensates for this attenuation. The intensity of the returning echoes is amplified by the receiver, displaying a crisper image. Gain can be adjusted for the near field, far field, or the entire field (overall gain), changing the amount of white, black, and gray displayed on the monitor. Excessive gain may add noise to the image.

Focus

Beam focus, and thus image quality, is optimized in the focal zone. Most transducers provide electronic focus that can be adjusted for depth. It is important to position the focal zone at or slightly deep to the structure of interest. The focus function available on most US machines may help to improve visualization of the targeted structure; it is rarely needed for superficial structures if the depth is set correctly (see below).

Depth Settings

It is helpful to scan initially at higher depths, decreasing depth when the structure of interest is identified. For US-guided injection, the depth should be set approximately 1 cm deeper than the target of interest. To improve safety, when structures of importance (eg, blood vessel or lung) are situated below the target, the depth should be adjusted to provide a full view of these structures. Ideal screen position allows optimal estimation of target depth and angle of approach, facilitating more precise needle advancement before direct visualization.

Probe Orientation and Manipulation

Probe orientation and manipulation is a matter of personal preference. The US probe can be rotated 180 degrees easily while the monitor position remains unchanged to provide the examiner an alternate orientation; each probe has a marker that orients the sonographer to a corresponding side on the monitor. Manipulation of the US probe may provide variable image characteristics of the same structures—both good and bad. Keys to manipulation of the transducer include pressure, alignment, rotation, and tilt.

Adequate and even *pressure* provides better image quality by directly increasing echogenicity of most tissues and reducing attenuation. It may be helpful to apply more pressure to one side of the probe, directing the US beam to a desired structure, but excessive pressure can be detrimental. It may compress anatomical structures of interest (eg, a vein or bursa) in the area of intervention, masking pathology or obscuring structures that should be avoided.

Probe *alignment* allows the sonographer to position structures differently on the image in preparation for the planned procedure. The typical alignment for out-of-plane approach is to position the structure of interest in the middle of the screen. ■

For an in-plane approach, one can position the desired structure on one end of the screen to allow better visualization of the needle's approach.

Rotation of the transducer allows varying degrees of axial visualization after a structure has been identified. As the long axis of the structure remains parallel to the surface and the US probe is gradually rotated, the round, cross-sectional view will be replaced by a more oval shape. Additionally, rotation also allows versatility in evaluating needle trajectory during intervention. In particular, rotation is vital in monitoring the needle tip and trajectory, allowing the interventionalist to visualize needle approach.

The *tilt* of the probe is also vital in both diagnostic and interventional imaging. Reflection and refraction of the beam can produce artifacts (detailed below), which can be corrected by varying the degree of tilt. Angling the transducer along its axis to one end more than the other, known as the *heel-toe* maneuver, can accomplish this correction. This is best exemplified in structures running obliquely to the US beam, where tilt allows the orientation of the beam so that it approaches structures of interest at a perpendicular angle, minimizing anisotropy. Similarly, varying degrees of tilt may better visualize the needle as it runs obliquely beneath the skin. In both cases, a buildup of gel between the skin and transducer may be necessary to maintain a continuous medium through which the beam can travel (see Figure 2-3 below for example).

Common Artifacts

The term *artifact* is used to describe imaging findings that do not accurately represent the anatomic structures being evaluated. The physics of US imaging make this modality

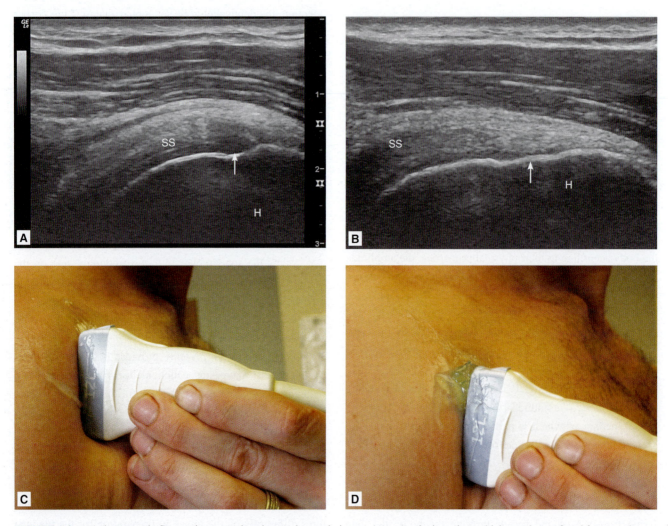

FIGURE 2-3 ■ Anisotropy. **A.** Supraspinatus tendon shows a hypoechoic area (*arrow*) at its insertion, which may be confused for an undersurface tear. **B.** The hypoechoic area disappears after performing a heel-toe maneuver with the probe, indicating that it is due to anisotropy. **C.** Probe position corresponding to Figure 2-3A. **D.** Probe position after performance of heel-toe maneuver to correct anisotropic artifact. Note the buildup of gel to maintain a continuous medium through which the US beam can travel without interruption. H, humerus; SS, supraspinatus tendon.

particularly prone to artifact, even when carefully observing the techniques above for image optimization.

One should be prepared to recognize artifacts when they occur and adjust technique to minimize their effects on diagnosis and treatment.

Anisotropy

Anisotropy is the property of tissues to vary in their appearance depending on the angle of the US beam. Tendons, nerves, and muscles are particularly prone to anisotropy and may appear markedly different with changes in orientation of the US beam. This is troublesome in image interpretation and treatment, especially in tendons where the appearance suggests injury. The presence of homogenous fluid in the tendon, as in inflammation, appears relatively isotropic compared to the hyperechoic structure of the adjacent tendon. Thus, anisotropy can be easily mistaken for pathology.

Two core principles related to anisotropy are important to understand. First, the echogenicity of an anisotropic tissue is dependent on the angle of the US beam. For example, when examining a curved tendon such as the supraspinatus, those portions of the tendon that are not perpendicular to beam may appear hypoechoic (Figure 2-3). Hypoechoic areas may be related to a technical factor—the angle of the beam—and not a true injury to the tissue (tendinopathy). One must visualize the hypoechoic area after adjusting the angle and orientation of the beam to affirm that it is true pathology.

Second, the clinician can use the anisotropic properties of various tissues to help distinguish different tissue types. For example, when evaluating the carpal tunnel, the median nerve can easily be confused with the neighboring finger flexor tendons. By adjusting the tilt of the US beam, the median nerve can be easily distinguished from the more anisotropic finger flexor tendons (Figure 2-4).

Shadowing

As noted above, the nature of US beam reflection, and thus image production, is determined primary by tissue impedances and the AOI as the beam approaches tissue interfaces. Naturally, if the beam encounters interfaces that are highly reflective, there is little remaining US beam to penetrate into deeper tissues. The result is shadowing. In musculoskeletal imaging, this typically happens where soft tissue transitions to bone or calcifications, for example when evaluating for sacro iliac (SI) joint injection or evaluation of tendon insertion onto bone. Abnormal calcifications within muscles and tendons, such as calcific tendonitis or myositis ossificans, can also create shadowing (Figure 2-5). Finally, this may also occur when gas or air is present within soft tissue, given the great difference in acoustic impedance.

Refractile Shadowing

Refractile shadowing is similar in appearance but occurs when the US beam approaches a tissue interface at an oblique angle. It is typically observed when objects with highly curved surfaces are imaged, such as the diaphysis of a long bone or tendon observed in a short-axis plane (Figure 2-5B).

Shadow is observed at the lateral margins of the object where the sound beam contacts the interface at a critical angle, beyond which the beam can no longer be refracted (refer to Snell's law above). Thus, much of the sound beam cannot penetrate into deeper tissues and return to the transducer, resulting in an acoustic shadow. This is a common finding at the ends of torn, retracted tendons, where refractile shadowing will almost invariably signify a full-thickness tear.

Posterior Acoustic Enhancement

Posterior acoustic enhancement, or enhanced through transmission, occurs as a result of image processing after the

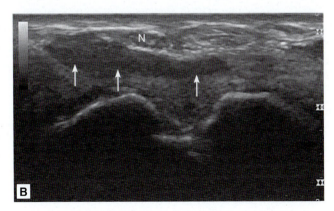

FIGURE 2-4 ■ Anisotropy. **A.** The flexor tendons of the carpal tunnel are easily confused with the median nerve given similar echogenicity (*arrows show hyperechoic flexor tendons*). **B.** By tilting the transducer, the operator uses the anisotropic property of tendon to distinguish the tendons from the still isotropic nerve (*arrows show same flexor tendons, now hypoechoic due to anisotropy*). N, median nerve.

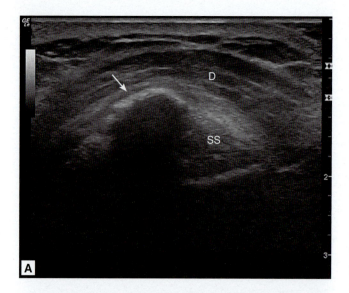

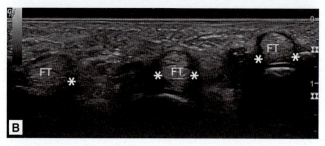

FIGURE 2-5 ■ Shadowing. **A.** Calcific structures, in this case within the supraspinatus tendon, produce a shadow deep to it (*arrow* points to large calcification within tendon with shadowing). D, deltoid muscle; SS, supraspinatus tendon. **B.** Refractile shadowing occurs here with evaluation of multiple flexor tendons of the fingers in short-axis view around the level of the A1 pulley. FT, flexor tendon; asterisk, areas of refractile shadowing.

US beam has been received by the transducer. As the beam penetrates into deeper tissues, an exponential proportion of the beam's energy is absorbed by the tissues or *attenuated* (see "Ultrasound Physics" section above for further detail). This is corrected by TGC to produce an image that preserves consistent image intensity among various tissue depths. This image processing system assumes that the beam is attenuated by various tissues equally, which is not the case; some tissues absorb more US wave energy than others. Thus, when the beam travels through less absorptive tissues, most commonly, simple fluid-filled structures such as the diaphysis of a long bone or tendon observed in a short-axis plane. The image produced will have more intense structures deep to the fluid when compared to adjacent structures at that same depth. Accordingly, this artifact is quite useful in the identification of simple cysts or fluid-filled bursae, a useful trick for the interventionalist.

Reverberation Artifacts

Reverberation artifact is best thought of as a series of echoes that are produced by the same structure but appear at increasing depths on the resulting image. The initial echo returns to the transducer after a single reflection and conveys the proper depth of the structure. However, sequential echoes can be produced when the echo again reflects back into the tissue from the skin–transducer interface or from other interfaces' large differences in impedance within the body (eg, gas–tissue or foreign bodies including needles). These subsequent echoes will take longer to return to the receiving crystals and, thus, will be displayed erroneously at greater tissue depths. Reverberation artifact is typically seen as a repeated, equally spaced linear array pattern extending deep to the true position of the imaged structure (Figure 2-6).

Comet tail artifact is a useful form of reverberation artifact. In this artifact, the two reflective interfaces and resulting sequential echoes are closely spaced; as a result, it is very useful in identifying small, dense foreign bodies or implanted hardware composed of metal. These sequential echoes may be so close together that individual signals are not perceivable and typically decrease in width with greater depth. Thus, this reverberation artifact is typically displayed as a triangular, tapered shape (Figure 2-7).

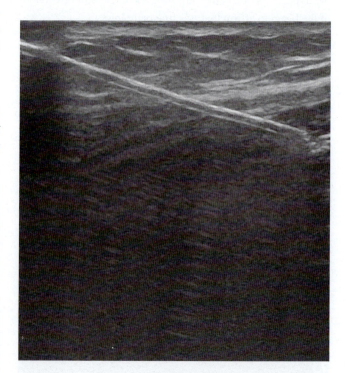

FIGURE 2-6 ■ Reverberation. Echoes are reflected back and forth between tissue–needle interfaces, creating reverberation artifact deep to the needle.

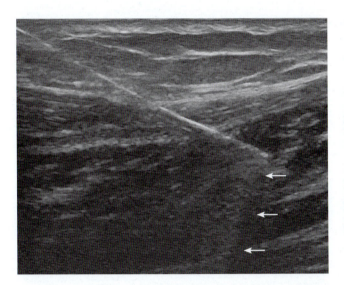

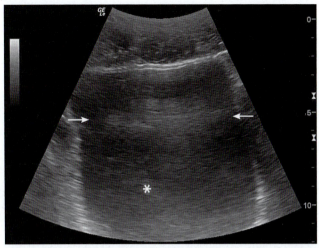

FIGURE 2-7 ■ Comet tail. Reverberation extending deep to the needle tip is tightly spaced and tapers with increasing depth, creating a "comet tail" appearance (*arrows indicate comet tail artifact*).

FIGURE 2-8 ■ Mirror and beam width artifact. A mirror image of the skin is evident as a hyperechoic band within the urinary bladder (*between arrows*). Deeper within the bladder, a hyperechoic area represents beam width artifact (*asterisk*). Echoes from the bladder wall are erroneously displayed within the lumen of the bladder, which could be mistakenly be interpreted as soft tissue.

Mirror image artifact is essentially a very well-defined reverberation artifact, so much so that it may be misconstrued as true anatomic structure. In this case, the US beam encounters a highly reflective interface surrounding the structure, causing it to reflect back and forth before returning to the transducer. As a result, the display shows a duplicate image equidistant from but deep to the strongly reflective interface. In musculoskeletal imaging, mirror image artifact is most relevant to imaging of the pelvis and tibia where structures adjacent to the highly reflective bone cortex may be duplicated (Figure 2-8).

Beam Width Artifact

As the US beam exits the transducer at approximately the same width as the transducer, it narrows slightly as it approaches the focal zone and widens again distal to the focal zone. Despite this variation in true beam width, the image produced is of uniform width, necessitating volume averaging of the echo data received by the transducer.

This may display structures in erroneous locations. Clinically, beam width artifact may be recognized as an anechoic structure with hyperechoic intensities within (see Figure 2-8).

These hyperechoic structures are anatomically located adjacent to the anechoic structure. This classically occurs with fluid-filled structures such as the bladder or distended bursae. This "volume averaging" may also obscure the classical shadowing artifact that helps to identify small calcifications or foreign bodies; thus, one cannot exclude these structures in the absence of shadowing. When beam width artifact is recognized during scanning, one can improve image quality by tuning the focal zone to the level of interest and centering the beam over the object of interest.

References

1. Bianchi S, Martinoli C, Abdelwahad IF, Baert AL, Derchi LE. *Ultrasound of the Musculoskeletal System.* New York, NY: Springer-Verlag Berlin Heidelberg; 2007.
2. van Holsbeeck MT, Introcaso JH, eds. *Musculoskeletal Ultrasound,* 2nd ed. St. Louis, MO: Mosby; 2001.
3. Jacobson JA. *Fundamentals of Musculoskeletal Ultrasound.* Philadelphia, PA: Saunders; 2007.

Paul H. Lento, MD

Ultrasound (US)-guided musculoskeletal procedures are performed for various purposes including instillation of medications and biologics, aspiration of fluid, or needling of tissues. Although there are many acceptable ways to perform these procedures, basic setup and stepwise preparation is vital for the success and safety of the injection. A well-planned procedure will also optimize comfort for both the patient and the clinician. This chapter will describe the general setup prior to performing US-guided musculoskeletal procedures. It will also provide tips on ergonomics as well as discuss appropriate skin and probe preparation.

Although there is no absolute way to proceed with US-guided interventions, an organized approach will be helpful in successfully and safely carrying out the procedure. Although individual variations exist and may be considered perfectly acceptable, the following steps may be useful when preparing to perform these interventions.

Step 1. **History and physical.** Perform an appropriate history and physical examination including a review of previous diagnostic tests.

Step 2. **Obtain consent.** It may be helpful to explain to the patient that US-guided procedures typically require more time than the standard palpation-guided injection. Patients may become anxious when realizing the extent of preparation that often occurs with these procedures. Patients can be reassured that with proper technique, these injections target the area more accurately than non-image-guided injections.

Step 3. **Assemble appropriate equipment (Table 3-1).** Consider using a sterile field on a table top or stand where supplies may be placed sterilely (Figure 3-1).

Step 4. **Position the patient and US machine.** It is highly recommended that the patient be placed in a position of comfort while also allowing proper visualization of the targeted structure. To prevent a vasovagal episode, a recumbent position is recommended.

Attention to proper ergonomics is an important and often overlooked component of US procedures. In one survey, a large proportion of sonographers complained of significant musculoskeletal complaints.[1] Of these, neck and back complaints lead

TABLE 3-1 ▪ EQUIPMENT FOR ULTRASOUND PROCEDURES
Essential Equipment Ultrasound machine Appropriate transducer and gel Skin prep (ie, ChloraPrep®) Probe (prepared appropriately) Sterile gel Appropriate-size needles and syringes Medications/biologics Gauze Bandages **Optional Equipment** Sterile condom cover Drapes Needle guide Extension tubing

the list. To limit these complaints, the US machine should be located directly in front of the individual at eye level so that excessive strain not be placed on the cervical spine (Figure 3-2). Prolonged flexed posture through the lumbar spine should be avoided as well. A comfortable chair and correct position of the body has been shown to reduce the incidence of neck and back pain.[1] To reduce strain and fatigue on the upper limb, the probe should not be held with excessive force. Maintaining contact with the patient using the ulnar two

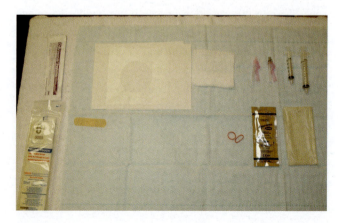

FIGURE 3-1 ▪ Sterile field with supplies used during an ultrasound-guided procedure (tubing not shown).

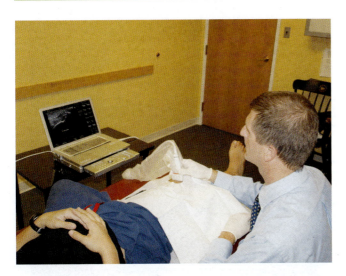

FIGURE 3-2 ■ The ultrasound machine should be in direct view at eye level so as to avoid cervical strain.

digits serves to provide a sense of tactile feedback for the clinician as well as anchors one's hand to the patient. Routinely, the nondominant hand holds the probe while the dominant hand places the needle, although many experienced clinicians can use either hand for either task. This technique is referred to as the *freehand technique*. Alternatively, a needle guide attached to the transducer may be used, which will anticipate the trajectory of the needle and allows one hand not to have to constantly hold the needle. Because both hands are often used during the procedure, it is usually recommended that an assistant be present. The assistant can make US setting adjustments, store images, retrieve additional supplies, and assist with drawing up of medications.

Step 5. Proceed with a preliminary scan. This scan helps confirm the diagnosis as well as identifies relevant structures that are to be avoided during the procedure. It is recommended that a picture of the targeted image be archived. During this time an appropriate technique (in-plane vs out-of-plane) as well as needle length and gauge can be ascertained.

Step 6. Demarcate the overlying skin once the appropriate starting position is confirmed. Marking the skin with an indelible marker or indenting the skin on either side of the probe helps relocate where the probe should be replaced after the skin is prepared (Figure 3-3). The nonsterile gel that was used during the preliminary scan should then be completely removed from the skin.

Step 7. Don sterile gloves.

Step 8. Prepare the skin with appropriate cleaning agent. It has been shown that prior to some interventional procedures, skin preparation with the use of alcohol-based chlorhexidine compared with the use of povidone iodine lowered the incidence of bacterial skin colonization.[2]

Step 9. Draw up appropriate medications and provide local anesthetic if needed. The local anesthetic can be instilled without US guidance or later after appropriate skin and probe preparation. Placing local anesthetic under direct US visualization ensures that the appropriate subcutaneous tissues are anesthetized and also provides a way to test needle trajectory.

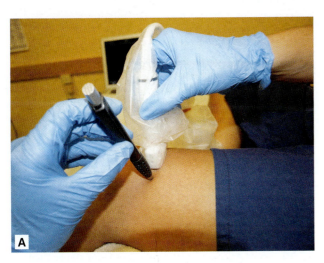

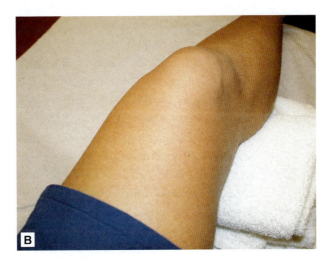

FIGURE 3-3 ■ Demarcating the skin with an indentation helps mark the skin where the probe is to be placed. Ink is often washed away during skin preparation and thus not recommended for skin marking.

Step 10. Prepare probe. There is tremendous controversy as well as variability regarding preparation of the transducer prior to any US-guided procedure. Although the risk of infection is extremely low with appropriate skin preparation during palpation-guided peripheral injections, every effort should be made to maintain sterile technique during US-guided procedures.[3,4] Contamination of the US gel, skin, or transducer may increase the risk of infection. More importantly, contact with bodily fluid that remains on the transducer could theoretically be spread from one patient to another if proper technique and disinfecting of the probe do not occur. The practitioner must ensure that the skin around the needle entry point remain sterile throughout the procedure. This can be accomplished through several methods:

The "no touch" technique implies that the probe and gel are placed in a location on the patient such that they do not contaminate the sterile field. This technique should only be employed by individuals experienced in performing US-guided procedures because of the higher risk of sterile field contamination from unintentional transducer movements in less experienced individuals.[5]

If it is possible that the transducer or US gel will contaminate the sterile field, then it is recommended to use sterile US gel and to sterilize the transducer with antiseptic cleanser before and after every use. The sonographer should consult with the manufacturer of their US machine to identify the manufacturer's recommended antiseptic cleanser. A sterile drape can also be used, when appropriate in this setting.

If strict sterility is required because of a higher-risk procedure or higher-risk patient, in addition to the above measures, one should use a sterile cover for the transducer. An assistant can hold the transducer that has nonsterile gel on the head. A sterile condom cover can then be placed over the transducer head and secured in placed with rubber bands (Figure 3-4). Alternatively a Tegaderm® dressing can be placed directly on the probe (Figure 3-5). One should check first with the US manufacturer to determine what substances or covers should be placed on the probe as damage may occur if recommendations are not followed.

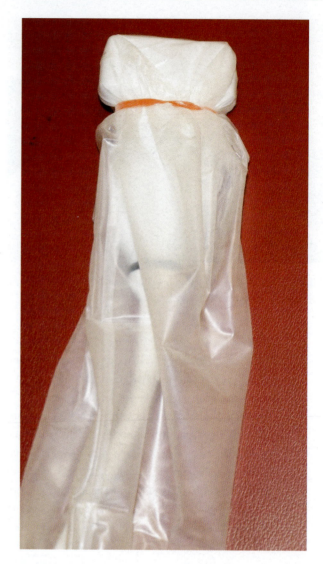

FIGURE 3-4 ■ Placing a sterile condom cover over the probe is an excellent way to provide a sterile interface during an ultrasound-guided procedure.

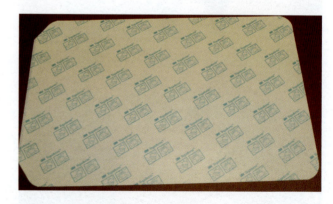

FIGURE 3-5 ■ Alternatively, a sterile Tegaderm® can be used over the probe. One should check with the manufacturer to see that this will not damage the probe.

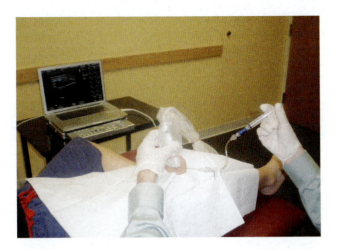

FIGURE 3-6 ■ Ultrasound-guided procedure showing the use of extension tubing while performing an injection.

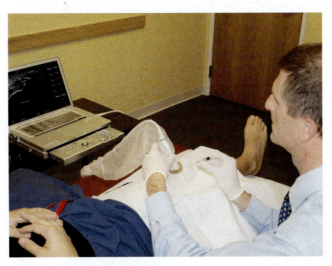

FIGURE 3-7 ■ Having the ultrasound machine, probe, and needle all in direct visualization will reduce the strain on the cervical spine and makes placing the needle under the middle of the probe easier.

Sterile gel, which often comes prepackaged with the sterile condom cover, can then be placed on the skin to serve as an appropriate interface.

Step 11. Attach syringe directly to needle. Alternatively the syringe can be attached to extension tubing, which is then secured to the needle. This technique is useful because the plunger of the syringe can be depressed without moving the tip of the needle. Also the injecting hand can be alternatively moved between the syringe and the needle without having the weight of the syringe alter the position of the needle. (Figure 3-6).

Step 12. Place needle under probe into tissue while in direct view (Figure 3-7). Having the needle entry point placed within direct view ensures that the needle is placed midline under the probe. It also will lessen strain on the cervical spine. Proceed with in-plane or out-of-plane approach.

Summary

Although modification to these recommendations may be acceptable, following a stepwise approach to the setup and preparation of any musculoskeletal US-guided procedures will help ensure that these interventions are carried out safely and comfortably for both patient and clinician.

References

1. Magnavita N, Bevilacqua L, Mirk P, et al. Work-related musculoskeletal complaints in sonologists. *J Occup Environ Med*. 1999 Nov;41(11):981-988.
2. Krobbuaban B, Diregpoke S, Prasan S, et al. Alcohol-based chlorhexidine vs. povidone iodine in reducing skin colonization prior to regional anesthesia procedures. *J Med Assoc Thai*. 2011 Jul;94(7):807-812.
3. Nazarian L, et al. AIUM practice guideline for the performance of the musculoskeletal ultrasound examination. 2007;1–13.
4. Baima J, Isaac Z. Clean versus sterile technique for common joint injections: a review from the physiatry perspective. *Curr Rev Musculoskelet Med*. 2008;1:88–91.
5. Sites B, Spence B, Gallagher J, Wiley CW, Bertrand ML, Blike GT. Characterizing novice behavior associated with learning ultrasound-guided peripheral regional anesthesia. *Reg Anesth Pain Med*. 2007;32:107–115.

Gerard A. Malanga, MD / Matthew Axtman, DO / Kenneth R. Mautner, MD

Musculoskeletal injections are a routinely used treatment for a variety of conditions. Treatment often includes injections into joints, bursa, tendon sheaths, or perineural spaces performed in an office setting. Traditionally, most of these injections are performed in a palpation-guided manner, that is, without image guidance using palpation of surface anatomy and directing the needle into the suspected area of pathology. There are concerns using palpation of the area for injection, which include whether the injectate has been effectively delivered to the target area and safety concerns regarding inadvertent penetration of the other nearby structures such as nerves and blood vessels. In some cases, fluoroscopy has been used to increase the efficacy and accuracy of injections; however, the use of this technology has the disadvantages of lack of portability, radiation exposure, relatively high cost, and lack of visualization of soft tissue structures. Recent advances in musculoskeletal ultrasound have now allowed for the clinician to be able to perform various types of musculoskeletal injections while directly visualizing needle position into these structures.

The use of musculoskeletal ultrasound has rapidly increased for both diagnostic and therapeutic purposes. Physicians of many specialties are increasingly using ultrasound to guide injection procedures to improve the accuracy and thereby enhance the efficacy of these injections. The benefits of ultrasound include portability, lack of ionizing radiation, low cost, capability of dynamic evaluation, time efficiency, and visualization of soft tissues. Recent research has demonstrated the superior accuracy of ultrasound guidance to palpation-guided techniques and in many studies, an associated improvement in outcomes, which will be cited in this chapter.

Accuracy

There are now multiple studies that have demonstrated improved accuracy of ultrasound guidance for injections versus standard palpation-guided or fluoroscopically guided injections of various musculoskeletal structures and peripheral nerves (Tables 4-1 and 4-2).[1-10]

Shoulder

The acromioclavicular (AC) joint is a joint that is injected for pain relief in sprains, osteoarthritis, and osteolysis. The

TABLE 4-1 ■ UPPER EXTREMITY INJECTION ACCURACY COMPARISON

Location	Ultrasound (%)	Palpation (%)	Fluoroscopy (%)
AC joint[1]	100	40	
GH joint[2]	95	79	
GH joint[3]	94		72
SA-SD bursa[2,4]	100	63	60
Biceps sheath[13]	100	66	

joint is a superficial joint, suggesting an injection of the AC joint would be considered simple and effective with palpation. Recent literature would contradict this assumption. Peck et al. compared injection of the AC joint with palpation versus ultrasound guidance.[1] They noted a 100% accuracy rate with ultrasound guidance and only a 40% accuracy rate with palpation of the AC joint.

The glenohumeral joint (GH) is injected in cases of shoulder pain from osteoarthritis, joint effusions, and prior to contrast-enhanced imaging studies such as magnetic resonance imaging. This joint is a deeper structure and therefore difficult to palpate, which would suggest that

TABLE 4-2 ■ LOWER EXTREMITY INJECTION ACCURACY COMPARISON

Location	Ultrasound (%)	Palpation (%)	Fluoroscopy (%)
Knee joint[5]		71–93	
Knee joint[2]	99	79	
Knee joint[6]	100	55	
Knee joint[7]	96	83	
Pes anserine[8]	92	17	
Hip joint[9,10]	97		51
Piriformis[11]	95		30
Tibiotalar joint[12]	100	85	
Sinus tarsi[12]	90	35	
Peroneal sheath[14]	100	60	

image guidance such as ultrasound would likely increase the accuracy of a glenohumeral joint injection. Daley et al. noted that ultrasound guidance had a 95% success rate of being injected into the glenohumeral joint, while palpation demonstrated a 79% success rate.[2] Fluoroscopic guidance has also been used to ensure an accurate injection. When comparing ultrasound to fluoroscopic guidance, Rutten et al. found a 94% success rate with ultrasound on the first attempt at injection as compared to a 72% success rate with fluoroscopic guidance.[3]

The subacromial-subdeltoid (SA-SD) bursa is a common structure of the shoulder that is injected for various diagnoses that include impingement, rotator cuff tendinopathy, adhesive capsulitis, and bursitis. Daley et al. found that injection of the SA-SD bursa was successful in 100% of injections with ultrasound compared to only 63% with palpation.[2] Matthews et al. used fluoroscopic guidance and, only had successful injection of the SA-SD bursa on 60% of the procedures.[4]

Knee

The knee is another common area of pain that is treated with injections. This can include intraarticular knee joint injections as well as injection of the pes anserine bursa and other soft tissues about the knee. For knee joint injections, corticosteroids and viscosupplementation injections are often used in treating knee pain secondary to osteoarthritis. An accurate injection of the knee would appear to be quite important to provide effective pain relief and treatment of underlying causes of the pain. Jackson et al. demonstrated that with palpation alone, the rate of intraarticular knee injection was only 71% with an anterolateral approach, 75% with an anteromedial approach, and 93% with a lateral midpatellar approach.[5] Multiple studies have also shown that there is an increased accuracy rate with a superolateral approach to injection of the knee joint. Daley et al. established that with palpation there was a 79% accuracy rate that increased to 99% with ultrasound guidance. Curtiss et al. demonstrated a 55% accuracy rate with palpation as compared to a 100% accuracy rate with ultrasound guidance. Finally, Park et al. found an 83% accuracy rate with palpation versus 96% accuracy with ultrasound-guidance.[2,6,7]

Another source of knee pain is pes anserine bursitis. This structure lies between the medial collateral ligament and the semitendinosus, gracilis, and sartorius tendons. The bursa is a superficial structure and it would be suspected that the bursa would be easily and accurately injected with palpation. Finnoff et al. found a high rate of inaccuracy with palpation-guided injections of only 17% into the pes anserine bursa versus a 92% success rate with ultrasound-guided injection.[8]

Hip

Intraarticular hip injections are performed in cases that cause pain such as osteoarthritis, joint effusions, and labral pathology. These injections may be completed using fluoroscopic guidance; however, Diracoglu et al. demonstrated only a 51% accuracy rate using fluoroscopic guidance.[9] In contrast, Smith et al. demonstrated that ultrasound-guided hip joint injection was successful in 97% of the procedures performed.[10]

Piriformis syndrome is an irritation of the sciatic nerve as it passes under or through the piriformis muscle. This condition is commonly treated with physical therapy, medication, and injections. Piriformis injections are commonly performed with fluoroscopic guidance with use of contrast to ensure accurate placement. Finnoff et al. performed a study to compare the accuracy of ultrasound-guided injections versus fluoroscopic-guided injections. They found that ultrasound guidance had 95% accuracy rate into the piriformis muscle versus a 30% accuracy with fluoroscopic-guided injections, which tended to be injected more superficially into the gluteus maximus.[11]

Foot and Ankle

Ankle joint arthritis is relatively common and can result in considerable pain and functional impairment. Patients often seek pain control wishing to defer joint replacement. Tibiotalar joint injections are commonly performed in the office using palpation guidance. Wisniewski et al. revealed a 100% accuracy with ultrasound-guided injection of the tibiotalar joint and only an 85% accuracy rate with nonguided injections.[12]

The sinus tarsi can also be an area of pain in various patients including running athletes. In the same study by Wisniewski et al., they found a 90% success rate with injections using ultrasound guidance into the sinus tarsi versus a 35% success rate with palpation.[12]

Tendon Injections

Tendonitis (more properly referred to as *tendinosis*) and tenosynovitis are common diagnoses, especially in repetitive and overuse syndromes that can involve various tendons of the upper and lower extremities. Patients are treated with injections into the tendon sheath to decrease inflammation surrounding the tendon and reduce pain. It is accepted that when performing these injections, the clinician should avoid direct injection into the tendon with steroid to avoid damage to the tendon, which may lead to tendon rupture from the injection.

Ultrasound guidance allows for increased accuracy of injecting into the tendon sheath around the tendon, while avoiding injecting directly into the tendon or surrounding tissues. Various studies have been performed to demonstrate significantly improved accuracy often associated with improved clinical outcomes.

Hashiuchi et al. found a 100% accuracy of biceps tendon sheath injection with ultrasound as compared to a 66% accuracy rate with palpation guidance.[13] Likewise, Muir et al. noted 100% accuracy with injection of the peroneal tendon versus 60% accuracy with palpation.[14]

Efficacy

The main goal of most injections is to alleviate pain and increase function. Therefore, the most important aspect of an injection is the efficacy of the injection, which is driven by accuracy. Ultrasound-guided injections for the diagnoses of the shoulder, knee, inflammatory arthritis, and plantar fascia have not only been shown to give a greater response rate for pain relief, but have also demonstrated decreased procedural pain and a greater duration of pain relief.

Several studies have shown that there is a decrease in the visual analog scale score and increased range of motion of the shoulder with ultrasound-guided versus palpation-guided injections following injection of the SA-SD bursa. Chen et al. evaluated the improvement in range of motion of the shoulder 1 week after subacromial injection in patients with a diagnosis of subacromial bursitis using palpation-guided versus ultrasound-guided corticosteroid injections. The group who received a palpation-guided injection increased their range of motion in abduction from an average of 71–100 degrees, which was not considered statistically significant ($P > 0.05$). This was compared to the group who underwent a subacromial injection with ultrasound guidance and improved their range of motion from an average of 69–139 degrees ($P < 0.05$).[15]

Zufferey et al. evaluated pain reduction after subacromial bursa injection and demonstrated that there was significantly less pain at 2 and 6 weeks in the group who received the injection with ultrasound guidance versus the group who had palpation-guided injection. In addition, the patients who were injected under ultrasound guidance had a higher response rate of 81% at 2 weeks as compared to 54% in the palpation-guided injection group.[16]

Naredo et al. investigated the change in visual analog scale (VAS) and shoulder function assessment (SFA) 6 weeks after injection of corticosteroid into the subacromial bursa with ultrasound-guided or palpation-guided directed injection. The ultrasound-guided injection group demonstrated a decreased VAS of 34.9 and increased SFA of 15 versus the palpation-guided injected group, which had a decreased VAS of 7.1 and increased SFA of 5.6, both statistically significant.[17]

Studies also examined the efficacy and outcomes of ultrasound-guided injections of the knee. Sibbit et al. performed studies on the outcomes from injections in the knee with and without effusions. The study found that patients who had the procedure using ultrasound guidance had a 48% reduction in procedural pain, 42% reduction in pain scores at outcomes of 2 weeks and 6 months, 107% increase in responder rate, 52% reduction in nonresponder rate, and 36% increase in therapeutic duration when compared to the group treated with palpation-guided injections.[18] In a separate study of patients with knee osteoarthritis and knee effusions, there was 48% less procedural pain (based on VAS), improved clinical outcomes at 2 weeks based on VAS, and 183% increase in aspirated volumes aspirated from the knee effusion.[19]

Hip intraarticular steroid injection using ultrasound guidance has been shown to increase functional status in patients affected by osteoarthritis of the hip. Micu et al. found that patients who received an intraarticular steroid injection had a decreased VAS from baseline (8.17), at 1 month (2.77) and 3 months (3.66) as compared to a control group at baseline (8.66), 1 month (8.66), and 3 months (7.02) who did not have any intervention.[20]

Plantar fascia injection has also been studied with improved outcomes noted in studies using ultrasound guidance. Tsai et al. compared the benefit of corticosteroid injection into the proximal plantar fascia using palpation versus ultrasound guidance. They found that there was a significant decrease in pain in both groups; however, there was only an 8% recurrence rate in the ultrasound-guided group versus a 46% recurrence rate in the palpation-guided group. There was also noted to be a decrease in thickness of the plantar fascia and decrease in proximal plantar fascia hypoechogenic signal in the patients who were injected with ultrasound guidance.[21]

Inflammatory arthritis can be a very debilitating process, and it is important that any corticosteroid injections into the arthritic joint be properly placed for improved clinical outcome. Arthritic joints may become small and difficult to direct injections into because of the destructive process, and ultrasound guidance can help establish proper placement. Sibbit et al. injected joints affected with inflammatory arthritis (shoulder, elbow, wrist, finger, knee, and ankle joints) comparing ultrasound-guided and palpation-guided techniques. When compared to palpation-guided injections, ultrasound-guided injections resulted in a 35% greater reduction in pain outcomes, 81% reduction in procedural pain, 34% reduction in the nonresponder rate, and 32% increase in duration of the injection.[22]

Cost

The current healthcare system is faced with ever increasing costs and health insurance carriers are continuing to see ways to reduce cost. Because of these issues, the modern practitioner is required to make decisions that are based on providing the most cost-efficient care while delivering evidence-based, practical, and effective treatments.

For example, let us consider a patient with hip osteoarthritis and pain who is electing to have a corticosteroid injection into the intraarticular space performed for pain relief. Often, this is performed with fluoroscopic guidance. This procedure requires advanced planning and scheduling. In addition, it often requires the use of a surgical suite, nurse, fluoroscopic C-arm, and radiology technician. By comparison, the use of ultrasound guidance for this procedure requires only an ultrasound machine and physician, who completes the procedure in an office-based examination room. When comparing total costs, the ultrasound-guided procedure will cost significantly less than the fluoroscopic procedure and decrease burden and cost for both the patient and healthcare system.

There are arguments that ultrasound-guided injections only add to the cost of these procedures and that ultrasound guidance is not necessary for most of the injections performed. As we have previously noted, improved accuracy and efficacy with ultrasound guidance will likely result in decreased costs and improved patient satisfaction. For example, Sibbit et al. compared intraarticular injections using palpation versus ultrasound guidance to evaluate clinical outcomes. They concluded that the use of ultrasound resulted in a 25.6% increase in responder rate (reduction in VAS score ≥50% from baseline) and 62% decrease in nonresponder rate (reduction in VAS score <50% from baseline). They noted a 58.8% reduction in absolute pain scores at 2 weeks, increased detection of effusion by 200%, and increase in volume of aspirated fluid by 337% as compared to palpation-only injections and procedures.[23] These data would demonstrate reduction in cost and time savings for both the patient and physician by reduction of unnecessary follow-up visits, repeated injections, improved resolution of pain, and overall greater clinical outcomes.

Viscosupplementation is another injection that requires specific placement into the joint for effectiveness. The majority of times these injections are done with palpation, but in certain cases, body habitus may hinder the approach,

and surrounding soft tissues may be injected instead of the intended joint. Ultrasound guidance with this procedure may not only increase efficacy, but possibly decrease costs because of enhanced accuracy driving improved efficacy, while decreasing complications from inaccurate medication placement into soft tissues, and so forth.

Recently, platelet-rich plasma (PRP) has been used to enhance healing of both acute and chronic injuries as research continues to support the procedure. It would appear logical that directing the injectate into the area of pathology is of utmost importance to maximize the efficacy of this treatment. Performing an injection by palpation guidance may not result in depositing the PRP into the intended target tissue and therefore may affect the outcome of this costly procedure and reduce its potential benefits; however, there is no literature comparing the effectiveness of palpation-only versus ultrasound-guided injections using PRP.

Conclusion

Ultrasound-guided injections have been proven to enhance the accuracy of injection for a variety of musculoskeletal structures. Many studies have also demonstrated how this improved accuracy has resulted in improvement in pain and clinical outcome. The benefits of improved accuracy, efficacy, pain reduction, and decreased costs appear to support ultrasound guidance in maximizing outcome for a variety of musculoskeletal conditions.

References

1. Peck E, Lai JK, Pawlina W, Smith J. Accuracy of ultrasound-guided versus palpation-guided acromioclavicular joint injections: a cadaveric study. *PM&R*. 2010 Sep;2(9):817–821.
2. Daley E, Bajaj S, Bisson L, Cole B. Improving injection accuracy of the elbow, knee, and shoulder: does injection site and imaging make a difference? A systemic review. *Am J Sports Med*. 2011;39:656–662.
3. Rutten M, Collins J, Maresch B, et al. Glenohumeral joint injection: a comparative study of ultrasound and fluoroscopically guided techniques before MR arthrography. *Eur Radiol*. 2009;19:722–730.
4. Mathews P, Glousman R. Accuracy of subacromial injection: anterolateral versus posterior approach. *J Shoulder Elbow Surg*. 2005;14(2)145–148.
5. Jackson D, Evans M, Thomas B. Accuracy of needle placement into the intra-articular space of the knee. *J Bone Joint Surg Am*. 2002; 84:1522–1527.
6. Curtiss H, Finnoff J, Peck E, Hollman J, Muir J, Smith J. Accuracy of ultrasound-guided and palpation-guided knee

injections by an experienced and less-experienced injector using a superolateral approach: a cadaveric study. *PM&R.* 2011 Jun;3:507–515.

7. Park Y, Choi W, Kim Y, Lee S, Lee J. Accuracy of blind versus ultrasound-guided suprapatellar bursal injection. *J Clin Ultrasound.* 2012:40(1)20–25.

8. Finnoff J, Nutz D, Henning P, Hollman J, Smith J. Accuracy of ultrasound-guided versus unguided pes anserinus bursa injections. *PM&R.* 2010 Aug;8:732–739.

9. Diracoglu D, Alptekin K, Dikici F, et al. Evaluation of needle positioning during blind intra-articular hip injections for osteoarthritis: fluoroscopy versus arthrography. *Arch Phys Med Rehabil.* 2009 Dec;90(12):2112–2115.

10. Smith J, Hurdle M, Weingarten T, et al. Accuracy of sonographically guided intra-articular injections in the native adult hip. *J Ultrasound Med.* 2009;28(3):329–335.

11. Finnoff J, Hurdle M, Smith J. Accuracy of ultrasound-guided versus fluoroscopically guided contrast-controlled piriformis injections. *J Ultrasound Med.* 2008 Aug;8:1157–1163.

12. Wisniewski S, Smith J, Patterson D, Carmichael S, Wojciech P. Ultrasound-guided versus nonguided tibiotalar joint and sinus tarsi injections: a cadaveric study. *PM&R.* 2010 Apr;4:277–281.

13. Hashiuchi T, Sakurai G, Morimoto M, Komei T, Yoshinori T, Tanaka Y. Accuracy of the biceps tendon sheath injection: ultrasound-guided or unguided injection? A randomized controlled trial. *J Shoulder Elbow Surg.* 2011;20(7):1069–1073.

14. Muir J, Curtiss H, Hollman J, Smith J, Finnoff J. The accuracy of ultrasound-guided and palpation-guided peroneal tendon sheath injections. *Am J Phys Med Rehabil.* 2011;90:564–571.

15. Chen M, Lew H, Hsu T, et al. Ultrasound-guided shoulder injections in the treatment of subacromial bursitis. *Am J Phys Med Rehabil.* 2006 Jan;1:31–35.

16. Zufferey P, Revaz S, Degailler X, Balaque F, So A. A controlled trial of the benefits of ultrasound-guided steroid injection for shoulder pain. *Joint Bone Spine.* 2012 Mar;79(2):166–169.

17. Naredo E, Cabero F, Beneyto P, et al. A randomized comparative study of short-term response to blind injection versus sonographic-guided injection of local corticosteroids in patients with painful shoulder. *J Rheumatol.* 2004;31(2):308–314.

18. Sibbit W, Band P, Kettwich L, Chavez-Chiang N, DeLea S, Bankhurst A. A randomized controlled trial evaluating the cost-effectiveness of sonographic guidance for intra-articular injection of the osteoarthritic knee. *J Clin Rheumatol.* 2011 Dec;17(8):409–415.

19. Sibbit W, Kettwich L, Band P, et al. Does ultrasound guidance improve the outcomes of arthrocentesis and corticosteroid injection of the knee? *Scand J Rheumatol.* 2012 Feb;41(1)66–72.

20. Micu M, Bogdan G, Fodor D. Steroid injection for hip osteoarthritis: efficacy under ultrasound guidance. *Rheumatology (Oxford).* 2010;49(8):1490–1494.

21. Tsai W, Hsu C, Chen C, Chen M, Yu T, Chen Y. Plantar fasciitis treated with local steroid injection: comparison between sonographic and palpation guidance. *J Clin Ultrasound.* 2006 Jan;34(1);12–16.

22. Sibbit W, Band P, Chavez-Chiang N, DeLea S, Norton H, Bankhurst A. A randomized controlled trial of the cost-effectiveness of ultrasound-guided intra-articular injection of inflammatory arthritis. *J Rheumatol.* 2010 Nov;38(2):252–263.

23. Sibbit W, Peisajovich A, Michael A, et al. Does sonographic needle guidance affect the clinical outcome of intraarticular injections? *J Rheumatol.* 2009;36:9:1892–1902.

SECTION II

Shoulder

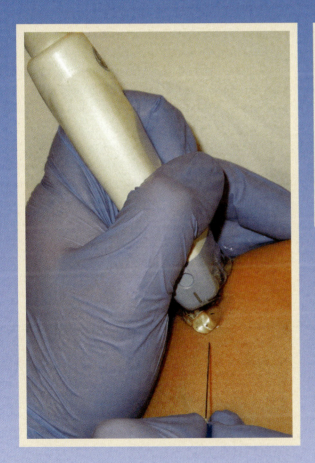

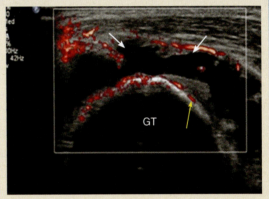

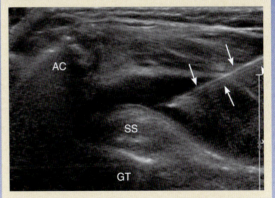

Troy Henning, DO

Pertinent Anatomy

The glenohumeral joint (GHJ) is a diarthrodial joint where the humeral head articulates with the glenoid fossa of the scapula. The joint is stabilized statically by intrinsic ligaments, joint capsule, the glenoid labrum, and dynamically by the rotator cuff group (Figure 5-1).

Common Pathology

The GHJ can be injured by acute traumatic events such as a fall on an outstretched arm resulting in an anterior shoulder dislocation or via repetitive overuse injuries associated with impaired biomechanics such as internal impingement in overhead athletes. Degenerative changes can also occur with aging, which can become symptomatic with movement in virtually all planes. Also, the joint can be affected by inflammatory processes such as rheumatoid arthritis or adhesive capsulitis.

Ultrasound Imaging Findings

The GHJ is best visualized in long axis using a low-frequency curvilinear array transducer. Common findings include cortical irregularities, osteophytes, joint effusions, and labral tears/degeneration.

Indications for Injections of the Glenohumeral Joint

Injection of the GHJ can be performed for patients with recalcitrant pain that is unresponsive to rest, icing, antiinflammatories, and physical therapy. Injection of the GHJ has been described based on palpation (ie, unguided).[1,2] The success rate of these unguided injections has been found to be 10%–99%.[2,3] Ultrasound-guided injection of the GHJ from an anterior and posterior approach has been described by Valls and Zwar et al., respectively.[4,5] More recently, Souza et al. described an approach through the rotator cuff interval.[6] A randomized control trial performed by Sibbitt et al. comparing cost-effectiveness of nonguided to ultrasound-guided joint injections found that the guided injections were more clinically effective and reduced patient care cost per year.[7]

Equipment

- Needle: 22- to 25-gauge 2- to 3.5-inch needle depending on body habitus of patient
- Injectate: 4–9 mL of local anesthetic and 1 mL of an injectable corticosteroid
- Medium- to high-frequency transducer, curvilinear array probe often preferred

A Glenohumeral joint
Anterior view-Tendons and ligaments

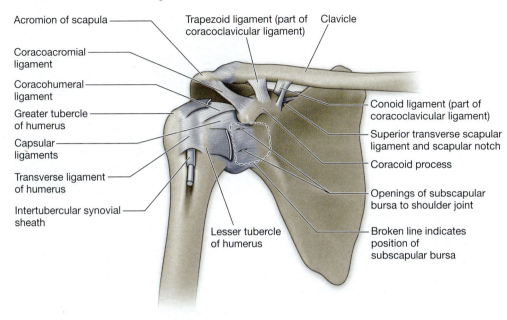

Acromion of scapula

Coracoacromial ligament

Coracohumeral ligament

Greater tubercle of humerus

Capsular ligaments

Transverse ligament of humerus

Intertubercular synovial sheath

Trapezoid ligament (part of coracoclavicular ligament)

Clavicle

Lesser tubercle of humerus

Conoid ligament (part of coracoclavicular ligament)

Superior transverse scapular ligament and scapular notch

Coracoid process

Openings of subscapular bursa to shoulder joint

Broken line indicates position of subscapular bursa

B Normal shoulder anatomy
Posterior view-Muscles

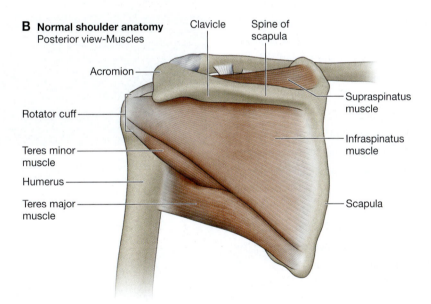

Clavicle

Spine of scapula

Acromion

Rotator cuff

Teres minor muscle

Humerus

Teres major muscle

Supraspinatus muscle

Infraspinatus muscle

Scapula

FIGURE 5-1 ■ **A.** Anterior view of the glenohumeral joint depicting ligamentous structures. **B.** Posterior view of rotator cuff muscles and respective insertion on humeral tuberosities.

Author's Preferred Technique

a. Patient position (Figure 5-2)
    i. Lateral recumbent position, affected side up
    ii. Arm at patient's side in neutral rotation, may have bolster under arm for patient comfort
b. Transducer position
    i. Anatomic axial oblique plane (parallel to fibers of infraspinatus tendon) over the posterior aspect of the GHJ
c. Needle orientation relative to the transducer
    i. In plane
d. Needle approach (Figure 5-3)
    i. Posterior lateral to anterior medial
    ii. Needle directly visualized entering down into joint space between humeral head and glenoid labrum
e. Target
    i. Posterior GHJ; ideally needle tip is positioned between humeral head and glenoid labrum.
f. Pearls/Pitfalls
    i. Anesthetizing needle can be used to determine trajectory before performing intraarticular injection.
    ii. Needle trajectory is fairly steep; a shallow needle entry into the skin will make proper placement of the needle more challenging.
    iii. Needle bevel should be facing articular surface of the humerus to avoid gouging the articular cartilage.
    iv. The solution should be visualized flowing into the joint space to ensure accurate placement. Accumulation of fluid in one area suggests extraarticular placement of the needle tip, and the procedure should be halted until the needle tip is repositioned.
    v. Placement of the needle superficial and medial to the GHJ poses risk of injury to the neurovascular structures within the spinoglenoid notch.

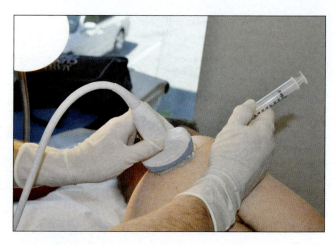

FIGURE 5-2 ▪ Patient positioned lateral recumbent position with affected side up. Transducer is placed in the oblique axial plane to optimize visualization of the posterior glenohumeral joint.

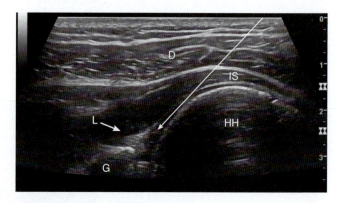

FIGURE 5-3 ▪ Sonographic view of posterior aspect of the glenohumeral joint. Top, superficial; bottom, deep; left, lateral; right, medial; G, glenoid; HH, humeral head; IS, Infraspinatus; L, labrum.

Alternate Technique

a. Patient position (Figure 5-4)

    i. Supine, arm neutral rotation to slightly externally rotated

b. Transducer position (Figure 5-4)

    i. Anatomic axial plane directly over the anterior GHJ

c. Needle orientation relative to transducer

    i. In plane

d. Needle approach (Figure 5-5)

    i. Lateral to medial

e. Target

    i. Anterior GHJ space

    ii. Needle directly visualized entering down between subscapularis tendon and articular cartilage or anterior glenoid labrum and articular cartilage

f. Pearls/Pitfalls

    i. Slight external rotation of the arm reduces needle angle trajectory, thereby improving visualization of the needle.

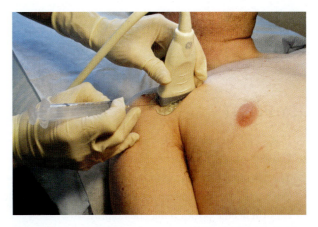

FIGURE 5-4 ■ Anterior approach to glenohumeral joint injection from lateral to medial.

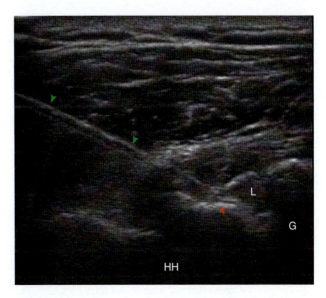

FIGURE 5-5 ■ Sonographic view of anterior approach to glenohumeral joint injection. Top, superficial; bottom, deep; left, lateral; right, medial; green arrow head, needle shaft; red arrow head, needle tip; G, glenoid; HH, humeral head; L, glenoid labrum.

References

1. Hegedus EJ, Zavala J, Kissenberth M, et al. Positive outcomes with intra-articular glenohumeral injections are independent of accuracy. *J Shoulder Elbow Surg.* 2010;19(6):795–801.

2. Porat S, Leupold JA, Burnett KR, Nottage WM. Reliability of non-imaging-guided glenohumeral joint injection through rotator interval approach in patients undergoing diagnostic MR arthrography. *AJR Am J Roentgenol.* 2008;191(3):W96–W99.

3. Esenyel CZ, Ozturk K, Demirhan M, et al. Accuracy of anterior glenohumeral injections: a cadaver study. *Arch Orthop Trauma Surg.* 2009;130(3):297–300.

4. Valls R, Melloni P. Sonographic guidance of needle position for MR arthrography of the shoulder. *AJR Am J Roentgenol.* 1997:845–847.

5. Zwar R, Read J, Noakes J. Sonographically guided glenohumeral joint injection. *AJR Am J Roentgenol.* 2004:48–50.

6. Souza PCME, de Aguiar ROC, Marchiori E, Bardoe SAW. Arthrography of the shoulder: a modified ultrasound guided technique of joint injection at the rotator interval. *Eur J Radiol.* 2010;74(3):e29–e32.

7. Sibbitt WL, Band PA, Chavez-Chiang NR, et al. A randomized controlled trial of the cost-effectiveness of ultrasound-guided intraarticular injection of inflammatory arthritis. *J Rheumatol.* 2011;38(2):252–263.

Evan Peck, MD

KEY POINTS

- Use a high-frequency linear array transducer.
- Use a 25-gauge, 1.5-inch needle, or equivalent, for injection.
- The acromioclavicular joint is widest anteriorly.
- Changing the transducer axis during the injection to confirm needle position may be helpful.

- If out-of-plane technique is chosen, use additional caution and proper technique to avoid advancement of the needle tip beyond the desired location.

Pertinent Anatomy

The acromioclavicular joint (ACJ) is a diarthrodial joint consisting of the articulation between the distal clavicle and the acromion (Figure 6-1). The ACJ is stabilized by three major ligaments: the acromioclavicular ligament (consisting of the superior acromioclavicular ligament and the inferior acromioclavicular ligament), which attaches the acromion to the clavicle; the coracoacromial ligament, which attaches the coracoid process to the acromion; and the coracoclavicular ligament (consisting of the conoid ligament and the trapezoid ligament), which attaches the coracoid process to the clavicle. The ACJ may contain an intraarticular disk, although this is commonly absent. The joint is wider anteriorly than posteriorly.

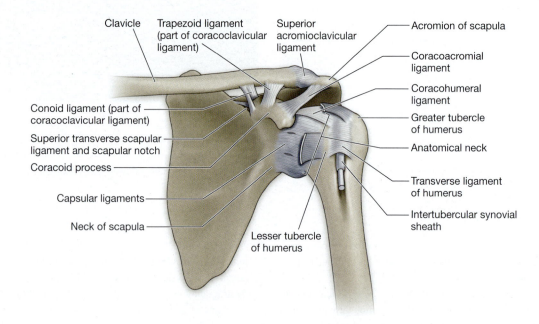

FIGURE 6-1 ■ The acromioclavicular joint.

Common Pathology

The ACJ may be injured by a direct blow to the shoulder, causing an ACJ separation. In addition, ACJ separation may occur with a fall on an outstretched hand. ACJ separation is common in collision sports such as football, hockey, lacrosse, and rugby. Osteoarthritis frequently affects the ACJ. Pain in the ACJ may also be caused by osteolysis of the distal clavicle, often seen in powerlifters, weightlifters, and others who may engage in a significant volume of strength training.

Ultrasound Imaging Findings

The ACJ is best sonographically visualized in its long axis, perpendicular to the joint line, using a high-frequency linear array transducer. The joint is typically easily located by palpation prior to transducer placement. Up to 3 mm of hypoechoic ACJ capsule distension is considered normal.[1] The intraarticular disk may be visualized as a hypoechoic structure within the joint; increasing the ultrasound's gain setting may accentuate its appearance.

Pathology that may be visualized sonographically includes cortical irregularities, widening or instability of the joint (examined statically or dynamically), joint effusion with capsular distension, and associated ganglion cysts. In the setting of a chronic full-thickness rotator cuff tear, fluid from the glenohumeral joint may track into the ACJ, producing capsular distension, a ganglion cyst associated with the ACJ, and the resultant sonographic "geyser sign" (Figure 6-2).

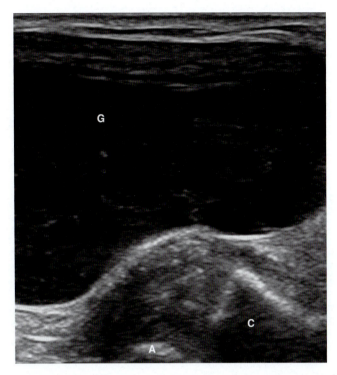

FIGURE 6-2 ■ Ultrasound image in long axis of a "geyser sign" associated with the acromioclavicular joint (ACJ) due to a chronic full-thickness rotator cuff tear. In this scenario, fluid tracks from the glenohumeral joint to the ACJ, producing capsular distension and, in this case, a large ganglion cyst. Left, lateral; top, superficial; A, acromion; C, clavicle; G, ganglion cyst.

Indications for Acromioclavicular Joint Injection

Injection of the ACJ may be considered for patients with recalcitrant pain resulting from an ACJ-associated pain generator that is unresponsive to appropriate activity modifications, oral or topical medications, therapeutic modalities, therapeutic exercises, and protection or bracing where indicated. In addition, ACJ injection may be used for diagnostic purposes if the primary pain generator is uncertain based on history, physical examination, and imaging findings.

Palpation-guided ACJ injection has been described, with accuracy documented to be 40%–72%.[2-7] Ultrasound-guided ACJ injections have been shown to achieve an accuracy rate of 95%–100%.[5,7] In two investigations, ACJ injections were shown to be significantly more accurate using ultrasound guidance versus palpation guidance.[5,7] The clinical outcomes of palpation-guided versus ultrasound-guided ACJ injections have been reported as similar at up to 3 weeks postinjection in one small study.[8]

Equipment

- ▥ Needle: 25-gauge, 1.5-inch
- ▥ Injectate: 0.5–1 mL of local anesthetic and 0.5–1 mL of an injectable corticosteroid
- ▥ High-frequency linear array transducer

Author's Preferred Technique

a. Patient position
   i. Seated or supine
   ii. Arm adducted in neutral rotation
b. Transducer position (Figure 6-3)
   i. Anatomic sagittal oblique plane over the anterior aspect of the ACJ
c. Needle orientation relative to the transducer (see Figure 6-3)
   i. In plane
d. Needle approach (Figure 6-4)
   i. Anterior to posterior
e. Target
   i. Anterior ACJ
f. Pearls/Pitfalls
   i. Because of ACJ degenerative changes or variability in orientation, the transducer may need to be tilted slightly (typically, adjusting the ultrasound beam such that it travels slightly lateral to medial as it exits the transducer) in order to optimally visualize the needle while using this approach.
   ii. The clinician may consider rotating the transducer axis by 90 degrees during the procedure (only when the needle is stationary) to confirm out-of-plane needle position (in short-axis view).

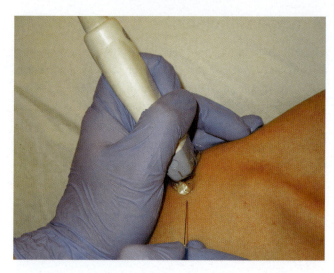

FIGURE 6-3 ■ Transducer position and needle orientation for an anterior approach, transducer short-axis to joint, needle in-plane ultrasound-guided ACJ injection. Sterile transducer cover not pictured.

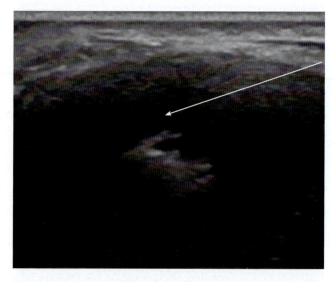

FIGURE 6-4 ■ Ultrasound image for an anterior approach, transducer short-axis to joint, needle in-plane ultrasound-guided ACJ injection. Arrow corresponds to needle position during injection. Left, anterior; top, superficial. Note there are no bony landmarks for this injection approach.

Alternate Technique 1

a. Patient position
   i. Seated or supine
   ii. Arm adducted in neutral rotation

b. Transducer position (Figure 6-5)
   i. Anatomic coronal oblique plane over the anterior aspect of the ACJ

c. Needle orientation relative to the transducer (see Figure 6-5)
   i. Out of plane

d. Needle approach (Figure 6-6)
   i. Anterior to posterior
   ii. Walk-down technique

e. Target
   i. Anterior ACJ

f. Pearls/Pitfalls
   i. As with all ultrasound-guided injections in which the needle is out of plane, be certain to stop advancement of the needle as soon as the tip is visible on the ultrasound monitor as described in the introductory chapters in this book.
   ii. The clinician may consider rotating the transducer axis by 90 degrees during the procedure (only when the needle is stationary) to confirm in-plane needle position (in long-axis view).

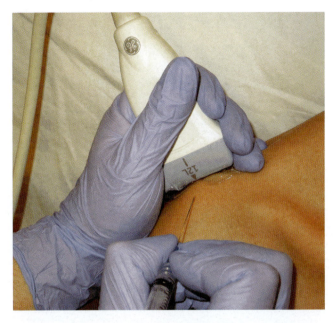

FIGURE 6-5 ■ Transducer position and needle orientation for an anterior approach, transducer long-axis to joint, needle out-of-plane ultrasound-guided ACJ injection. Sterile transducer cover not pictured.

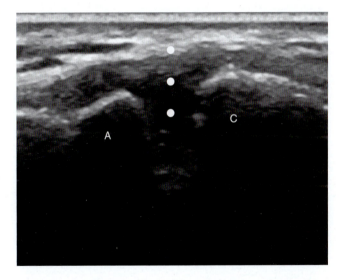

FIGURE 6-6 ■ Ultrasound image for an anterior approach, transducer long-axis to joint, needle out-of-plane ultrasound-guided ACJ injection. Dots correspond to needle position during injection using a step-down technique. Left, lateral; top, superficial; A, acromion; C, clavicle.

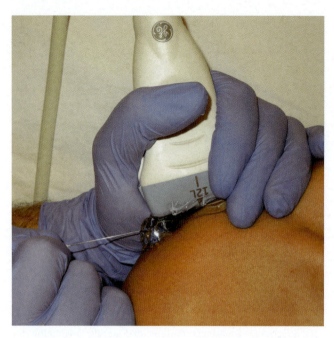

FIGURE 6-7 ■ Transducer position and needle orientation for a lateral approach, transducer long-axis to joint, needle in-plane ultrasound-guided ACJ injection. Note oblique stand-off technique, with additional ultrasound gel stacked laterally. Sterile transducer cover not pictured.

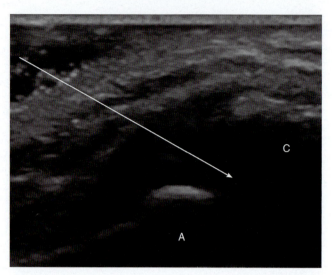

FIGURE 6-8 ■ Ultrasound image for a lateral approach, transducer long-axis to joint, needle in-plane ultrasound-guided ACJ injection. Arrow corresponds to needle position during injection. Note oblique stand-off technique, with additional ultrasound gel stacked laterally. This is visible in the upper left corner of the image. Left, lateral; top, superficial; A, acromion; C, clavicle.

Alternate Technique 2

a. Patient position
   i. Seated or supine
   ii. Arm adducted in neutral rotation
b. Transducer position (Figure 6-7)
   i. Anatomic coronal oblique plane over the lateral aspect of the ACJ
c. Needle orientation relative to the transducer (see Figure 6-7)
   i. In plane
d. Needle approach (Figure 6-8)
   i. Lateral to medial
e. Target
   i. Lateral ACJ
f. Pearls/Pitfalls
   i. An oblique stand-off technique may be necessary, wherein additional sterile ultrasound gel is placed on the patient's skin over the ACJ and the acromion. This is particularly true if a large step-off deformity exists from ACJ injury.

References

1. Alasaarela E, Tervonen O, Takalo R, Lahde S, Suramo I. Ultrasound evaluation of the acromioclavicular joint. *J Rheumatol.* 1997;24(10):1959–1963.
2. Bain GI, Van Riet RP, Gooi C, Ashwood N. The long-term efficacy of corticosteroid injection into the acromioclavicular joint using a dynamic fluoroscopic method. *Int J Shoulder Surg.* 2007;1(4): 104–107.
3. Bisbinas I, Belthur M, Said H, Green M, Learmonth DJ. Accuracy of needle placement in ACJ injections. *Knee Surg Sports Traumatol Arthrosc.* 2006;14(8):762–765.
4. Partington PF, Broome GH. Diagnostic injection around the shoulder: hit and miss? A cadaveric study of injection accuracy. *J Shoulder Elbow Surg.* 1998;7(2):147–150.
5. Peck E, Lai JK, Pawlina W, Smith J. Accuracy of ultrasound-guided versus palpation-guided acromioclavicular joint injections: a cadaveric study. *PM&R.* 2010 Sep;2(9):817–821.
6. Pichler W, Weinberg AM, Grechenig S, et al. Intra-articular injection of the acromioclavicular joint. *J Bone Joint Surg Br.* 2009;91(12):1638–1640.
7. Sabeti-Aschraf M, Lemmerhofer B, Lang S, et al. Ultrasound guidance improves the accuracy of the acromioclavicular joint infiltration: a prospective randomized study. *Knee Surg Sports Traumatol Arthrosc.* 2011 Feb;19(2):292–295.
8. Sabeti-Aschraf M, Ochsner A, Schueller-Weidekamm C, et al. The infiltration of the AC joint performed by one specialist: ultrasound versus palpation a prospective randomized pilot study. *Eur J Radiol.* 2010;75(1):e37–e40.

Evan Peck, MD

KEY POINTS

- Use a high-frequency linear array transducer.
- Use a small-gauge (eg, 25) and relatively short (eg, 1.5-inch) needle.
- Use caution to avoid passing the needle posterior to the joint, where it may injure vital structures.

Pertinent Anatomy

The sternoclavicular joint (SCJ) is a diarthrodial joint consisting of the articulation between the manubrium sterni, the proximal clavicle, and the cartilage of the first rib (Figure 7-1). The SCJ is stabilized by three major ligaments: the sternoclavicular ligament (consisting of the anterior, posterior, superior, and inferior sternoclavicular ligaments), which attaches the manubrium sterni to the clavicle; the costoclavicular ligament, which attaches the cartilage of the first rib to the clavicle; and the interclavicular ligament, which attaches the proximal end of one clavicle to that of the other, and also attaches to the superior manubrium sterni. The joint contains an intraarticular disk. Several vital structures are situated directly posterior to the SCJ, including the subclavian vessels, trachea, and esophagus.

Common Pathology

The SCJ may be injured by a direct impact to the joint, or indirectly from a blow to the shoulder. SCJ injuries may be classified into sprains, partial ligamentous tears, and complete ligamentous tears with resultant subluxations and dislocations. Subluxations and dislocations of the SCJ may be anterior or posterior. Posterior dislocations are of increased concern because of the vital structures that exist directly posterior to the joint. Osteoarthritis may also affect the SCJ.

Ultrasound Imaging Findings

The SCJ is best sonographically visualized in its long axis, perpendicular to the joint line, using a high-frequency linear array transducer, generally with a top frequency of no less than 10 MHz. The joint is typically easily located by direct palpation prior to transducer placement. The intraarticular disk may be visualized as a hypoechoic structure within the joint; increasing the ultrasound's gain setting may accentuate its appearance.

Pathology that may be visualized sonographically includes cortical irregularities, widening or instability of the joint (examined statically or dynamically), and joint effusion with capsular distension.

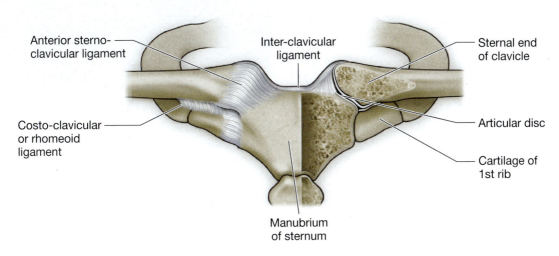

Anterior sterno-clavicular ligament

Inter-clavicular ligament

Sternal end of clavicle

Costo-clavicular or rhomeoid ligament

Articular disc

Cartilage of 1st rib

Manubrium of sternum

FIGURE 7-1 ■ The sternoclavicular joint.

Indications for Sternoclavicular Joint Injection

Injection of the SCJ may be considered for patients with recalcitrant pain resulting from an SCJ-associated pain generator that is unresponsive to appropriate activity modifications, oral or topical medications, therapeutic modalities, therapeutic exercises, and protection or bracing where indicated. In addition, SCJ injection may be used for diagnostic purposes if the primary pain generator is uncertain based on history, physical examination, and imaging findings.

Palpation-guided SCJ injection has been described, with accuracy documented to be 78% in one study.[1] Neither the accuracy of ultrasound-guided SCJ injections, nor a comparison of clinical outcomes between palpation-guided and ultrasound-guided SCJ injections, have been reported in the literature.

Equipment

- Needle: 25-gauge, 1.5-inch
- Injectate: 0.5–1 mL of local anesthetic and 0.5–1 mL of corticosteroid
- Ultrasound machine with high-frequency linear-array transducer

Author's Preferred Technique

a. Patient position
   i. Seated or supine
   ii. Arm adducted in neutral rotation
b. Transducer position (Figure 7-2)
   i. Anatomic sagittal oblique plane over the anterior aspect of the SCJ
c. Needle orientation relative to the transducer (see Figure 7-2)
   i. In plane
d. Needle approach (Figure 7-3)
   i. Anterior to posterior
e. Target
   i. Anterior SCJ
f. Pearls/Pitfalls
   i. Caution should be taken to avoid advancement of the needle beyond the SCJ, where it may injure vital structures.

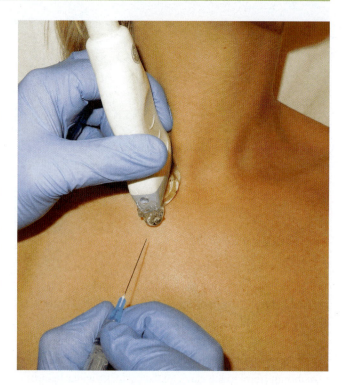

FIGURE 7-2 ■ Transducer position and needle orientation for an anterior approach, transducer short-axis to joint, needle in-plane ultrasound-guided SCJ injection. Sterile transducer cover not pictured.

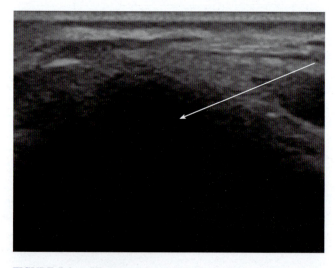

FIGURE 7-3 ■ Ultrasound image for an anterior approach, transducer short axis to joint, needle in-plane ultrasound-guided SCJ injection. *Arrow* corresponds to needle position during injection. Left, posterior; top, superficial. Note there are no bony landmarks for this injection approach.

Alternate Technique

a. Patient position
   i. Seated or supine
   ii. Arm adducted in neutral rotation
b. Transducer position (Figure 7-4)
   i. Anatomic coronal oblique plane over the medial aspect of the SCJ
c. Needle orientation relative to the transducer (see Figure 7-4)
   i. In plane
d. Needle approach (Figure 7-5)
   i. Medial to lateral
e. Target
   i. Medial SCJ
f. Pearls/Pitfalls
   i. Caution should be taken to avoid advancement of the needle beyond the SCJ, where it may injure vital structures.
   ii. An oblique stand-off technique may be necessary, wherein additional sterile ultrasound gel is placed on the patient's skin over the SCJ and the manubrium sterni, in order to maintain continuous visualization of the needle while using this injection approach. This is particularly true if a large step-off deformity exists from SCJ injury.

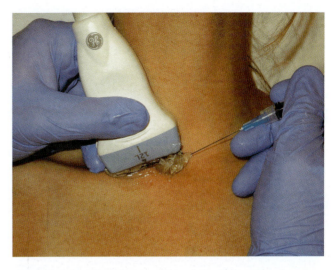

FIGURE 7-4 ■ Transducer position and needle orientation for a medial approach, transducer long-axis to joint, needle in-plane ultrasound-guided SCJ injection. Sterile transducer cover not pictured.

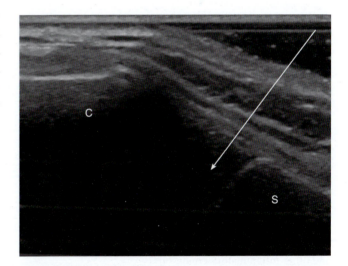

FIGURE 7-5 ■ Ultrasound image for a medial approach, transducer long axis to joint, needle in-plane ultrasound-guided SCJ injection. *Arrow* corresponds to needle position during injection. Note oblique stand-off technique, with additional ultrasound gel stacked medially. This is visible in the upper right corner of the image. Left, lateral; top, superficial; C, clavicle; S, sternum.

Reference

1. Weinberg AM, Pichler W, Grechenig S, et al. Frequency of successful intra-articular puncture of the sternoclavicular joint: a cadaver study. *Scand J Rheumatol.* 2009;38(5):396–398.

Gregory R. Saboeiro, MD

KEY POINTS

- A high-resolution linear array probe with a small footprint is best for visualizing and injecting this superficial structure.
- A 25-gauge, 1.5-inch needle is often ideal for this procedure.

- The bursa is often best visualized and injected as it passes superficial to the supraspinatus tendon beneath the acromion process.

Pertinent Anatomy

The subacromial-subdeltoid (SA-SD) bursa, as its name implies, lies beneath the acromion process and deltoid muscle and superficial to the rotator cuff tendons, glenohumeral joint, and upper aspect of the biceps tendon sheath.

Common Pathology

Subacromial bursitis is a common cause of shoulder pain and limited range of motion. Classically, the patient's symptoms are greatest with elevation of the arm. The pain results from inflammation and distension of the SA-SD bursa and is exacerbated with arm elevation as the bursa slides beneath the acromion process of the scapula. Subacromial bursitis may arise independently but is commonly seen in conjunction with impingement syndromes and rotator cuff pathology, including rotator cuff tears and tendinosis. The incidence is increased in patients with osseous narrowing of the subacromial interval. It is also associated with rheumatoid arthritis and other inflammatory conditions.

This condition is often diagnosed clinically, due to the character of the patient's presenting pain and also signs on physical examination. Differential diagnostic possibilities include rotator cuff pathology, glenohumeral joint arthrosis, and adhesive capsulitis.

Ultrasound Imaging Findings

The SA-SD bursa is best evaluated using a high-resolution linear array probe, as this structure is very superficial. It is generally well seen with the same linear array probe used for evaluation of the rotator cuff tendons. The normal bursa is a thin hypoechoic structure measuring approximately 1 mm in thickness located between the subdeltoid fat plane and a slender fat plane superficial to the rotator cuff (Figure 8-1).

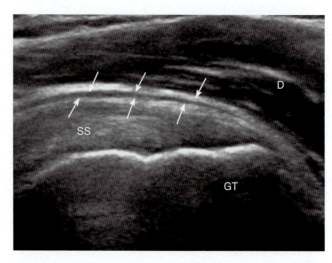

FIGURE 8-1 ■ Normal long-axis ultrasound (US) image of the subacromial-subdeltoid SA-SD bursa (*arrows*). D, deltoid; GT, greater tuberosity of humerus; SS, supraspinatus tendon.

Ultrasound imaging in the setting of bursitis demonstrates enlargement of the bursa. The bursa may be distended with fluid (Figure 8-2) or may be thickened and filled with soft tissue material (Figure 8-3). Often, the bursa is distended with both fluid and inflamed synovium and hyperemia may be seen with power Doppler imaging (Figure 8-4). In addition, provocative maneuvers are performed with elevation of the arm while visualizing the SA-SD bursa as it slides beneath the acromion, evaluating for bunching of the thickened bursa or fluid accumulation beneath the acromion and superficial to the supraspinatus tendon.

Indications for Injection of the Subacromial-Subdeltoid Bursa

Treatment options for confirmed cases of SA-SD bursitis include nonsteroidal antiinflammatory medications, physical therapy, and ice or heat to the area. These are often of limited value.

Injection of the SA-SD bursa with anesthetic and corticosteroid is performed in the setting of clinical and/or sonographic evidence of bursitis, using the criteria for pathology noted above. Additionally, in cases where the diagnosis is uncertain, the SA-SD bursa may be injected with anesthetic alone and repeat physical examination can be performed to assess for symptom resolution after the injection, thus confirming or excluding the diagnosis of bursitis.

Palpation-guided injections into the bursa have been demonstrated to be suboptimal, with only 49% of injections filling the bursa and with 87% also infiltrating regional structures

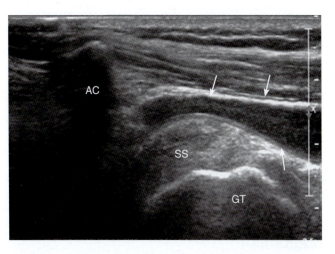

FIGURE 8-2 ■ Fluid distention of the subacromial-subdeltoid SA-SD bursa (*arrows*) extending superficial to the rotator cuff and deep to the deltoid muscle and acromion process. AC, acromion process of scapula; GT, greater tuberosity of humerus; SS, supraspinatus tendon.

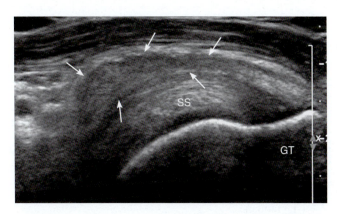

FIGURE 8-3 ■ Thickened and distended subacromial-subdeltoid SA-SD bursa (*arrows*) filled with hypoechoic material. GT, greater tuberosity of humerus; SS, supraspinatus tendon.

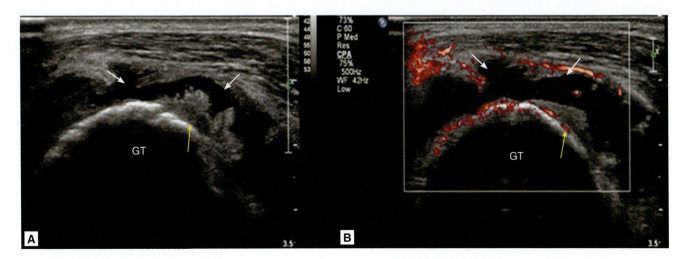

FIGURE 8-4 ■ **A.** subacromial-subdeltoid SA-SD bursa containing fluid (*white arrows*) and extensive synovial debris (*yellow arrows*). **B.** Power Doppler imaging demonstrating bursal hyperemia consistent with active inflammation.

in one study.[1] Henkus et al. confirmed the relatively poor accuracy of palpation-guided injections and also showed that only accurate injections into the SA-SD bursa resulted in pain relief.[2] Chen et al. confirmed this improved clinical response with ultrasound-versus palpation-guided injections,[3] as did Hashiuchi et al.[4] Although using fluoroscopy can help to confirm the accuracy of a palpation-guided injection, it requires both iodinated contrast and ionizing radiation. SA-SD bursa injection is thus most accurately and safely performed using ultrasound guidance.

Equipment

■ Needle: 25-gauge, 1.5-inch needle
■ Injectate: 1 mL of local anesthetic and 0.5–1.0 mL of corticosteroid
■ High-frequency linear array transducer

Author's Preferred Technique

a. Patient position
    i. Seated, lateral decubitus, or supine
    ii. Arm at side
b. Transducer position (Figure 8-5)
    i. Anatomic coronal oblique plane or sagittal plane, or wherever the bursa is best visualized
c. Needle orientation relative to transducer
    i. In plane
d. Needle approach
    i. Lateral to medial
e. Target (Figure 8-6)
    i. SA-SD bursa just lateral to the acromion process
f. Pearls/Pitfalls
    i. The normal bursa is thin and nearly imperceptible (<1 mm).
    ii. The injectate may rapidly pass away from the needle and into the more dependent (usually anterior) aspect of the bursa (Figure 8-7).
    iii. In cases of marked bursal distention, in which the enlarged bursa may extend anteroinferiorly anterior to the proximal biceps tendon, a supine position may be used.
    iv. When the needle is seen to enter the bursa, a small amount of anesthetic is injected. If the needle is within the bursa, the injection should be free of significant resistance and the bursa will be seen to distend with the injected anesthetic.

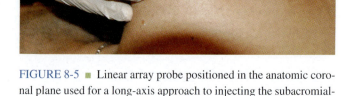

FIGURE 8-5 ■ Linear array probe positioned in the anatomic coronal plane used for a long-axis approach to injecting the subacromial-subdeltoid SA-SD bursa.

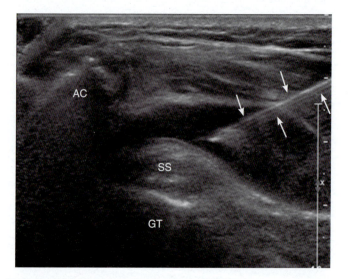

FIGURE 8-6 ■ Ultrasound (US) image demonstrating a long-axis in-plane approach with the needle (*arrows*) entering the distended subacromial-subdeltoid SA-SD bursa. AC, acromion process of scapula; GT, greater tuberosity of humerus; SS, supraspinatus tendon.

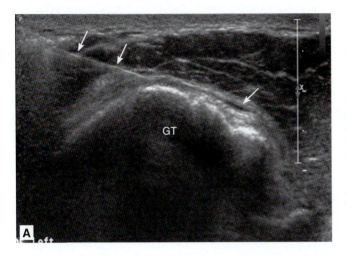

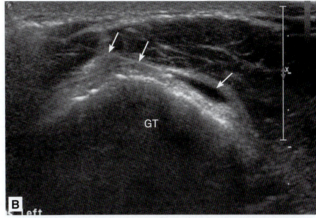

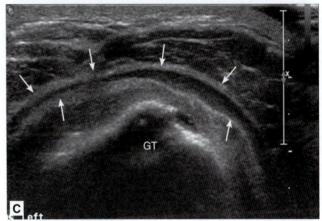

FIGURE 8-7 ■ **A–C.** Sequential images during injection and distention of the subacromial-subdeltoid SA-SD bursa. Note the progressive widening of the bursa during injection (*arrows*) and filling of the anterior and posterior aspects of the bursa. GT, greater tuberosity of humerus.

References

1. Park JY, Siti HT, O KS, Chung KT, Lee JY, Oh JH. Blind subacromial injection from the anterolateral approach: the ballooning sign. *J Shoulder Elbow Surg*. 2010;19(7): 1070–1075.
2. Henkus HE, Cobben LP, Coerkamp EG, Nelissen RG, van Arkel ER. The accuracy of subacromial injections: a prospective randomized magnetic resonance imaging study. *Arthroscopy*. 2006;22(3):277–282.
3. Chen MJ, Lew HL, Hsu TC, et al. Ultrasound-guided shoulder injections in the treatment of subacromial bursitis. *Am J Phys Med Rehabil*. 2006;85(1):31–35.
4. Hashiuchi T, Sakurai G, Sakamoto Y, Takakura Y, Tanaka Y. Comparative survey of pain-alleviating effects between ultrasound-guided injection and blind injection of lidocaine alone in patients with painful shoulder. *Arch Orthop Trauma Surg*. 2010; 130(7):847–852.

Sean N. Martin, DO / Joshua G. Hackel, MD, FAAFP

KEY POINTS

- Use a high-frequency linear array transducer.
- Use a 23–25 gauge, 1.5– 2-inch needle, or equivalent, for injection.
- The biceps tendon is most easily located by imaging in short axis over the greater and lesser tuberosity.

- Use the long axis to guide needle to appropriate depth, but short axis to confirm appropriate placement within sheath.
- Be wary of the anterior circumflex artery as it lies just lateral to the biceps tendon within the sheath.

Pertinent Anatomy (Figure 9-1)

The two heads of the biceps muscle are each attached to the scapula via their own tendons. For the purposes of this chapter, the focus will be on the tendon to the long head of the biceps, commonly called the "biceps tendon." From a pathologic perspective, it is most commonly the tendon to the long head that is of concern. Fibers of the biceps tendon originate from the supraglenoid tubercle, superior labrum, and the joint

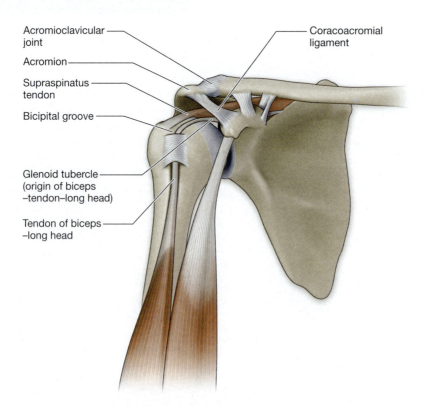

Acromioclavicular joint

Acromion

Supraspinatus tendon

Bicipital groove

Glenoid tubercle (origin of biceps –tendon–long head)

Tendon of biceps –long head

Coracoacromial ligament

FIGURE 9-1 ■ Schematic of anatomy pertinent to ultrasound examination and ultrasound-guided interventions to the biceps tendon sheath. Note the relationship of the proximal biceps tendon to the greater and less tuberosity as it courses after originating from the superior glenoid tubercle.

capsule before traversing the rotator cuff interval, the space between the subscapularis and the supraspinatus. At this point in its course, the tendon is considered intraarticular as it is invested in the capsule of the glenohumeral joint. It is stabilized in this position by the coracohumeral ligament, the superior glenohumeral ligament, and peripheral fibers of the supraspinatus and subscapularis tendons.

As the biceps tendon continues out of the joint distally, it curves in contour with the humeral head. It then remains intrasynovial for approximately 3–4 cm within a sheath that it shares with a branch of the anterior circumflex artery. The tendon courses through the groove formed by the greater tuberosity (laterally) and lesser tuberosity (medially) at the level of the proximal humerus, the biceps tendon is maintained within this intertubercular groove by the transverse humeral ligament as well as overlying fibers of the subscapularis tendon, which inserts on the greater tuberosity. Distal to the tuberosities, the biceps tendon is stabilized by bridging fibers of the pectoralis major tendon.

Common Pathology

Isolated pain within the region of the proximal biceps tendon can be caused from a variety of conditions. Rupture of the long head of the biceps, from either overuse or trauma, often occurs concomitantly with rotator cuff tears and accounts for approximately 95% of all biceps tendon tears.[1] The site of rupture is typically at the biceps–labral junction. The biceps tendon can also be partially torn or congenitally split within the sheath. Localized tenosynovitis can occur within the tendon sheath and easily confused with diffuse tendon sheath effusion. The latter condition is generally secondary to intraarticular pathology. In fact, isolated tenosynovitis of the biceps tendon has been reported to occur only 5% of the time.[1] Being that the glenohumeral joint is congruent with the origin of the biceps tendon sheath, excessive fluid accumulation from within this joint can easily leak into the biceps tendon sheath. Finally, some patients experience subluxation and/or dislocation of their biceps tendon secondary to slack stabilizing structures. This can occur from forced external rotation against resistance.

Ultrasound Imaging Findings

The origin of the biceps tendon is not able to be seen with ultrasound because of shadowing from the acromion. The tendon, rounded proximally and transitioning to an oval shape as it courses distally, is most easily visualized on short axis as it sits within the intertubercular groove between the hyperechoic greater (rounded) and lesser (pointed) tuberosity (Figure 9-2).

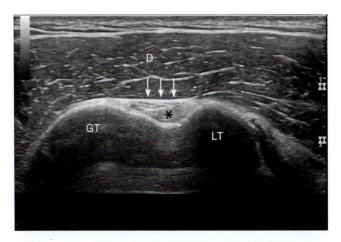

FIGURE 9-2 ■ Short-axis view of proximal biceps tendon between greater (GT) and lesser (LT) tuberosities. Asterisk, biceps tendon; thin arrows, transverse humeral ligament.

Here, the transverse humeral ligament is seen as a thin, slightly hyperechoic linear array structure course immediately superficial to the tendon. Any amount of fluid, which is usually anechoic, that fully encircles the tendon is considered abnormal. Because of the tendon's variable course, care should be taken to ensure that hypoechoic signaling is from fluid and not anisotropy. Differentiation between fluid within the sheath from localized tenosynovitis versus an effusion from the glenohumeral joint can often be made with sonography. Tenosynovitis will display localized swelling of the sheath (Figure 9-3) and the patient will report pain when the ultrasound probe is pressed firmly into the skin at this location. On short-axis imaging, the fluid within the biceps sheath is seen as a hypoechoic ring around the isoechoic biceps tendon, which is a finding

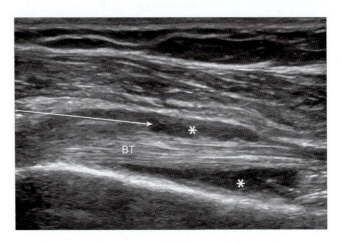

FIGURE 9-3 ■ Long-axis scan of biceps tendon (BT) with hypoechoic tenosynovitis (asterisk). *Arrow* indicates path and target of needle for longitudinal, in-plane approach.

classically called the "ring sign" (Figure 9-4). A glenohumeral effusion with extension into the biceps tendon sheath will appear as a diffuse swelling that courses a large portion of the biceps tendon sheath and the patient generally does not endorse localized pain with ultrasound probe pressure. The fluid from an effusion is usually anechoic.[2] The anterior circumflex artery can be seen within the synovial sheath immediately adjacent to the lateral edge of the biceps tendon.

The biceps tendon suffering from tendinosis appears diffusely enlarged and hypoechoic. On both short and long axis, the tendon can be traced distally until it reaches the myotendinous junction, located at the junction of the proximal and middle third portions of the humerus. The tendon can be examined within the groove for signs of partial tears, seen as linear array anechoic disruptions. Care should be taken not to confuse the easily anisotropic appearance of the biceps tendon with the presence of a partial tear. A ruptured biceps tendon will appear as a hypoechoic empty intertubercular groove. Conversely, hemorrhage following a complete biceps tendon rupture can appear either isoechoic or hyperechoic. This finding should not be misinterpreted as the presence of the biceps tendon.[2] Finally, absence of the biceps tendon within the groove may indicate that it has dislocated. Dynamic ultrasound imaging can be used to evaluate presence of a subluxing or dislocation biceps tendon.

Indications for Injections of the Biceps Tendon Sheath

Biceps tendon sheath injections should be considered for patients who have pain isolated to the biceps tendon region and accompanying ultrasound findings who have failed more conservative treatment. Ultrasound-guided biceps tendon sheath injection has been shown to have an accuracy of 86.7% with regards to placement of medicine within the sheath, versus 26.7% using landmark-based techniques.[3] The use of ultrasound has also been shown to result in a statistically significant higher degree of pain relief.[4]

Equipment

- Needle: 23- or 25-gauge, 1.5–2 inch needle
- Injectate: 0.5–1.0 mL of local anesthetic and 1 mL of corticosteroid

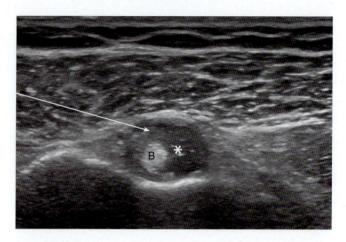

FIGURE 9-4 ■ The "ring sign" short-axis scan of biceps tendon (B) with hypoechoic tenosynovitis (asterisk). *Arrow* indicates path and target of needle for short-axis, in-plane approach.

Author's Preferred Technique

a. Patient position
   i. Supine with arm in neutral position, palm up
   ii. Alternate position
      1. Seated with hand supinated, elbow flexed to 90 degrees, resting on thigh
b. Transducer position
   i. Short axis to biceps tendon to identify isoechoic rounded biceps within sheath
c. Needle orientation relative to the transducer
   i. In plane
d. Needle approach (Figure 9-5)
   i. Lateral to medial
e. Target (see Figure 9-4)
   i. Space between tendon sheath and tendon
f. Pearls/Pitfalls
   i. Based on the size of the patient, a spinal needle may be required to reach the biceps tendon to avoid a steep needle approach.
   ii. Care should be taken to not penetrate the tendon itself.
   iii. It is important to identify the anterior circumflex artery, lateral to biceps tendon, so that it can be avoided during procedure.
   iv. The tendon and its sheath should be viewed in long axis, both during and after the procedure, to assure spread of injectate in the correct tissue space.

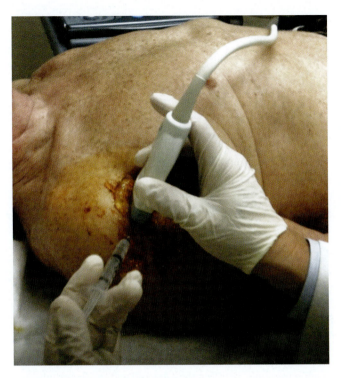

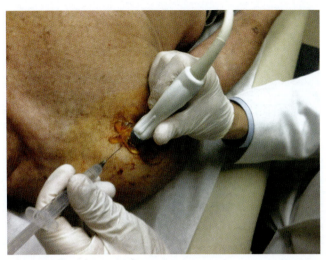

FIGURE 9-6 ■ Proximal to distal approach to injection of the biceps tendon sheath using long-axis approach.

FIGURE 9-5 ■ Lateral to medial approach to injection of the biceps tendon sheath using short-axis approach.

Alternate Technique

a. Patient position
   i. Supine with arm in neutral position, palm up
b. Transducer position
   i. Sagittal plane, parallel to long head of biceps tendon fibers
c. Needle orientation relative to the transducer
   i. In plane
d. Needle approach (Figure 9-6)
   i. Proximal to distal
e. Target (see Figure 9-3)
   i. Space between tendon sheath and tendon
f. Pearls/Pitfalls
   i. Following placement using a long-axis view, short-axis imaging in the axial plane is used to confirm needle placement within the tendon sheath.
   ii. Care should be taken not to penetrate the tendon itself.

References

1. Patton WC, McClusky GM III. Biceps tendinitis and subluxation. *Clin Sports Med.* 2001;20(3):505–529.
2. Jacobson J. *Fundamentals of Musculoskeletal Ultrasound.* Philadelphia, PA: Saunders; 2007.
3. Hashiuchi T, Sakurai G, Morimoto M, et al. Accuracy of the biceps tendon sheath injection: ultrasound-guided or unguided injection? A randomized controlled trial. *J Shoulder Elbow Surg.* 2011;20(7): 1069–1073.
4. Zhang J, Ebraheim N. Lause GE. Ultrasound-guided injection for the biceps brachii tendinitis: results and experience. *Ultrasound Med Biol.* 2011;37(5):729–733.

Joshua G. Hackel, MD, FAAFP

KEY POINTS

- Use a high-frequency linear array transducer.
- A 25-gauge, 1.5–2.0-inch needle can be used for most body types.
- Injection of the subcoracoid bursa can be used diagnostically for suspected subcoracoid impingement syndrome.
- Arm should be in external rotation to better visualize the bursa.

Pertinent Anatomy (Figure 10-1)

There is often confusion regarding the synovial-lined structures in the subcoracoid space. The term *subcoracoid bursa* refers to the bursa located anterior to the subscapularis muscle and deep in relation to the coracoid process, which does not communicate with the glenohumeral joint. The anterior recess of the glenohumeral joint, which may saddlebag the subscapularis tendon, is sometimes referred to as a bursa; however, the term *subscapularis recess* more accurately describes this entity and prevents confusion between the two structures.[1,2]

Common Pathology

Pathology of the subscapularis tendon is infrequently encountered as a major source of shoulder pain and dysfunction.[3] However, isolated subcoracoid bursitis has been implicated as a source of shoulder pain.[2,4] This entity can lead to, or be the result of, subcoracoid impingement, where the subscapularis tendon impinges between the coracoid and the lesser tuberosity. Subcoracoid bursitis may also be associated with rotator cuff and interval tears.

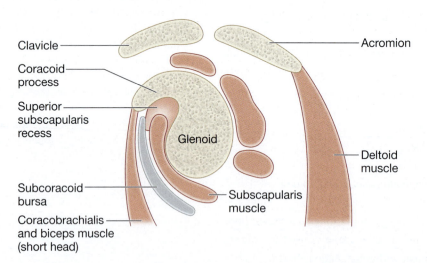

FIGURE 10-1 ■ Drawing shows subcoracoid space in oblique sagittal plane. Note superior subscapularis recess and subcoracoid bursa located anterior to subscapularis muscle. Also note saddlebag appearance of subscapularis recess over subscapularis muscle.

Ultrasound Imaging Findings

The subscapularis tendon and subcoracoid bursa are best visualized with a high-frequency linear array transducer. Typically, a pathologic subcoracoid bursa will contain a hypoechoic fluid collection (Figure 10-2). Passive internal and external rotation of the arm may cause bursal fluid distension and pooling, similar to that seen in the subacromial bursa in the setting of external impingement.

Indications for Injection of the Subcoracoid Bursa

Suspected anterior shoulder pain due to subcoracoid bursitis or impingement is an indication for a diagnostic and therapeutic injection of the bursa, especially in those who have failed more conservative treatments to the area.

Equipment

■ Needle: 25-gauge, 1.5–2-inch needle
■ Injectate: 1 mL of local anesthetic and 1 mL of injectable corticosteroids
■ High-frequency linear array transducer

Author's Preferred Technique

a. Patient position (Figure 10-3)
　i. Supine with elbow at side, glenohumeral joint in external rotation
b. Transducer position (see Figure 10-3)
　i. Anatomic coronal, long axis to the subscapularis tendon
c. Needle orientation relative to transducer
　i. In plane
d. Needle approach
　i. Lateral to medial
e. Target
　i. Subcoracoid bursa just superficial to the subscapularis tendon (see Figure 10-2)
f. Pearls/Pitfalls
　i. Note the distance from the lateral side of the image to the target fluid collection.
　ii. The needle entry must be close enough to the target to reach with your chosen needle length.
　iii. As with all ultrasound-guided injections, always use Doppler to identify vascular structures prior to needle entry.

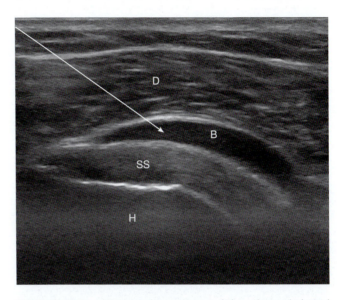

FIGURE 10-2 ■ Ultrasound appearance of the subscapularis and overlying subcoracoid bursa in a patient with anterior shoulder pain. Arrow, needle approach to aspirate/inject bursa; B, subscapularis bursa; D, deltoid muscle; H, humerus; SS, subscapularis tendon.

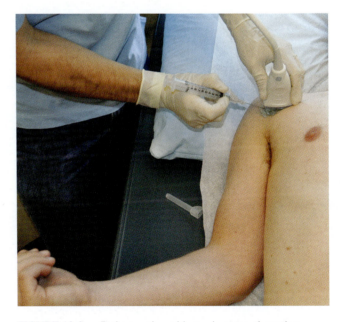

FIGURE 10-3 ■ Patient supine with arm in external rotation.

References

1. Horowitz MT, Tocantins LM. An anatomical study of the role of the long thoracic nerve and the related scapular bursae in the pathogenesis of local paralysis of the serratus anterior muscle. *Anat Rec.* 1938;71:375–385.

2. Schraner AB, Major NM. MR imaging of the subcoracoid bursa. *AJR Am J Roentgenol.* 1999;172:1567–1571.

3. Lyons RP, Green A. Subscapularis tendon tears. *J Am Acad Orthop Surg.* Sept 2005;13:353–363.

4. Mens J, van der Korst JK. Calcifying supracoracoid bursitis as a cause of chronic shoulder pain. *Ann Rheum Dis.* 1984;43: 758–759.

Johan Michaud, MD, FRCPC

KEY POINTS

- Use a high-frequency linear array transducer with a depth of approximately 4 to 5 cm.
- Use a 3.5-inch-long, 22-gauge needle with an in-plane, medial to lateral, approach.
- The transducer must be parallel to the spine of the scapula, over the suprascapular fossa.
- Identify the suprascapular nerve and artery, deep to the supraspinatus muscle, close to the suprascapular notch.

Pertinent Anatomy

The suprascapular nerve (SSN) is a mixed nerve with motor and sensory fibers, mainly formed by the cervical nerve roots C5 and C6 that branch from the upper trunk of the brachial plexus. The SSN courses deep to the trapezius muscle before entering the supraspinous fossa, passing through the suprascapular notch below the superior transverse scapular ligament (STSL), giving motor branches to the supraspinatus muscle and sensory fibers to some shoulder ligaments and to the acromioclavicular and glenohumeral joints.[1] The SSN then passes to the infraspinous fossa through the spinoglenoid notch to give terminal motor branches to the infraspinatus muscle. The SSN is followed in its course by the suprascapular artery and veins that passes above the superior transverse scapular ligament[1] (Figure 11-1).

Common Pathology

SSN neuropathy is a rare cause of shoulder pain caused by traction or compression of the nerve resulting from trauma, repetitive movements, or space-occupying lesions at either the suprascapular or spinoglenoid notch. The patient usually presents with a dull aching shoulder pain and possible weakness and atrophy of supraspinatus and infraspinatus muscles when the SSN is compressed at the suprascapular notch or isolated infraspinatus atrophy when compressed at the spinoglenoid notch. The diagnosis can be confirmed by imaging modality and electrophysiology testing after exclusion of other common causes of shoulder pain. Suprascapular nerve block (SSNB) is commonly used for a wide variety of painful shoulder pathologies other than proper SSN neuropathy.[2]

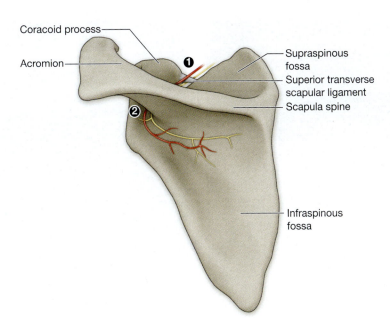

FIGURE 11-1 ■ Anatomy of the suprascapular nerve (*yellow*) and artery (*red*) in relation to the suprascapular notch ❶ and spinoglenoid notch ❷. Ac, acromion; CP, coracoid process; ISf, infraspinatus fossa; SS, spine of the scapula; SSf, supraspinatus fossa; STSL, superior transverse scapular ligament.

Ultrasound Imaging Finding

The SSNB is performed using a high-frequency linear array transducer at a depth between 3 and 5 cm. Except in cases of space-occupying lesions, pathology is rarely seen in ultrasound (US)-guided SSNB. The nerve is not always visible, depending on equipment quality and patient echogenicity. It can be seen in short axis as a round hyperechoic structure located close to the cortical line of the supraspinous fossa, close to the suprascapular notch and deep to the STSL. In the area of the suprascapular notch, power Doppler can be used to identify the suprascapular artery above the STSL, a useful landmark that runs along with SSN.

Indications for Suprascapular Nerve Block at the Suprascapular Notch

In the acute pain setting, SSNB is mainly used for postoperative pain control and bupivacaine 0.5% is usually used as lone injectate. For chronic shoulder pain SSNB has been used in a large variety of painful shoulder pathologies such as rheumatoid arthritis, osteoarthritis, adhesive capsulitis, hemiplegia shoulder, and chronic rotator cuff lesion, where conservative treatments or other type of injections have failed.[3] SSNB for chronic conditions will usually mix bupivacaine and methylprednisolone even if there is no clear evidence of added value to cortisone.[4] SSN neurolysis using radio-frequency, cryolesion,

and phenol for long-lasting effect have also been described.[3] The SSNB based on palpation was described in 1941[5] and multiple modifications have been published since. The few studies on the accuracy of palpation-guided techniques for SSNB seem to show a great variability in the distance between the tip of the needle and the suprascapular notch.[3] US-guided SSNB[6] has been described by Peng with his cadaveric study showing that US-guided SSNB technique is actually targeting the SSN at the level of the supraspinatus fossa, between the suprascapular and the spinoglenoid notches, rather than at the suprascapular notch itself.[7] Comparing the efficacy of palpation-guided versus US-guided SSNB showed better analgesic effect at 1 month and fewer complications for US-guided technique.[8] Rare but potential complications of SSNB are pneumothorax, intravascular injection, residual motor block, and local soft tissue trauma.[3]

Equipment

■ Needle: 22-gauge, 2.5–3.5-inch needle
■ Injectate: 4 mL of local anesthetic and 1 mL of an injectable corticosteroid

Author's Preferred Technique

a. Patient position
    i. Seated (Figure 11-2A)
    ii. Hand of the patient resting on the contralateral shoulder

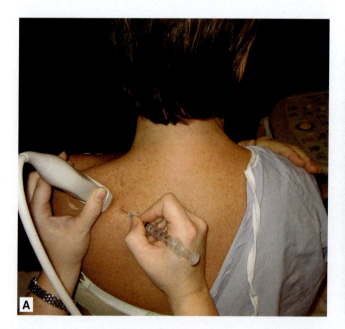
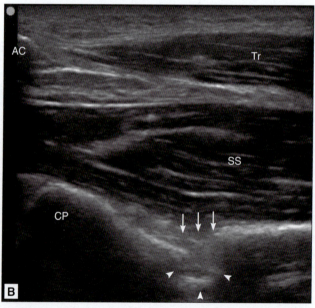

FIGURE 11-2 ■ **A.** Patient position with hand resting on contralateral shoulder. Probe is over the supraspinatus muscle, parallel to the spine of the scapula. Injection is shown using an in-plane approach with a medial to lateral entry point of the needle. **B.** Corresponding ultrasound image. Left, lateral; right, medial; Ac, acromion; CP, coracoid process; SS, supraspinatus muscle; Tr, trapezius muscle; white arrows, STSL; white arrowheads, suprascapular notch.

b. Transducer position (Figure 11-2B)
    i. Anatomical coronal oblique plane. Probe is parallel to the spine of the scapula and over the suprascapular fossa.
c. Needle orientation relative to the transducer
    i. In plane
d. Needle approach
    i. Medial to lateral (Figure 11-3) or lateral to medial
e. Target
    i. The SSN at the level of the suprascapular notch or fossa
f. Pearls/Pitfalls
    i. Use the heel-toe maneuver with the probe for a better needle visualization.
    ii. Patient can also be lying prone with the arm hanging down.

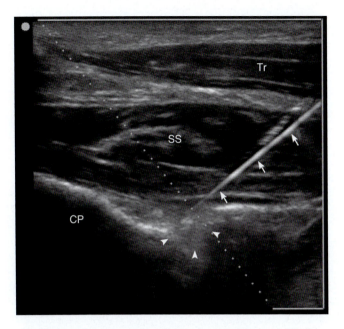

FIGURE 11-3 ▪ Same ultrasound image as in Figure 11-2B showing the needle at the level of the suprascapular notch using. Left, lateral; right, medial; CP, coracoid process; SS, supraspinatus muscle; Tr, trapezius muscle; white arrows, needle; white arrowheads, suprascapular notch.

References

1. Schuenke M, Schutle E, Schumacher U. *Thieme Atlas of Anatomy*. Germany: Thieme Verlag; 2006.
2. Piasecki DP, Romeo AA, Bach BR Jr, Nicholson GP. Suprascapular neuropathy. *J Am Acad Orthop Surg*. 2009 Nov;17(11):665–676.
3. Chan CW, Peng PW. Suprascapular nerve block: a narrative review. *Reg Anesth Pain Med*. 2011 Jul-Aug;36(4):358–373.
4. Gado K, Emery P. Modified suprascapular nerve block with bupivacaine alone effectively controls chronic shoulder pain in patients with rheumatoid arthritis. *Ann Rheum Dis*. 1993 Mar;52(3):215–218.
5. Wertheim HM, Rovenstein EA. Suprascapular nerve block. *Anesthesiology*. 1941;2:541–545.
6. Harmon D, Hearty C. Ultrasound-guided suprascapular nerve block technique. *Pain Physician*. 2007 Nov;10(6):743–746.
7. Peng PW, Wiley MJ, Liang J, Bellingham GA. Ultrasound-guided suprascapular nerve block: a correlation with fluoroscopic and cadaveric findings. *Can J Anaesth*. 2010 Feb;57(2):143–148.
8. Gorthi V, Moon YL, Kang JH. The effectiveness of ultrasonography-guided suprascapular nerve block for perishoulder pain. *Orthopedics*. 2010 Apr 16:238–241.
9. Feigl GC, Anderhuber F, Dorn C, et al. Modified lateral block of the suprascapular nerve: a safe approach and how much to inject? A morphological study. *Reg Anesth Pain Med*. 2007 Nov-Dec; 32(6):488–494.

Elbow

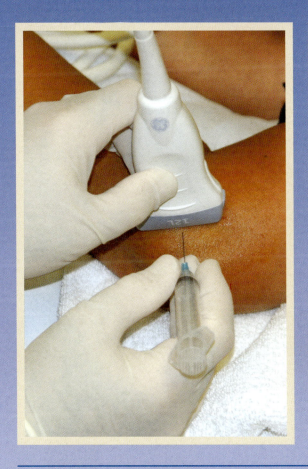

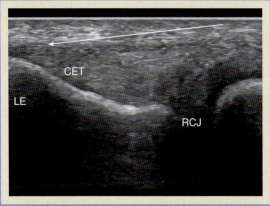

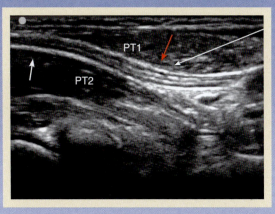

Jonathan S. Halperin, MD

KEY POINTS

- It is best to use a high-frequency linear array transducer.
- The radio-capitellar joint is best accessed using a small-gauge (eg, 25) and relatively short (eg, 1.5 inch) needle.
- The elbow joint can be accessed for aspiration or injection by both the lateral and the posterior approaches using ultrasound guidance.
- Relief of pain from a tense effusion after aspiration can be dramatic.

Pertinent Anatomy

The elbow joint is formed by articulations between three bones: the proximal radius (radial head), the proximal ulna (the anterior coronoid process and posterior olecranon), and the distal humerus (the lateral capitellum and medial trochlea). There are three joints in the elbow. The proximal radio/ulnar joint and the radio/humeral (capitellar) joint allow forearm rotation. The humeral/ulnar joint allows elbow flexion and extension and functions as a hinge type joint. These three joints are encased by a single joint capsule that is loose in flexion and tight in extension (Figure 12-1).

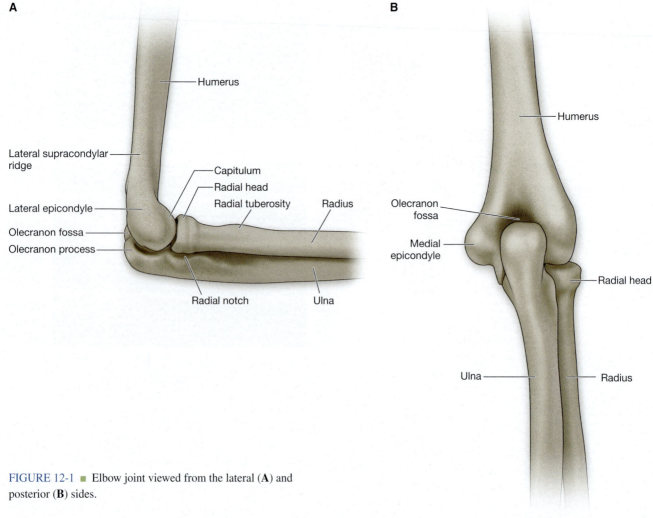

A

- Humerus
- Lateral supracondylar ridge
- Capitulum
- Radial head
- Radial tuberosity
- Radius
- Lateral epicondyle
- Olecranon fossa
- Olecranon process
- Radial notch
- Ulna

B

- Humerus
- Olecranon fossa
- Medial epicondyle
- Radial head
- Ulna
- Radius

FIGURE 12-1 ■ Elbow joint viewed from the lateral (**A**) and posterior (**B**) sides.

Common Pathology

The elbow joint can be injured by direct trauma such as a fracture and/or dislocation. A painful elbow joint may also be related to an intrinsic process such as infection, osteoarthritis, rheumatoid disease, crystal-induced arthropathy, or hemarthrosis secondary to coagulopathy. The joint can also be injured and become painful from repetitive stress and overuse. These conditions may present clinically as a stiff, swollen, and painful joint.

Ultrasound Imaging Findings

The elbow joint can be visualized using a high-frequency linear array transducer. Different aspects of the elbow joint can be visualized from all directions with the ultrasound machine (anterior, lateral, medial, and posterior). In the anterior view, joint space changes to the cartilage interface between the radio-capitellar joint and the ulnar-humeral trochlear joint can be seen in both long-axis and short-axis views. Subtle erosions and cartilage irregularities may indicate pathology. In the lateral view, the radio-capitellar joint can be accessed. Joint effusion (hypoechoic signal anterior to the joint) and abnormalities of the radial head can be seen. In the posterior view, the triceps tendon insertion and fluid in the olecranon bursa and posterior joint space may be seen. Increased signal on color or power Doppler may indicate acute inflammation and/or increased vascularization.

The elbow joint can be accessed using ultrasound guidance at the radio-capitellar articulation and at the posterior elbow lateral to the triceps insertion into the olecranon. Studies or clinical outcome measurements that compare ultrasound versus palpation-guided or fluoroscopically guided injections are limited.

Indications for Injection/ Aspiration of the Elbow Joint

In general, a painful and swollen joint of uncertain etiology will benefit from diagnostic ultrasound-guided aspiration. Evaluation of joint fluid can determine if accumulation is from inflammatory or noninflammatory arthritic disease, infection, subacute fracture, or crystal-induced arthropathy. Evaluation of joint fluid can also be used to monitor the effect of systemic treatment of joint infection (Gram stain, culture, and complete blood count). Therapeutic aspiration can be used to drain a septic joint or to relieve pain from increased joint pressure from traumatic hemarthrosis. Injection of lidocaine or bupivacaine (Marcaine) can anaesthetize the joint to rule out a true locked joint that may require further definitive imaging. Injection with corticosteroid may be used to treat pain from inflammatory arthritic conditions such as osteoarthritis and rheumatoid arthritis and from crystal-based arthropathy such as gout.

Equipment

- Needle: 25-gauge, 1.5-inch needle
- Injectate: 1.0 mL of local anesthetic and 1 mL of injectable corticosteroids
- High-frequency linear array transducer

Author's Preferred Technique

a. Patient position
    i.   Prone, elbow over head propped on pillow
    ii. Elbow flexed to 40 degrees
    iii. Palm down; forearm pronated
b. Alternate position
    i.   Sitting, elbow resting on table with palm down, forearm pronated
c. Transducer position (Figure 12-2)
    i.   Transverse to radio-capitellar joint in line with long axis of the radius
d. Needle orientation relative to transducer (see Figure 12-2)
    i.   Out of plane
e. Needle approach (Figure 12-3)
    i.   Posterior to anterior
    ii. Use walk-down technique
f. Target (see Figure 12-3)
    i.   Radio-capitellar joint
g. Pearl/Pitfalls
    i.   It may be difficult to access the radio-capitellar aspect of the elbow joint if moderate-to-severe arthritis is present.
    ii. For this technique, it is ideal to switch to long axis to confirm needle position prior to injecting.

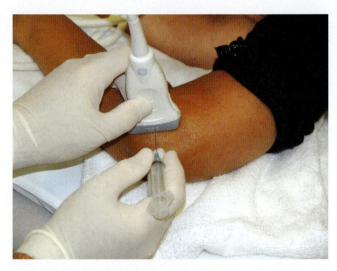

FIGURE 12-2 ■ Patient and transducer position for lateral elbow joint injection with out-of-plane approach.

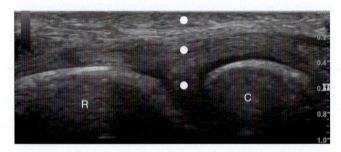

FIGURE 12-3 ■ Ultrasound appearance of lateral view of radio-capitellar joint with out-of-plane, walk-down approach; *dots* represent the needle path to the target area. Left, distal; right, proximal; C, capitellum; R, radius.

Alternate Technique 1

a. Patient position
   i. Prone, elbow over head propped on pillow
   ii. Elbow flexed to 40 degrees with palm down, forearm pronated
b. Alternate position (Figure 12-4)
   i. Sitting, elbow resting on table with palm down, forearm pronated
c. Transducer position
   i. Transverse to radio-capitellar joint in line with long axis of the radius
d. Needle orientation relative to transducer (see Figure 12-4)
   i. In plane
e. Needle approach (Figure 12-5)
   i. Distal to proximal
   ii. Stand-off oblique technique
f. Target (see Figure 12-5)
   i. Radio-capitellar joint
g. Pearl/Pitfalls
   i. It may be difficult to access the radio-capitellar aspect of the elbow joint if moderate-to-severe arthritis is present.
   ii. This technique requires a relatively steep angle of entry and use of stand-off oblique technique to approach the target area.

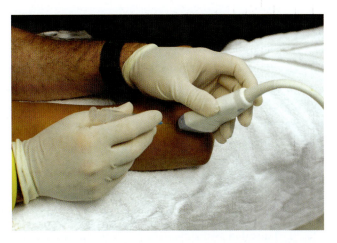

FIGURE 12-4 ▪ Patient and transducer position for lateral elbow joint injection in-plane approach.

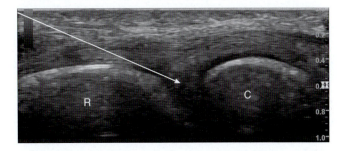

FIGURE 12-5 ▪ Ultrasound appearance of lateral view of radio-capitellar joint with in-plane, oblique stand-off technique. *Arrow* represents needle path to the target area. Left, distal; right, proximal; C, capitellum; R, radius.

Alternate Technique 2

a. Patient position (Figure 12-6)
    i. Prone, elbow over edge of examination table
    ii. Elbow flexed to 90 degrees with arm hanging over edge of table
b. Transducer position (see Figure 12-6)
    i. Short axis to triceps tendon and long axis of humerus and over the olecranon fossa
c. Needle orientation relative to transducer
    i. In plane
d. Needle approach (Figure 12-7)
    i. Lateral to medial, passing below triceps tendon
e. Target (see Figure 12-7)
    i. Posterior elbow joint through the olecranon fossa
f. Pearl/Pitfalls
    i. Visualize the ulnar nerve at the medial epicondyle prior to injection to avoid nerve puncture.
    ii. The long-axis (parallel to triceps tendon insertion), in-plane approach can also be used. For this approach, it is recommended that the needle approach through the triceps tendon or just lateral to it to access the joint space.

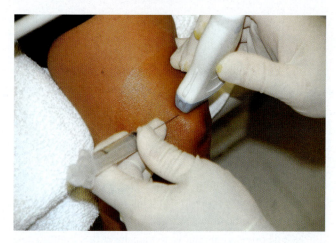

FIGURE 12-6 ■ Patient and transducer position for posterior injection to the elbow joint with an in-plane approach.

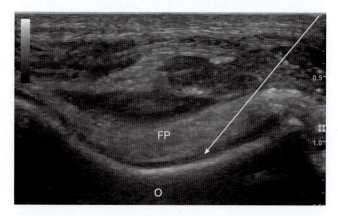

FIGURE 12-7 ■ Ultrasound appearance of posterior elbow joint short-axis view with in-plane approach. *Arrow* represents needle path to the target area. Left, medial; right, lateral; FP, fat pad; O, olecranon.

References

1. Barr LL, Babcock DS. Sonography of the normal elbow. *AJR Am J Roentgenol*. 1991;157:793–198.
2. Cardone DA, Tallia AF. Diagnostic and therapeutic injection of the elbow region. *Am Fam Physician*. 2002;66(11):2097–2100.
3. Cunnington J, Marshall N, Hide G, et al. A randomized, double blind, controlled study of ultrasound-guided cortisone injection into the joint of patients with inflammatory arthritis. *Arthritis Rheum*. 2010;62(7):1862–1869.
4. Martinoli C, Bianchi S, Giovagnorio F, et al. Ultrasound of the elbow. *Skeletal Radiol*. 2001;30:605–614.

Scott Jeffery Primack, DO, FAAPMR, FACOPMR

KEY POINTS

- A high-frequency linear array transducer is optimal.
- A 25-gauge, 1.5-inch needle is ideal for peritendinous procedure.
- Most common extensor tendinopathy occurs in the extensor carpi radialis brevis tendon deep to the extensor digitorum.

- The best approach is long axis and in plane.
- Although corticosteroids have traditionally been used to treat this condition with decent results, be aware that the pathology is more of tendon degeneration than inflammation.

Pertinent Anatomy

The common extensor tendon (CET) is composed of the extensor carpi radialis brevis, extensor digitorum communis, extensor digiti minimi, and extensor carpi ulnaris. These tendons originate at the lateral epicondyle. The extensor carpi radialis brevis tendon is the most anterior. The extensor carpi radialis longus and the brachioradialis originate proximal to the lateral epicondyle at the distal lateral humerus (Figure 13-1).

The function of the CET is wrist extension and radial/ulnar abduction.[1]

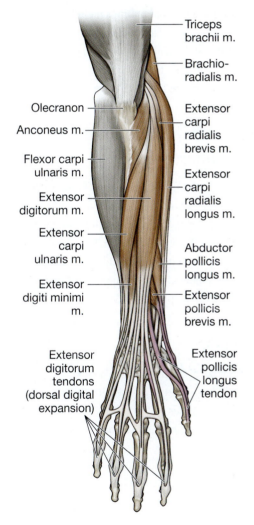

FIGURE 13-1 ■ Lateral compartment of the elbow demonstrating the muscles and tendons that attach at and around the lateral epicondyle. (Reproduced with permission from Morton DA, Foreman KB, Albertine KH, eds. *The Big Picture: Gross Anatomy.* New York: McGraw-Hill; 2011: figure 32-2.)

Common Pathology

Common extensor tendinopathy (commonly called tennis elbow) is normally caused by microtrauma and overuse injuries. The mechanism of injury is seen in occupational disorders as well as sport activities. Increased torque at the elbow, which can give lateral compartment pain, can also be seen in patients with tight internal rotation at the shoulder.[2]

Ultrasound Imaging Findings

The CET is best visualized using a high-frequency linear array transducer. The depth normally should be between 2 and 3 cm. The tendon is examined in long-axis and short-axis views. Common abnormal findings include cortical irregularities, focal loss of visualization, generalized hypoechogenicity, and thickening of the tendon itself. To optimize one's clinical acumen and appreciate the pathology, a side-to-side comparison often times can be useful (Figure 13-2).

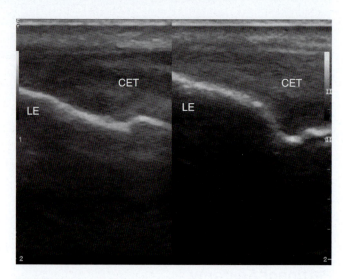

FIGURE 13-2 ▪ Side-by-side comparison demonstrating thickening and heterogenous signal of the CET on the left side compared to the normal right side. CET, common extensor tendon; LE, lateral epicondyle.

Indications for the Common Extensor Peritendinous Injection

An injection at the CET/lateral epicondyle interface can be performed for patients with recalcitrant pain that is unresponsive to relative rest, analgesics, icing, occupational, and/or physical therapy. Injection at the CET has been described by a point of maximum tenderness technique.[3] To date, there have not been any studies that have compared ultrasound-guided CET injections to palpation-guided ones.

Equipment

- Needle: 22–25-gauge, 1.5-inch needle
- Injectate: 1 mL of local anesthetic with 0.5–1 mL of injectable corticosteroids
- High-frequency linear array transducer

Author's Preferred Technique

a. Patient position (Figure 13-3)
   i. Seated or supine
   ii. Arm is on the table with the wrist in prone and lateral compartment is facing the clinician
b. Transducer position (see Figure 13-3)
   i. Long axis to the CET at the lateral epicondyle
c. Needle orientation relative to the transducer (Figure 13-4)
   i. In plane
d. Needle approach (Figure 13-5)
   i. Distal to proximal
e. Target
   i. Superficial to CET (in peritendinous region) at interface of lateral epicondyle
f. Pearls/Pitfalls
   i. It is important to attempt to keep steroid medication superficial to the CET in the peritendinous region.

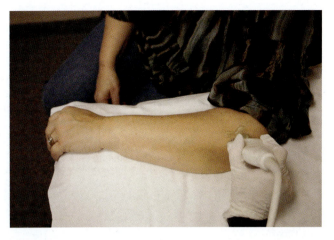

FIGURE 13-3 ▪ The position of the patient and the patient's arm for procedure. Note the linear array transducer long axis to the lateral epicondyle.

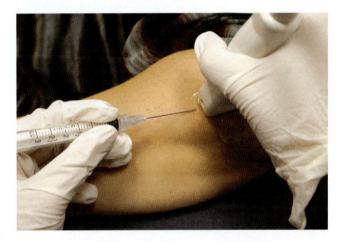

FIGURE 13-4 ▪ Close-up positioning of transducer with needle about to enter skin in-plane from distal to proximal.

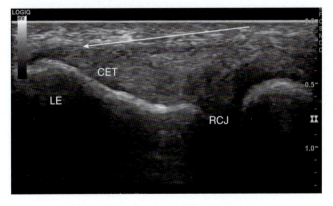

FIGURE 13-5 ▪ Long-axis, in-plane approach to the common extensor tendon from distal to proximal. *Arrow* indicates needle tract and location to place medication in peritendinous region. CET, common extensor tendon; LE, lateral epicondyle; left, anterior; right, posterior side of elbow.

Alternate Technique

a. Patient position (see Figure 13-3)
   i. Seated or supine
   ii. Arm is on the table with the wrist in prone and lateral compartment is facing the clinician
b. Transducer position (Figure 13-6)
   i. Short-axis view at the level of the lateral epicondyle
c. Needle orientation relative to the transducer (Figure 13-7)
   i. In plane
d. Needle approach (see Figure 13-7)
   i. Posterior to anterior
e. Target
   i. Superficial to CET (in peritendinous region) at interface of lateral epicondyle
f. Pearls/Pitfalls
   i. The probability of traumatizing normal tissue with this technique is lessened.

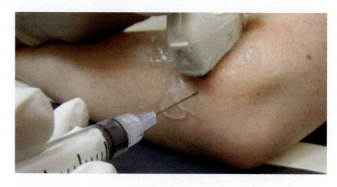

FIGURE 13-6 ■ Positioning of transducer short axis to common extensor tendon with needle about to enter skin in-plane from posterior to anterior.

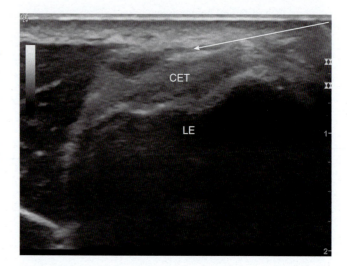

FIGURE 13-7 ■ Short-axis, in-plane approach to the common extensor tendon from posterior to anterior. *Arrow* indicates needle tract and location to place medication in peritendinous region. CET, common extensor tendon; LE, lateral epicondyle; left, anterior; right, posterior side of elbow.

References

1. Hollinshead WH, Jenkins DB. Extensor forearm. *Functional Anatomy of the Limbs and Back.* 5th ed. Philadelphia, PA: Saunders; 1981:147–157.
2. Kibler WB, Herring SA, Press JM. *Functional Rehabilitation of Sports and Musculoskeletal Injuries.* Gaithersburg, MD: Aspen; 1998:149–183.
3. Micheo WF, Rodriguez RA, Amy E. *Joint and Soft-Tissue Injections of the Upper Extremity,* Physical Medicine and Rehabilitation Clinics of North America. Philadelphia, PA: Saunders; 1995:830–832.

John M. McShane, MD

Pertinent Anatomy

The common extensor tendon originates at the lateral epicondyle of the elbow. It crosses the radio-capitellar (RC) joint and blends in to the extensor musculature of the dorsal forearm. As it passes over the RC joint, it lies superficial to the radial collateral ligament (Figure 14-1).

Common Pathology

Pain at the lateral elbow, often referred to as *tennis elbow*, usually results from chronic, repetitive stress to the common extensor tendon (CET). This results in a process of tendon degeneration, characterized by infiltration of the tendon by a matrix of disorganized and hypercellular tissue, along with immature fibroblasts and nonfunctional vascular buds.[1] Because of the microscopic appearance, Nirschl first used the term "angiofibroblastic tendinosis" to describe this tissue.[2] In addition, Nirschl's work also demonstrated that there are no markers of inflammation in this condition. As a result, tennis elbow is now understood to be a degenerative process, most appropriately termed *tendinosis*, rather than tendinitis.

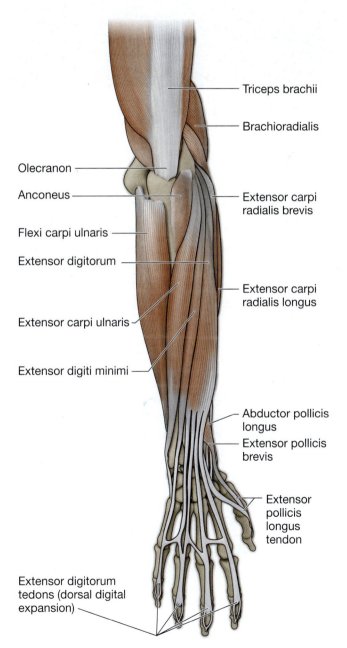

Triceps brachii

Brachioradialis

Olecranon

Anconeus

Flexi carpi ulnaris

Extensor digitorum

Extensor carpi ulnaris

Extensor digiti minimi

Extensor carpi radialis brevis

Extensor carpi radialis longus

Abductor pollicis longus

Extensor pollicis brevis

Extensor pollicis longus tendon

Extensor digitorum tedons (dorsal digital expansion)

FIGURE 14-1 ■ Lateral compartment of the elbow demonstrating the muscles and tendons that attach at and around the lateral epicondyle.

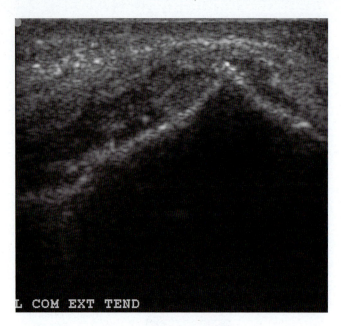

FIGURE 14-2 ■ Tendinopathic CET with thickening and heterogenous appearance under ultrasound. CET, common extensor tendon.

Ultrasound Imaging Findings

The CET should be visualized in both the long and short axes using a high-frequency linear array transducer. Typical findings include an enthesophyte at the apex of the epicondyle, and thickening and heterogeneity of the CET (Figure 14-2). Most tendinotic tendon will demonstrate interstitial tearing or tearing at the bone tendon interface. Only occasionally, however, will these interstitial tears be seen on initial scanning. More commonly, tears will only be seen after infiltration of anesthetic into the tendon. The injection of fluid will cause a separation of torn tendon fibers, allowing tears to become visible (Figure 14-3). Finally, color and/or power Doppler imaging almost always reveals increased flow within and around the CET (Figure 14-4).[3]

Indications for Ultrasound-Guided Percutaneous Tenotomy/Fenestration of the Common Extensor Tendon of the Elbow

Patients become candidates for this procedure if they have painful tendinosis of the CET that has failed both an adequate trial of rest from offending activities and an appropriately designed course of physical therapy. In addition, their level of pain and disability must be sufficiently high for them to

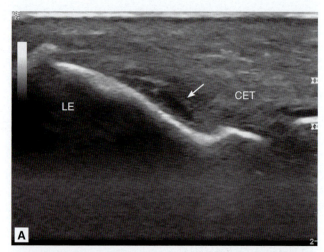

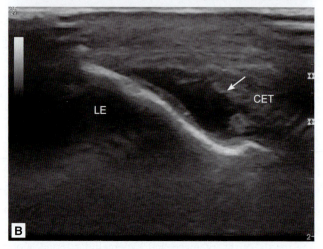

FIGURE 14-3 ■ **A.** Small undersurface tear seen at ECRB insertion to lateral epicondyle. **B.** Gapping of this same tear after administration of local anesthetic. *Arrow* demonstrates area of tear. CET, common extensor tendon; LE, lateral epicondyle.

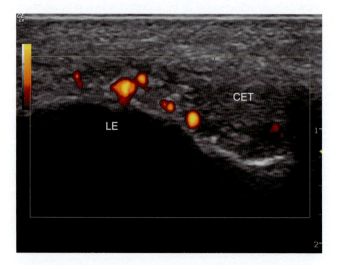

FIGURE 14-4 ■ Doppler flow within the CET. CET, common extensor tendon; LE, lateral epicondyle.

be willing to undergo the procedure and the required course of subsequent physical therapy. Patients will need to clearly understand that after this procedure, their symptoms will initially get worse, and then will slowly improve over a period of approximately 12 weeks. During this time they will have significant limitations of use of the affected limb. These limitations include avoidance of *any* activity that is repetitious and stressful to the CET. Although procedural technique is important, the physical therapy regimen after the procedure is also critical to a successful outcome. The outcomes for this procedure are quite favorable with McShane et al. reporting 92% of treated patients had "good" or "excellent" results.[4]

Equipment

- 25-gauge, 1.5-inch needle for local anesthesia
- Needle: 18- to 20-gauge, 1-5- to 3-inch needle for procedure
- Injectate: Limited amount of local anesthesia to allow for adequate pain control during needle fenestration of the tendon
- High-frequency linear array transducer or "hockey stick" transducer

Author's Preferred Technique

a. Patient position (Figure 14-5)
    i. Supine or seated with elbow on table, slightly bent
b. Transducer position (Figure 14-6)
    i. Longitudinal to the lateral epicondyle and RC joint so that CET is visualized in long axis
c. Needle orientation relative to the transducer (Figures 14-6 and 14-7)
    i. In plane
d. Needle approach (see Figure 14-7)
    i. Distal to proximal
e. Target
    i. Origin of the CET focusing on areas of tendinosis
f. Pearls/Pitfalls
    i. During the procedure it may be necessary to inject small amounts of fluid as the density of the tendinotic tissue may prevent spread of the fluid into certain small sections of the tendon.
    ii. The needle is passed repeatedly from superficial to deep and from medially to laterally, so that the entire abnormal region of the tendon has been repeatedly fenestrated. In addition, the periosteum should be diffusely abraded.

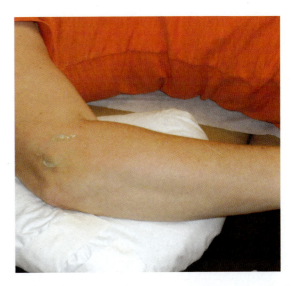

FIGURE 14-5 ■ Patient lying on examination table with right elbow at the side, resting on pad covered with chux.

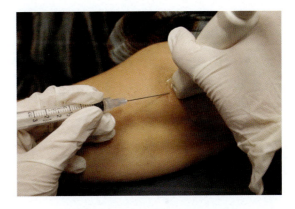

FIGURE 14-6 ■ Setup for long-axis, in-plane approach to CET. CET, common extensor tendon.

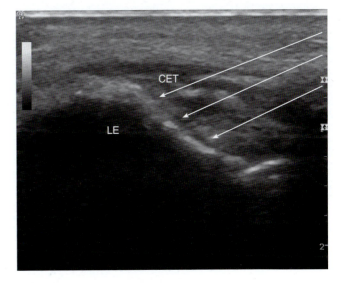

FIGURE 14-7 ■ *Arrows* demonstrate multiple areas that the needle should pass to ensure fenestration of entire tendinotic area. CET, common extensor tendon; LE, lateral epicondyle.

iii. There is no specific number of passes of the needle that must occur. Fenestration with the needle should continue until all regions of abnormal tendon have been addressed.

iv. At the completion of the procedure the needle should be able to be glided through the tendon with very little resistance.

References

1. Faro F, Wolf JM. Lateral epicondylitis: review and current concepts. *J Hand Surg Am.* 2007;32:1271–1277.
2. Nirschl RP, Pettrone F, et al. Tennis elbow: the surgical treatment of lateral epicondylitis. *J Bone Joint Surg Am.* 1979;61:832–841.
3. Levin D, Nazarian LN, et al. Lateral epicondylitis of the elbow: ultrasound findings. *Radiology.* 2005;237:230–234.
4. McShane JM, Shah VN, Nazarian LN. Sonographically guided percutaneous needle tenotomy for treatment of common extensor tendinosis in the elbow. *J Ultrasound Med.* 2008;27:1137–1144.

Scott Jeffery Primack, DO, FAAPMR, FACOPMR

KEY POINTS

- A high-frequency linear array transducer is best for this procedure.
- A 25-gauge, 1.0- to 1.5-inch needle is ideal for peritendinous procedure.
- The common flexor tendon is short and narrow with muscular fibers blending into the tendon proximally.

- The best approach is long axis and in plane.
- Although corticosteroids have traditionally been used to treat this condition with decent results, be aware that the pathology is more of tendon degeneration that inflammation.

Pertinent Anatomy (Figure 15-1)

The flexor muscles of the forearm can be divided into a superficial and a deep group. The common flexor tendon (CFT) is made up of four muscles within the superficial group: the pronator teres, the palmaris longus, the flexor carpi radialis, and the flexor carpi ulnaris. These muscles are fused together as tendons when they arise from the medial epicondyle and thus share a common origin. The function of the muscles of the CFT is forearm pronation (pronator teres), wrist flexion (flexor carpi radialis and palmaris longus), and flexion-adduction at the wrist (flexor carpi ulnaris).[1]

Common Pathology

Common flexor tendinopathy (commonly called golfer's elbow) is related to excess or repetitive stress. The condition can be seen in sports such as golf, racket sports, and weight training.[2] Also, there are many occupations where repetition and excessive gripping exist that can render a person with weakness and pain secondary to inflammation and degeneration at the medial epicondyle.[3]

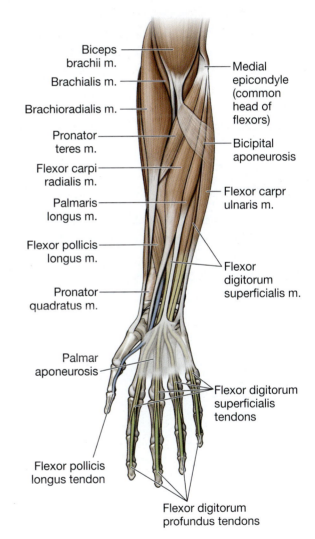

FIGURE 15-1 ■ Medial compartment of the elbow. (Reproduced with permission from Morton DA, Foreman KB, Albertine KH, eds. *The Big Picture: Gross Anatomy.* New York: McGraw-Hill; 2011: figure 32-1B.)

Ultrasound Imaging Findings

The CFT is best visualized using a high-frequency linear array transducer. The depth normally should be between 2 and 3 cm. The tendon is examined in long-axis and short-axis views. Common abnormal findings include cortical irregularities, focal loss of visualization, and generalized hypoechogenicity and thickening of the tendon.[4] To optimize one's clinical acumen and appreciate the pathology, a side-to-side comparison often times can be useful (Figure 15-2).

Indications for the Common Flexor Peritendinous Injection

An injection at the CFT/medial epicondyle interface can be performed for patients with recalcitrant medial compartment elbow pain that is unresponsive to relative rest, analgesics, icing, occupational and/or physical therapy. Injection at the CFT has been described by a point of maximum tenderness technique.[5] To date, there have not been any studies that have compared ultrasound-guided CFT injections to palpation-guided ones.

Equipment

- Needle: 22- to 25-gauge, 1.5-inch needle.
- Injectate: 1 mL of local anesthetic with 0.5–1 mL of injectable corticosteroid
- High-frequency linear array transducer

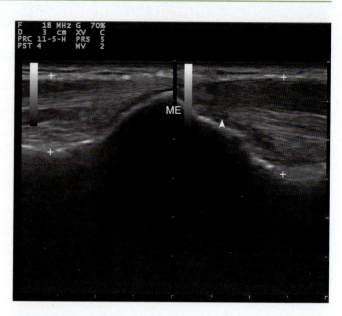

FIGURE 15-2 ■ Typical sonographic findings in common flexor tendinosis. The normal left side displays well-defined fibrillar pattern blending with relatively hypoechoic muscular fibers. The abnormal right side displays loss of that fibrillar pattern (*arrowhead*) and diffuse thickening of the musculotendinous junction. The distance between the calipers includes the CFT and anterior branch of the ulnar collateral ligament. ME, medial epicondyle.

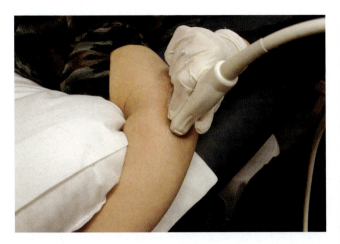

FIGURE 15-3 ▪ Patient is supine with arm abducted and externally rotated allowing the linear array transducer to be placed at the medial epicondyle for procedure.

Author's Preferred Technique

a. Patient position (Figure 15-3)
    i. Seated or supine
    ii. Arm is on the table with the wrist in supine and medial compartment facing the clinician
b. Transducer position (see Figure 15-3)
    i. Long axis to CFT at the medial epicondyle
c. Needle orientation relative to the transducer (Figure 15-4)
    i. In plane
d. Needle approach (Figure 15-5)
    i. Distal to proximal
e. Target
    i. CFT/medial epicondyle interface
f. Pearls/Pitfalls
    i. It is important to attempt to keep steroid medication superficial to the CFT in the peritendinous region.

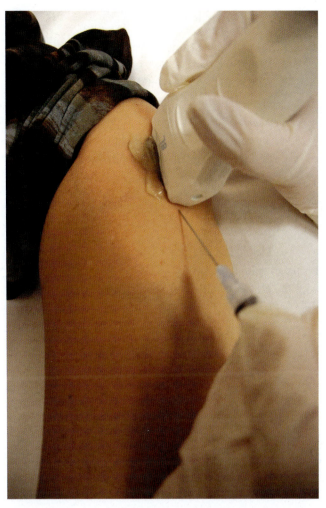

FIGURE 15-4 ▪ Close-up positioning of transducer with needle about to enter skin in plane from distal to proximal.

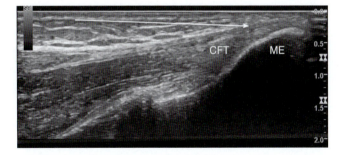

FIGURE 15-5 ▪ Ultrasound image demonstrating the long-axis view of a normal common flexor tendon with *arrow* representing needle approach to the peritendinous region.

Alternate Technique

a. Patient position (see Figure 15-3)
    i. Seated or supine
    ii. Arm is on the table with the wrist in supine and me-
        dial compartment facing the clinician
b. Transducer position (Figure 15-6)
    i. Short-axis view at the level of the medial epicondyle
c. Needle orientation relative to the transducer (Figure 15-7)
    i. In plane
d. Needle approach (see Figure 15-7)
    i. Anterior to posterior
e. Target
    i. Medial epicondyle/CFT interface
f. Pearls/Pitfalls
    i. The probability of traumatizing normal tissue is
        lessened.

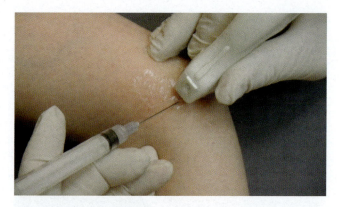

FIGURE 15-6 ▪ Positioning of transducer short axis to common flexor tendon at medial epicondyle with needle about to enter skin in plane from anterior to posterior.

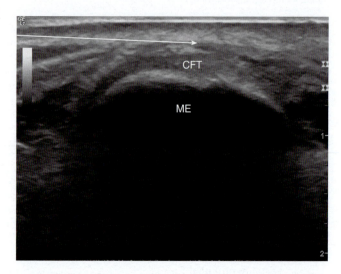

FIGURE 15-7 ▪ Short-axis, in-plane approach to the common flexor tendon from anterior to posterior. *Arrow* indicates needle tract and location to place medication in peritendinous region. CFT, common flexor tendon; ME, medial epicondyle; left, anterior; right, posterior side of elbow.

References

1. Hollinshead WH, Jenkins DB. Extensor forearm. In: *Functional Anatomy of the Limbs and Back*. 5th ed. Philadelphia, PA: Saunders; 1981:145–151.
2. Regan WD, et al. Tendinopathies around the elbow. In: Delee JC et al. *Delee and Drez's Orthopaedic Sports Medicine*. 3rd ed. Philadelphia, PA: Saunders; 2009.
3. Ranney D. Elbow, forearm, wrist and hand. In: *Chronic Musculoskeletal Injuries in the Workplace*. Philadelphia, PA: Saunders; 1997:145–167.
4. Finlay K, Ferr M, Friedman D. Ultrasound of the elbow. *Skeletal Radiol*. 2004,33:63–79.
5. Braddom RL. Upper limb musculoskeletal pain syndromes. In: *Physical Medicine & Rehabilitation*. Philadelphia, PA: Saunders; 1996:770–775.

Bradley D. Fullerton, MD

KEY POINTS

- A high-frequency linear array transducer is best for this procedure.
- A 18- to 20-gauge, 1.5-inch needle is ideal.
- The common flexor tendon is short and narrow with muscular fibers blending into the tendon proximally.

- The best approach is long axis and in plane.
- Be sure to rule out additional injury to the ulnar collateral ligament.

Pertinent Anatomy

The common flexor tendon (CFT) of the medial elbow arises from the medial epicondyle of the humerus. It is a blended origin of four flexor tendons: flexor carpi radialis, palmaris longus, flexor digitorum superficialis, and flexor carpi ulnaris (FCU). While their primary function is flexion of the wrist and fingers, they also assist in dynamic stability of the medial elbow. The ulnar nerve crosses the elbow posterior to the medial epicondyle/CFT origin and enters the forearm between the ulnar and humeral heads of the FCU (Figure 16-1).

Common Pathology

The most common pathology of the CFT is a tendinosis with degenerative changes of the tendon and adjoining muscular fibers. This is commonly termed *medial epicondylitis*, although the underlying pathology involves the tendon and is not inflammatory. The condition is also labeled "golfer's elbow," although the condition more commonly occurs in nongolfers.[1]

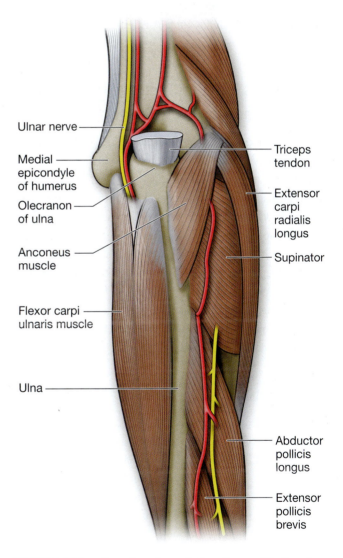

FIGURE 16-1 ■ Posterior view of the elbow with the ulnar nerve passing between the medial epicondyle (anterior and medial to the nerve) and olecranon process of the ulna (posterior and lateral to the nerve). The ulnar nerve enters the forearm between the humeral and ulnar origins of the flexor carpi ulnaris.

Ultrasound Imaging Findings

The CFT is best visualized in long axis using a high-frequency linear array transducer at a depth of 2–3 cm. Because of more proximal muscle fibers, the tendon is short and narrow compared to the common extensor tendon of the elbow. On ultrasonography, the region of the tendon appears more like a musculotendinous junction, rather than a well-formed, hyperechoic, fibrillar tendon. This makes ultrasonographic diagnosis of pathology more difficult than its lateral counterpart. Typical findings include thickening, hypoechoic signal, and more heterogenous echotexture compared to the asymptomatic side (Figure 16-2). Anechoic gaps consistent with partial tears can be seen. Cortical surface irregularities of the medial epicondyle and tendinous calcifications may also be observed.[2]

Indications for Percutaneous Tenotomy of the Common Flexor Tendon

Tenotomy of the CFT can be performed for patients with recalcitrant pain that is unresponsive to activity modification, icing, antiinflammatories, and physical therapy. Stahl and Kaufman reported reduced pain in corticosteroid-injected CFT at 6 weeks compared to placebo[3]; however, there was no difference at 3 months and 1 year. Randomized controlled trials with long-term follow-up (6–12 months) have shown unfavorable results of corticosteroid injection in lateral epicondylitis compared to no intervention.[4] Palpation-guided percutaneous fenestration and dextrose injection of the CFT (ie, prolotherapy) has been described.[5,6] The success rate of these unguided procedures has not been reported.

Equipment

- ■ Needle: 25-gauge, 1.5-inch needle for local anesthesia
- ■ 18- to 20-gauge, 1.5-inch needle for procedure
- ■ Injectate: Limited amount of local anesthetic to allow for adequate pain control during needle fenestration of the tendon
- ■ High-frequency linear array transducer

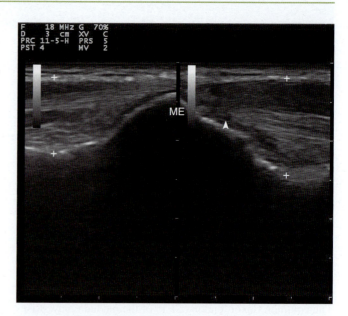

FIGURE 16-2 ■ Typical sonographic findings in common flexor tendinosis. The normal left side displays well-defined fibrillar pattern blending with relatively hypoechoic muscular fibers. The abnormal right side displays loss of that fibrillar pattern (at the *arrowhead*) and diffuse thickening of the musculotendinous junction. The distance between the calipers includes the common flexor tendon (CFT) and anterior branch of the ulnar collateral ligament (UCL). ME, medial epicondyle.

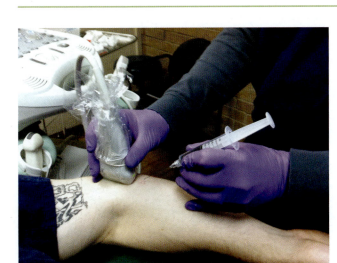

FIGURE 16-3 ■ Patient, transducer and needle position for common flexor tendon (CFT) fenestration and injection. Patient is prone with internally rotated shoulder, pronated forearm. The probe is oriented in the coronal plane, resting on the medial epicondyle with a long-axis view of the tendon.

Author's Preferred Technique

a. Patient position (Figure 16-3)
   i. Prone
   ii. Arm at patient's side with shoulder internally rotated and forearm pronated
b. Alternate position: (Figure 16-4)
   i. Supine
   ii. Hand over head with elbow/forearm resting on pillow (ie, shoulder in full flexion)
c. Transducer position
   i. Anatomic coronal plane (long axis to the flexor tendon) with proximal edge of probe at the medial epicondyle
d. Needle orientation relative to the transducer
   i. In plane
e. Needle approach (Figure 16-5)
   i. Distal to proximal
f. Target
   i. CFT and musculotendinous junction, including medial epicondyle origin
g. Pearls/Pitfalls
   i. Turning the probe to a short-axis, out-of-plane approach may be useful to assure the full width of the pathologic tendon is treated. With a short-axis view

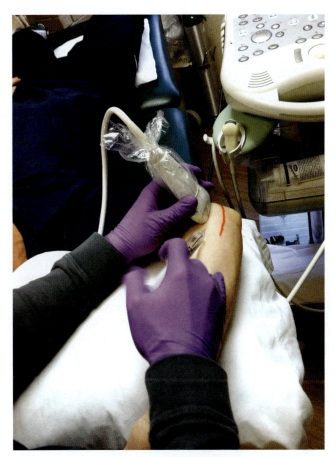

FIGURE 16-4 ■ Alternate position: patient is supine with shoulder flexed and externally rotated. The elbow and forearm rest on a pillow. Practitioner stands at the head of the examination table.

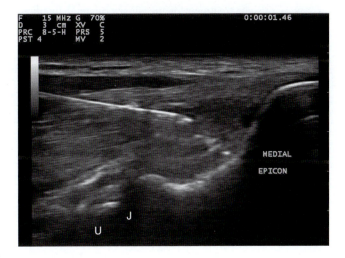

FIGURE 16-5 ■ Long-axis view of the common flexor tendon (CFT) with needle approaching approximately 20 degrees from parallel to the transducer. Needle approach from distal to proximal. J, medial joint line with overlying UCL fibers; U, ulna.

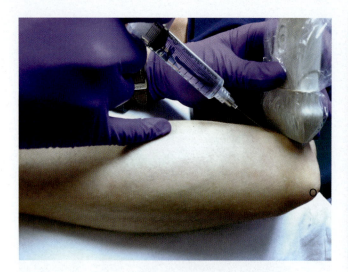

FIGURE 16-6 ▪ Transducer and needle position for out-of-plane approach to common flexor tendon (CFT)/medial epicondyle. A medial view of the ulna and flexor muscle mass. The probe rests on the CFT, just distal to the medial epicondyle. The patient is in alternate position (supine with shoulder externally rotated/fully flexed and forearm resting on pillow). O, olecranon process.

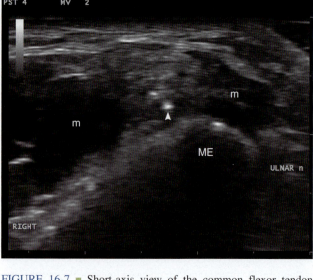

FIGURE 16-7 ▪ Short-axis view of the common flexor tendon (CFT) with needle tip (*arrowhead*) seen in out-of-plane approach as in Figure 16-6. The edge of the ulnar nerve can be seen to the right. m, muscular fibers.

of tendon, observe the ulnar nerve posteriorly at edge of ultrasound screen (Figures 16-6 and 16-7).

ii. The option of supine or prone position allows the practitioner to always inject with the syringe in the dominant hand.

iii. The prone position also allows better visualization of the course of the ulnar nerve through the cubital tunnel.

iv. Consider treatment of the ulnar collateral ligament (deep to the CFT) and pronator teres origin (at the superior edge of epicondyle) for recalcitrant cases.

References

1. Ciccotti MG, Ramani MN. Medial epicondylitis. *Tech Hand Up Extrem Surg*. 2003;7(4):190–196.
2. Park G-Y, Lee S-M, Lee MY. Diagnostic value of ultrasonography for clinical medial epicondylitis. *Arch Phys Med Rehabil*. 2008;89(4):738–742.
3. Stahl S, Kaufman T. The efficacy of an injection of steroids for medial epicondylitis. A prospective study of sixty elbows. *J Bone Joint Surg Am*. 1997;79(11):1648–1652.
4. Coombes BK, Bisset L, Vicenzino B. Efficacy and safety of corticosteroid injections and other injections for management of tendinopathy: a systematic review of randomised controlled trials. *Lancet*. 2010;376(9754):1751–1767.
5. Reeves KD. Prolotherapy: regenerative injection therapy. In: Waldman, ed. *Atlas of Pain Management Injection Techniques*. 2nd ed. Philadelphia, PA: Saunders; 2007:1106–1127.
6. Fullerton BD, Reeves KD. Ultrasonography in regenerative injection (prolotherapy) using dextrose, platelet-rich plasma, and other injectants. *Phys Med Rehabil Clin N Am*. 2010;21(3):585–605.

Mederic M. Hall, MD

KEY POINTS

- A high-frequency linear array transducer is recommended.
- The posterior approach is recommended for injection.
- The technique for aspiration varies depending on size and location of the bursa and neurovascular structures.
- Use a 25-gauge, 2-inch needle, or equivalent, for injection.

- Use an 18-gauge, 2-inch needle, or equivalent, for aspiration.
- Identify the regional neurovascular structures during the preprocedural planning.
- Do not inject into the tendon.

Pertinent Anatomy

At the distal aspect of the biceps muscle two fibrous bands are formed: the lacertus fibrosus (or bicipital aponeurosis) extending medially to insert on the fascia of the forearm, and the distal biceps tendon, which courses laterally and deep to insert on the bicipital tuberosity of the ulnar aspect of the proximal radius (Figure 17-1).[1-4] Unlike the proximal biceps, there is no distal tenosynovial sheath, but rather a paratenon. Classically, the distal biceps tendon has been described as a single flat tendon that rotates 90 degrees externally as it moves obliquely from anterior to posterior and from medial to lateral toward its insertion site.[2,5,6] More recently, the complex anatomy of the distal biceps tendon has been better defined, demonstrating that there are often distinct short-head and long-head components contributing to a bifurcated tendon.[2,3,7,8] These findings are important for diagnostic imaging and surgical repair; however, for the purposes of the injection techniques described below, we will consider the distal biceps tendon as a single entity.

The distal biceps tendon attaches to the ulnar (or posterior) aspect of the radial tuberosity.[9] When the arm is in full supination, the attachment site is oriented in an ulnar direction and the tendon lies medial to the extensor musculature of the forearm and the supinator muscle. The brachial artery and median nerve lie medial to the distal biceps tendon, whereas

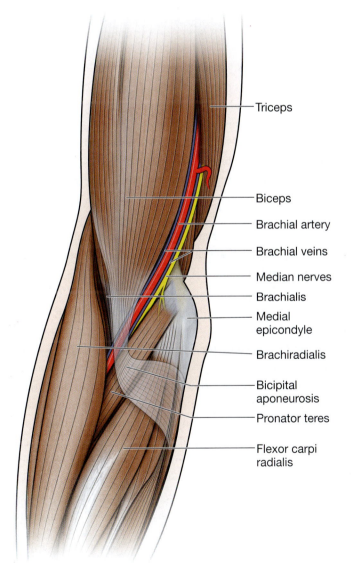

FIGURE 17-1 ■ Anatomy of the cubital fossa. Note the relationship between the distal biceps tendon, bursa, and the adjacent neurovascular structures.

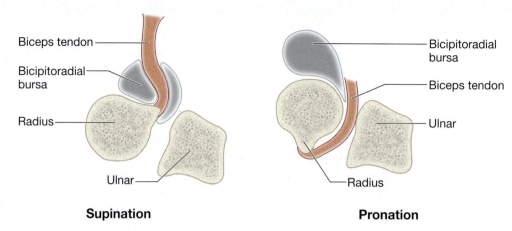

Supination **Pronation**

FIGURE 17-2 ■ Diagram shows the position of the bicipitoradial bursa during pronation and supination. With pronation, the interval between the radius and ulna is decreased, resulting in increased intrabursal pressure.

the lateral antebrachial cutaneous nerve and radial nerve are positioned laterally. With pronation, the distal biceps tendon attachment moves posterior and superficial between the proximal radius and ulna. In this position, the anconeus muscle lies superficially on the lateral side of the ulna with the supinator positioned deep to the anconeus and overlying the most distal fibers of the biceps tendon.[10]

The cubital fossa contains two bursa, the interosseous bursa and the bicipitoradial bursa, neither of which are seen in normal patients during ultrasound or magnetic resonance imaging studies[11] (Figure 17-2). Communication may occur between these two bursa, but no communication has been reported with the joint.[11,12] The bicipitoradial bursa is located between the distal biceps tendon anteriorly and the radial tuberosity posteriorly.[13,14] It lies along the medial cortex of the radius and partially envelops the distal biceps tendon (occasionally ensheathing the tendon).[14] The role of the bicipitoradial bursa is friction reduction between the distal biceps tendon and proximal radius during pronation and supination. Enlargement of the bursae can impair flexion and extension of the elbow as well as compress the adjacent neurovascular structures. The bicipitoradial bursa may compress the superficial or deep branches of the radial nerve resulting in sensory or motor symptoms, respectively.[14] The interosseous bursa lies medial (ie, ulnar) to the biceps tendon and may compress the median nerve when enlarged.[11,12] Compressive symptoms may worsen with pronation, which increases the tension within the bursae.[11,13]

Common Pathology

Injury to the distal biceps tendon is relatively uncommon. Pathology seen in the region includes tendinosis, partial rupture, complete rupture, and other causes of antecubital fossa pain such as bicipitoradial bursitis and pronator syndrome.[6] Most acute injuries occur by means of an eccentric load applied to a flexed load-bearing elbow.[6,10] These injuries are most common in the dominant arm of male manual laborers and athletes.[9,10]

Two factors may predispose the distal biceps tendon to injury. First, a 2-cm hypovascular zone approximately 1–2 cm proximal to the radial tuberosity has been identified that corresponds with tendon degenerative changes seen at microscopy.[4,6,15] Second, as the forearm moves through pronation and supination, mechanical impingement of the distal biceps tendon has been demonstrated between the lateral border of the ulna and the radial tuberosity.[4,6]

Cubital bursitis is an even more rare condition with few reports in the literature.[11-14,16,17] Clinical findings are painful swelling in the cubital fossa, which may be accompanied by neurologic complaints if there is mechanical compression of the radial or median nerves. The most common cause of cubital bursitis is felt to be mechanical trauma due to repetitive pronation and supination; however, infection, inflammatory arthropathy, chemical synovitis, bone proliferation, synovial chondromatosis, and lipoma arborescens have also been implicated.[14,17]

Ultrasound Imaging Findings

Multiple techniques have been described to image the distal biceps tendon. A high-frequency linear array transducer should be used for all of the described techniques. The anterior approach allows both short- and long-axis views of the distal biceps tendon, but often provides inadequate visualization of the most distal aspect of the tendon because of its oblique posterior course and susceptibility to anisotropy. It is useful in identifying the proximity of the adjacent neurovascular structures. The posterior approach (described below) provides an excellent window for both peritendinous injection and, at times, injection of the bicipitoradial bursa; however, only the distal most aspect of the biceps tendon attachment is seen, thus providing limited diagnostic utility. Both the lateral[1] and medial (or pronator window) approaches[9] provide excellent diagnostic information regarding tendon characteristics (tendinosis) and integrity (rupture), but are of limited use interventionally because of lack of visualization of important neurovascular structures adjacent to the needle trajectory. Findings are those typical of tendinosis (hypoechogenicity, focal thickening, calcification, neovascularity, etc). Distinguishing tendinosis from rupture is important as the latter may benefit from surgical consultation.

Regarding the bicipitoradial bursa, sonographic findings are similar to those seen in bursopathy of other locations, including regular walls containing anechoic fluid or a mix of anechoic fluid and hypoechoic septae and debris.[11,12] Dystrophic calcification, represented as scattered hyperechoic foci, has also been reported.[14] Vascularity may be appreciated with Doppler imaging and has been suggested to represent active inflammation.[14]

Indications for Aspiration/Injection of the Distal Biceps Tendon and Bicipitoradial Bursa

Peritendinous injection of the distal biceps tendon can be considered in patients with pain and dysfunction nonresponsive to rest, activity modification, oral analgesics, and physical therapy. Because of the deep location and proximity to important neurovascular structures, image guidance is recommended.

Aspiration or injection of the bicipitoradial bursa should be considered when enlargement of the bursa is compressing the regional neurovascular structures or the painful swelling in the cubital fossa does not respond to more conservative measures such as activity modifications and nonsteroidal antiinflammatory medications.

If aspiration is attempted, one must consider the regional anatomy and take care to note the position of the radial nerve as well as the lateral antebrachial cutaneous and median nerves, brachial artery, and multiple large veins present in the region. Optimal needle trajectory for aspiration varies considerably depending on the size and location of the bursa and its relation to the aforementioned sensitive structures. The posterior approach described below may be used to inject the bursa, but will often not provide an adequate window for aspiration (see Figure 17-2).

Equipment

- Needle: 25-gauge, 2-inch needle for local anesthesia and injection
- 18-gauge, 2-inch needle for aspiration
- Injectate: 2 mL of local anesthetic and 0.5–1.0 mL of corticosteroid
- High-frequency linear array transducer

Author's Preferred Technique

a. Patient position (Figure 17-3)
   i. Supine
   ii. Arm flexed at elbow and forearm hyperpronated
b. Transducer position
   i. Short-axis plane on the posterior forearm (3–4 cm distal to the olecranon) using the posterior approach[10]
c. Needle orientation relative to the transducer
   i. In plane
d. Needle approach (Figure 17-4)
   i. Radial to ulnar
e. Target
   i. For peritendinous placement, place just superficial to tendon, between the tendon and the overlying supinator muscle. This injection is placed in the vicinity of the interosseous space.
   ii. For bicipitoradial bursa, advance through tendon and place deep between distal biceps tendon and radius.
f. Pearls/Pitfalls
   i. Identify the regional neurovascular structures during the pre-procedural planning.
   ii. In the author's experience, superficial placement of injectate provides adequate peritendinous spread while avoiding advancement of the needle through the tendon. Unless the bicipitoradial bursa is being targeted, recommendation is for superficial placement only.
   iii. The contents of the bursa are often viscous and a large-gauge needle is required for aspiration. Occasionally, lavaging with either local anesthetic or sterile saline is required to yield aspirate.
   iv. There is no single reliable technique to aspiration of the bursa given the possible variations in relationship to the regional neurovascular structures and, thus, no such technique is described in this book. If aspiration is considered, careful identification of the neurovasculature during the pre-procedural planning is of utmost importance.

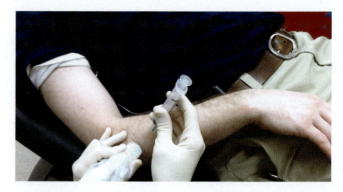

FIGURE 17-3 ■ Patient is positioned supine with arm flexed at the elbow and the forearm hyperpronated. The transducer is positioned in the short-axis plane on the posterior forearm. Approach is radial to ulnar, in plane with the transducer.

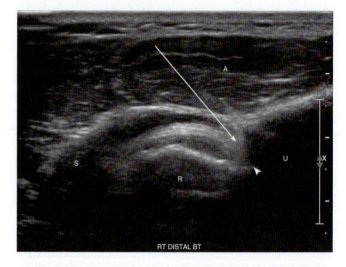

FIGURE 17-4 ■ Ultrasound image of the distal biceps tendon attachment to the radius (R) using the posterior approach. The forearm is hyperpronated to bring the tendon out from the posterior acoustic shadow of the ulna (U). The overlying supinator (S) and anconeus (A) are seen. The *arrow* identifies the target of the peritendinous injection, just superficial to the tendon in the vicinity of the interosseous space.

References

1. Kalume Brigido M, et al. Improved visualization of the radial insertion of the biceps tendon at ultrasound with a lateral approach. *Eur Radiol.* 2009;19(7):1817–1821.
2. Tagliafico A, et al. Ultrasound demonstration of distal biceps tendon bifurcation: normal and abnormal findings. *Eur Radiol.* 2010;20(1):202–208.
3. Athwal GS, Steinmann SP, Rispoli DM. The distal biceps tendon: footprint and relevant clinical anatomy. *J Hand Surg Am.* 2007;32(8):1225–1229.
4. Miyamoto RG, Elser F, Millett PJ. Distal biceps tendon injuries. *J Bone Joint Surg Am.* 2010;92(11):2128–2138.
5. Chew ML, Giuffre BM. Disorders of the distal biceps brachii tendon. *Radiographics.* 2005;25(5):1227–1237.

6. Quach T, et al. Distal biceps tendon injuries—current treatment options. *Bull NYU Hosp Jt Dis.* 2010;68(2):103–111.

7. Cho CH, et al. Insertional anatomy and clinical relevance of the distal biceps tendon. *Knee Surg Sports Traumatol Arthrosc.* 2011;19(11):1930–1935.

8. Jarrett CD, et al. Anatomic and biomechanical analysis of the short and long head components of the distal biceps tendon. *J Shoulder Elbow Surg.* 2012;21:942–948.

9. Smith J, et al. Sonographic evaluation of the distal biceps tendon using a medial approach: the pronator window. *J Ultrasound Med.* 2010;29(5):861–865.

10. Giuffre BM, Lisle DA. Tear of the distal biceps brachii tendon: a new method of ultrasound evaluation. *Australas Radiol.* 2005;49(5):404–406.

11. Liessi G, et al. The US, CT and MR findings of cubital bursitis: a report of five cases. *Skeletal Radiol.* 1996;25(5):471–475.

12. Sofka CM, Adler RS. Sonography of cubital bursitis. *AJR Am J Roentgenol.* 2004;183(1):51–53.

13. Kannangara S, et al. Scintigraphy of cubital bursitis. *Clin Nucl Med.* 2002;27(5):348–350.

14. Skaf AY, et al. Bicipitoradial bursitis: MR imaging findings in eight patients and anatomic data from contrast material opacification of bursae followed by routine radiography and MR imaging in cadavers. *Radiology.* 1999;212(1):111–116.

15. Tran N, Chow K. Ultrasonography of the elbow. *Semin Musculoskelet Radiol.* 2007;11(2):105–116.

16. Karanjia ND, Stiles PJ. Cubital bursitis. *J Bone Joint Surg Br.* 1988;70(5):832–833.

17. Le Corroller T, et al. Lipoma arborescens in the bicipitoradial bursa of the elbow: sonographic findings. *J Ultrasound Med.* 2011;30(1):116–118.

CHAPTER 18 Distal Biceps Tendon Percutaneous Tenotomy

Mederic M. Hall, MD

KEY POINTS

- A high-frequency linear array transducer is recommended.
- Use a 25-gauge, 1.5- to 2-inch needle for local anesthesia.
- Use a 18- to 20-gauge, 2-inch needle for tenotomy.
- Identify the regional neurovascular structures during the pre-procedural planning.
- Optimal technique remains to be defined.

Pertinent Anatomy (Figure 18-1)

At the distal aspect of the biceps muscle two fibrous bands are formed: the lacertus fibrosus (or bicipital aponeurosis) extending medially to insert on the fascia of the forearm, and the distal biceps tendon, which courses laterally and deep to insert on the bicipital tuberosity of the ulnar aspect of the proximal radius.[1-4] Unlike the proximal biceps, there is no distal tenosynovial sheath, but rather a paratenon. Classically, the distal biceps tendon has been described as a single flat tendon that rotates 90 degrees externally as it moves obliquely from anterior to posterior and medial to lateral toward its insertion site.[2,5,6] More recently, the complex anatomy of the distal biceps tendon has been better defined, demonstrating that there are often distinct short-head and long-head components contributing to a bifurcated tendon.[2,3,7,8] These findings are important for diagnostic imaging and surgical repair; however, for the purposes of the injection techniques described below, we will consider the distal biceps tendon as a single entity.

The distal biceps tendon attaches to the ulnar (or posterior) aspect of the radial tuberosity.[9] When the arm is in full supination, the attachment site is oriented in an ulnar direction and the tendon lies medial to the extensor musculature of the forearm and the supinator muscle. The brachial artery and median nerve lie medial to the distal biceps tendon, whereas the lateral antebrachial cutaneous nerve and radial nerve are positioned laterally (Figure 18-2). With pronation, the distal biceps tendon attachment moves posterior and superficial between the proximal radius and ulna. In this position, the anconeus muscle lies superficially on the lateral side of the ulna with the supinator positioned deep to the anconeus and overlying the most distal fibers of the biceps tendon.[10]

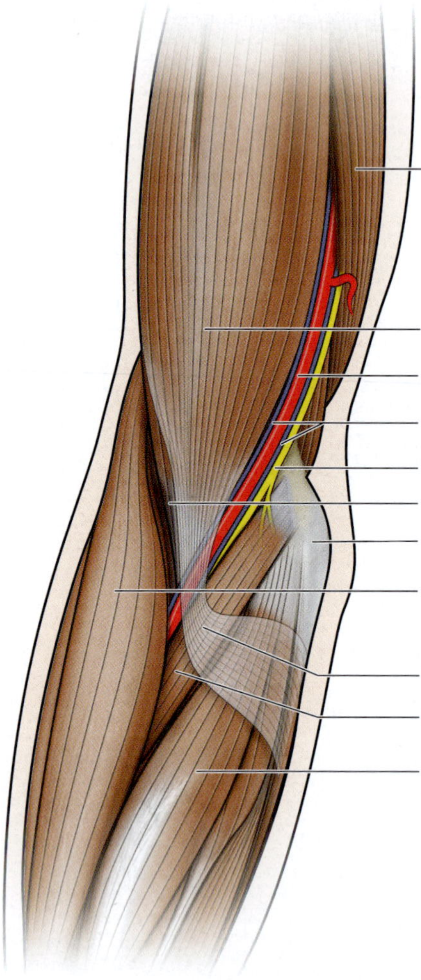

Triceps
Biceps
Brachial artery
Brachial veins
Median nerves
Brachialis
Medial epicondyle
Brachiradialis
Bicipital aponeurosis
Pronator teres
Flexor carpi radialis

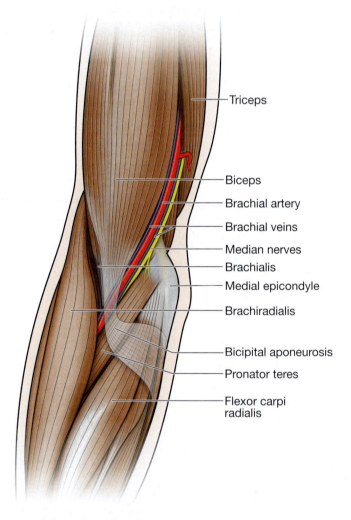

FIGURE 18-1 ■ Anatomy of the cubital fossa. Note the relationship between the distal biceps tendon and the adjacent neurovascular structures.

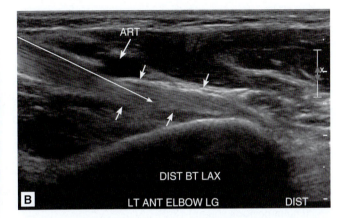

FIGURE 18-2 ■ **A.** Short-axis ultrasound image of the anterior elbow showing the relationship of the distal biceps tendon to the regional neurovascular structures. The brachial artery (ART) and median nerve (MED NV) lie medial to the distal biceps tendon (BT SAX); the radial nerve (RAD NV), lateral antebrachial cutaneous nerve (LACN), and cephalic vein (VEIN) lie laterally. **B.** Long-axis ultrasound image of the anterior elbow showing a long-axis view of the distal biceps tendon (*short arrows*) at the radial attachment (R). Note the proximity to the brachial artery (ART). The *long arrow* represents needle placement within the tendon.

Common Pathology

Injury to the distal biceps tendon is relatively uncommon. Pathology seen in the region includes tendinosis, partial rupture, complete rupture, and other causes of antecubital fossa pain such as bicipitoradial bursitis and pronator syndrome.[6] Most acute injuries occur by means of an eccentric load applied to a flexed load-bearing elbow.[6,10] These injuries are most common in the dominant arm of male manual laborers and athletes.[9,10]

Two factors may predispose the distal biceps tendon to injury. First, a 2-cm hypovascular zone approximately 1–2 cm proximal to the radial tuberosity has been identified that corresponds with tendon degenerative changes seen at microscopy.[4,6,11] Second, as the forearm moves through pronation and supination, mechanical impingement of the distal biceps tendon has been demonstrated between the lateral border of the ulna and the radial tuberosity.[4,6]

Ultrasound Imaging Findings

Multiple techniques have been described to image the distal biceps tendon. A high-frequency linear array transducer should be used for all of the described techniques. The anterior approach allows both short- and long-axis views of the distal biceps tendon, but often provides inadequate visualization of the most distal aspect of the tendon because of its oblique posterior course and susceptibility to anisotropy. It is useful in identifying the proximity of the adjacent neurovascular structures. The posterior approach provides an excellent window for both peritendinous injection and injection of the bicipitoradial bursa; however, only the distal most aspect of the biceps tendon attachment is seen, thus providing limited diagnostic utility. Both the lateral approach[1] and the medial (or pronator window) approach[9] provide excellent diagnostic information regarding tendon characteristics (tendinosis) and integrity (rupture), but are of limited use interventionally because of lack of visualization of important neurovascular structures adjacent to the needle trajectory. Findings are those typical of tendinosis (hypoechogenicity, focal thickening, calcification, neovascularity, etc). Distinguishing tendinosis from rupture is important as the latter often needs surgical consultation.

Indications for Percutaneous Tenotomy of the Distal Biceps Tendon

Percutaneous tenotomy of the distal biceps tendon has not been formally studied. As such, appropriate indications, safety and efficacy of the procedure, and optimal technique remain to be defined. It may be reasonable to consider this procedure in patients with chronic, recalcitrant pain and dysfunction, imaging findings consistent with distal biceps tendinosis, and having failed appropriate conservative therapies including rest, activity modification, oral analgesics, and physical therapy. One may also consider a peritendinous corticosteroid injection prior to proceeding with tenotomy. Because of the deep location and proximity to important neurovascular structures, image guidance is highly recommended.

Equipment

- Needle: 25-gauge, 1.5- to 2-inch for local anesthesia
- 18- to 20-inch, 2-inch needle for tenotomy
- Injectate: Limited amount of local anesthesia to allow for adequate pain control during needle fenestration of the tendon
- High-frequency linear array transducer

Author's Preferred Technique

a. Patient position (Figure 18-3)
   i. Supine
   ii. Arm extended at elbow and forearm supinated
b. Transducer position (see Figure 18-3)
   i. Sagittal plane over the antecubital fossa
   ii. May require small angulation of distal probe radially to best parallel biceps tendon fibers
c. Needle orientation relative to the transducer
   i. In plane
d. Needle approach (Figure 18-2B)
   i. Proximal to distal
e. Target
   i. Intratendinous
f. Pearls/Pitfalls
   i. The safety and efficacy of the procedure are unknown.
   ii. Identify the median nerve and brachial artery, which are just medial (ie, ulnar) to the distal biceps tendon.
   iii. There are several large veins typically in the region that should be avoided.
   iv. Anisotropy of the distal tendon is common with the anterior approach. A heel-toe maneuver with the distal end of the transducer will both improve the image of the tendon and allow for optimal trajectory of the needle. Ample acoustic coupling gel will be required.
   v. If, during procedure planning, there is no safe needle path that can clearly avoid the neurovascular structures in the area, then the author would advise a posterior approach to the tendon (as described below).

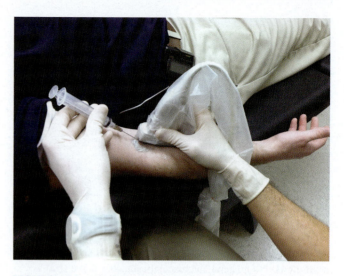

FIGURE 18-3 ▪ Patient is positioned supine with arm extended at the elbow and forearm supinated. The transducer is placed in the sagittal plane over the antecubital fossa. Approach is proximal to distal, in plane with the transducer.

Alternate Technique

a. Patient position (Figure 18-4)
    i.   Supine
    ii. Arm flexed at elbow and forearm hyperpronated
b. Transducer position
    i.   Short axis plane on the posterior forearm (3–4 cm distal to the olecranon) using the posterior approach[10]
c. Needle orientation relative to the transducer
    i.   In plane
d. Needle approach (Figure 18-5)
    i.   Radial to ulnar
e. Target
    i.   Intratendinous
f. Pearls/Pitfalls
    i.   The safety and efficacy of the procedure are unknown.
    ii. The posterior approach offers the safest window for the procedure, but the trade-off is only being able to address the distal most extent of the tendon.
    iii. Identify the radial nerve as it courses through the supinator during the pre-procedural scanning/planning.

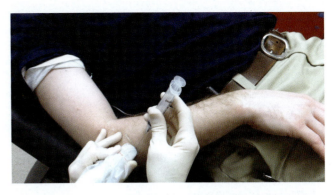

FIGURE 18-4 ■ Patient is positioned supine with arm flexed at the elbow and the forearm hyperpronated. The transducer is positioned in the short-axis plane on the posterior forearm. Approach is radial to ulnar, in plane with the transducer.

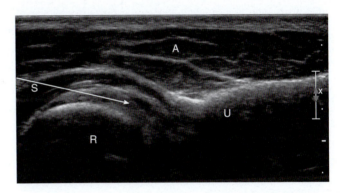

FIGURE 18-5 ■ Ultrasound image of the distal biceps tendon (*arrows*) attachment to the radius (R) using the posterior approach. The forearm is hyperpronated to bring the tendon out from the posterior acoustic shadow of the ulna (U). The overlying supinator (S) and anconeus (A) are seen. The *long arrow* represents intratendinous needle placement.

References

1. Kalume Brigido M, et al. Improved visualization of the radial insertion of the biceps tendon at ultrasound with a lateral approach. *Eur Radiol.* 2009;19(7):1817–1821.
2. Tagliafico A, et al. Ultrasound demonstration of distal biceps tendon bifurcation: normal and abnormal findings. *Eur Radiol.* 2010;20(1):202–208.
3. Athwal GS, Steinmann SP, Rispoli DM. The distal biceps tendon: footprint and relevant clinical anatomy. *J Hand Surg Am.* 2007;32(8):1225–1229.
4. Miyamoto RG, Elser F, Millett PJ. Distal biceps tendon injuries. *J Bone Joint Surg Am.* 2010;92(11):2128–2138.
5. Chew ML, Giuffre BM. Disorders of the distal biceps brachii tendon. *Radiographics.* 2005;25(5):1227–1237.
6. Quach T, et al. Distal biceps tendon injuries—current treatment options. *Bull NYU Hosp Jt Dis.* 2010;68(2):103–111.
7. Cho CH, et al. Insertional anatomy and clinical relevance of the distal biceps tendon. *Knee Surg Sports Traumatol Arthrosc.* 2011;19(11):1930–1935.
8. Jarrett CD, et al. Anatomic and biomechanical analysis of the short and long head components of the distal biceps tendon. *J Shoulder Elbow Surg.* 2012;21:942–948.
9. Smith J, et al. Sonographic evaluation of the distal biceps tendon using a medial approach: the pronator window. *J Ultrasound Med.* 2010;29(5):861–865.
10. Giuffre BM, Lisle DA. Tear of the distal biceps brachii tendon: a new method of ultrasound evaluation. *Australas Radiol.* 2005;49(5):404–406.
11. Tran N, Chow K. Ultrasonography of the elbow. *Semin Musculoskelet Radiol.* 2007;11(2):105–116.

Jose A. Ramirez-Del Toro, MD

KEY POINTS

- Use a high-frequency linear array transducer.
- Use a 22- to 25-gauge, 1.5- to 2-inch needle for peritendinous injection.
- Use an 18- to 20-gauge needle for tenotomy procedure.
- Be extremely cautious not to inject corticosteroids into tendon itself because of possibility of rupture.
- Pre-scan area to find radial nerve or other neurovascular structures that might be in path of needle.

Pertinent Anatomy

The triceps brachii muscle is the primary extensor of the elbow joint. It also acts as a shoulder adductor and extensor by way of the long head of the triceps, which crosses the shoulder joint. The triceps brachii muscle is composed of three heads that have separate origins but a common insertion. The long head of the triceps originates from the superolateral border of the scapula, at a bony prominence known as the infraglenoid tubercle, just inferior to the glenoid fossa of the scapula. The lateral head of the triceps brachii muscle originates from the proximal humerus and from the lateral intermuscular septum. These two heads, the long and lateral heads, unite about two-thirds of the way down the humerus to form the more superficial tendinous insertion of the muscle. The third head, the medial head, originates from the mid posterior humeral shaft and covers the entire posterior surface of the lower part of the humerus. It then joins the deep surface of the superficial tendon formed by the long and lateral heads.[1] These three heads then insert together on the proximal end of the olecranon of the ulna, although the medial head does have its own very short tendon attachment onto the proximal ulna prior to joining the more superficial tendon of the long and lateral heads.[2] This ends up being a an important distinction when it comes to sonography of the distal triceps brachii tendon, as it is this common insertion of all three heads that is the usual target for injections.

The insertion of the triceps tendon is over a wide area on the olecranon known as the triceps footprint.[2] Medially, the insertion extends to the posterior end of the ulna, and laterally, it inserts on the fascia of the extensor carpi ulnaris muscle (Figure 19-1).[2]

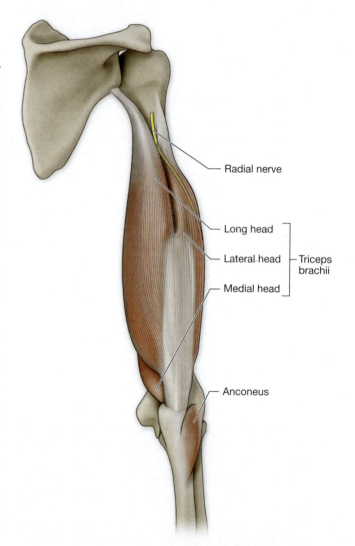

FIGURE 19-1 ■ The triceps brachii with its three heads.

Radial nerve

Long head

Lateral head

Medial head

Triceps brachii

Anconeus

Common Pathology

The triceps brachii tendon, like any other tendon, can be injured through overuse or through direct trauma. Overuse injury of the triceps tendon is most commonly seen in overhead athletes.[2,3] Such pathology presents with posterior elbow pain that is aggravated by repetitive and resisted elbow extension. This can clinically mimic posterior olecranon impingement syndrome, and in fact, it can be very difficult to differentiate the two on history and clinical examination alone.

Trauma to the triceps brachii tendon is actually quite rare when compared to the incidence and prevalence of all other tendon injuries.[4] When trauma to the triceps tendon does occur, it is usually through a fall on an outstretched hand mechanism while the triceps is actively contracting.[4] Such trauma can present as rupture of the muscle or of the tendon itself, but most commonly, an avulsion off of the olecranon is what is noted. This injury has also been reported in power lifters and in other activities that create a decelerating force on a contracting triceps.[4]

Ultrasound Imaging Technique and Findings

The distal triceps tendon is visualized in both long-axis and short-axis planes using a high-frequency linear array transducer at a depth of <3 cm. Much like other tendons in the body, the sonographic appearance of the triceps brachii tendon has a highly linear, very distinctly fibrillar and hyperechoic appearance in the long-axis view. The olecranon and the ulno-olecranon fossa are structures that should be noted when scanning the distal triceps tendon. In addition, the insertion of the tendon along the olecranon should be scanned and noted in its appearance.

There is scant literature on ultrasound imaging of the distal triceps brachii tendon. This is largely due to the rarity of the triceps tendon injuries as mentioned in the previous section. The ultrasound findings of triceps pathology is based on patients who present with complaints of distal elbow pain and who have history and physical examinations suggestive of triceps tendinopathy and/or posterior impingement. Downey et al. reviewed the ultrasound findings of partial-thickness tears of the distal triceps brachii and noted some common findings.[5]

The pathological findings of the triceps brachii tendon that can be noted under ultrasound include hypoechoic areas in the tendon suggestive of intratendinous tears, intratendon calcifications, tendon discontinuity, irregularity of the olecranon's bony cortex, presence of fracture fragments if an avulsion occurred, and signs of olecranon bursitis with increased fluid within the olecranon bursa.

Indications for Ultrasound-Guided Procedures of the Distal Triceps Tendon

Injections into the peritendinous area of the triceps brachii tendon should be considered when more conservative treatments, such as relative rest, physical therapy, and analgesics, have been tried. There is no literature regarding efficacy or failure of injections into the triceps brachii tendon.

Tenotomy or fenestration of the distal triceps tendon should be considered in the setting of tendinosis that has failed less-invasive treatments, including an eccentric strengthening program of the triceps tendon. There have been no studies to date that have examined the efficacy of such a treatment for this body region, although ultrasound-guided needle tenotomy has been found to be effective for other chronic tendon conditions.[6,7]

Much of the literature regarding distal triceps brachii tendon injuries focuses on tendon and muscle tears. Triceps tendon injuries have been described as possibly the rarest of all tendon injuries.[4] When traumatic injuries do occur, they usually involve avulsions off of the olecranon, or muscle tendon partial tears, or muscle belly partial tears.[2,4] These tears can be treated nonsurgically with splint immobilization, or they can also be treated surgically depending on the expectation of the patient.[2,4] Thus, partial- or full-thickness tears of the triceps tendon are not indications for injection.

In general, it is the person or athlete with overuse triceps tendinopathy who may benefit from an injection. It is imperative to rule out an avulsion fracture if significant weakness is noted during physical examination or if there is a history of anabolic steroid use or certain antibiotics use that can weaken the tendon attachment sites. To my knowledge, there are no data regarding triceps brachii tendon injection indications or efficacy, although there are some reports of possible triceps tendon rupture as a result of local steroid injections performed using palpation guidance.[8] However, there are no good studies to prove or disprove this possibility, and all case reports involved injections without any visual needle guidance.

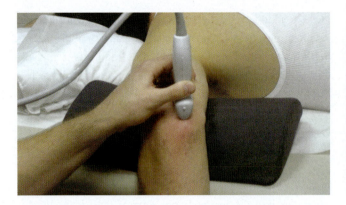

FIGURE 19-2 ■ Prone patient positioning for triceps brachii imaging.

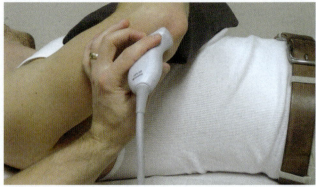

FIGURE 19-3 ■ Alternate supine positioning for triceps brachii imaging.

Equipment

- Needle: 22- to 25-gauge, 1.5- to 2-inch needle
- Injectate: 1 mL of local anesthesia and 1 mL of an injectable corticosteroid
- High-frequency linear array transducer

Author's Preferred Peritendinous Technique

a. Patient position
   i. Prone with the shoulder partially abducted and the elbow flexed at the edge of the examination table, allowing for the distal arm to hang off of the side. (Figure 19-2)
b. Alternate patient position
   i. Supine with the shoulder internally rotated and with about 30 degrees of shoulder flexion (Figure 19-3)
c. Transducer position
   i. Anatomic coronal plane transverse to the triceps tendon
d. Needle orientation relative to transducer (Figure 19-4)
   i. In plane
e. Needle approach (see Figure 19-4)
   i. Medial to lateral or lateral to medial
f. Needle target (Figure 19-5)
   i. Peritendinous tissue on the superficial side of triceps tendon
g. Pearls/Pitfalls
   i. You must account for the radial nerve prior to initiating injection.
   ii. Avoid intratendinous corticosteroid injection because of risk of potential rupture.
   iii. Counsel the patient on modification of activities following injection to avoid further injury to tendon.

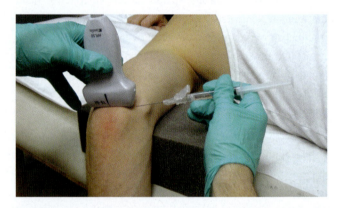

FIGURE 19-4 ■ Setup for a transverse (short-axis) injection, lateral to medial approach of needle.

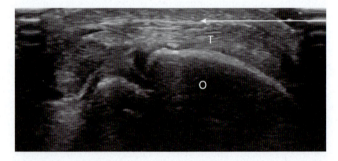

FIGURE 19-5 ■ Needle placement for peritendinous approach (*white arrow*). O, olecranon; T, triceps tendon; left, lateral; right, medial.

Equipment

- Needle: 25-gauge, 1.5-inch needle for local anesthesia
- 18- to 20-gauge, 1.5- to 2-inch needle for procedure
- Limited amount of local anesthetic to allow for adequate pain control during needle fenestrations
- High-frequency linear array transducer

Author's Preferred Tenotomy Technique

a. Patient position
   i. Prone with the shoulder partially abducted and the elbow flexed at the edge of the table for the distal arm to hang off of the side of the examination table (see Figure 19-2)
b. Alternate patient position
   i. Supine with the shoulder internally rotated and with approximately 30 degrees of shoulder flexion (see Figure 19-3)
c. Transducer position
   i. Anatomic sagittal plane longitudinal to the triceps tendon fibers
d. Needle orientation relative to transducer
   i. In plane (Figure 19-6)
e. Needle approach
   i. Proximal to distal (see Figure 19-6)
f. Needle target
   i. Intratendinous region of triceps tendon where pathology is noted (Figure 19-7)
g. Pearls/Pitfalls
   i. Locate and avoid the radial nerve prior to initiating the injection.
   ii. If the injection is performed too medially or laterally, there are local neurovascular structures that need to be avoided.
   iii. Patients should be cautioned that they may experience an increase in pain initially after injection and that it may take several weeks to note improvement in symptoms.

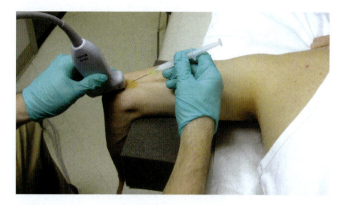

FIGURE 19-6 ■ Setup for a longitudinal (long-axis) injection, with proximal to distal approach.

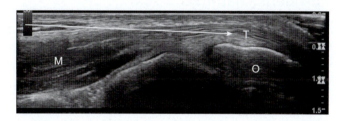

FIGURE 19-7 ■ Needle placement for intratendinous procedure (*white arrow*). M, triceps muscle; O, olecranon; T, triceps tendon.

References

1. Hollinshead WH, Jenkins DB. Chapter 5: the shoulder; Chapter 6: the arm. In: Hollinshead WH, Jenkins DB, eds. *Functional Anatomy of the Limbs and Back*. 5th ed. Philadelphia, PA: Saunders; 1981:72–126.
2. Yeh PC, Dodds SD, Smart LR, et al. Distal triceps rupture. *J Am Acad Orthop Surg*. 2010;18:31–40.
3. Grana WA, Boscardin JB, Schneider HJ, et al. Evaluation of elbow and shoulder problems in professional baseball pitchers. *Am J Orthop*. 2007;36(6):308–313.
4. Vidal AF, Drakos MC, Allen AA. Biceps tendon and triceps tendon injuries. *Clin Sports Med*. 2004;23(4):707–722.
5. Downey R, Jacobson AA, Fessell DP, et al. Sonography of partial-thickness tears of the distal triceps brachii tendon. *J Ultrasound Med*. 2011;30(10):1351–1356.
6. McShane JM, Nazarian LN, Harwood MI. Sonographically guided percutaneous needle tenotomy for treatment of common extensor tendinosis in the elbow. *J Ultrasound Med*. 2006; 25(10):1281–1289.
7. McShane JM, Shah VN, Nazarian LN. Sonographically guided percutaneous needle tenotomy for treatment of common extensor tendinosis in the elbow: is a corticosteroid necessary? *J Ultrasound Med*. 2008;27(8):1137–1144.
8. Lambert MI, St Clair Gibson A, Noakes TD. Rupture of the triceps tendon associated with steroid injections. *Am J Sports Med*. 1995;23(6):778.
9. Lee KS, Rosas HG, Craig JG. Musculoskeletal ultrasound: elbow imaging and procedures. *Semin Musculoskeletal Radiol*. 2010;14(4):449–460.

Joshua G. Hackel, MD, FAAFP

Pertinent Anatomy

The elbow joint is a hinged joint. The ulnar collateral ligament (UCL) is the medial stabilizer of the elbow joint (Figure 20-1). The UCL is a thick triangular band consisting of two portions, anterior and posterior, united by a thinner intermediate portion. The anterior portion, directed obliquely forward, is attached by its apex to the front part of the medial epicondyle of the humerus; and by its broad base to the medial margin of the coronoid process also called the sublime tubercle. It is the anterior band that causes the overhead athlete (ie, baseball and tennis players) and nonthrowing individual so much trouble with a simulated throwing motion or, in rare instances, pain with routine daily activities.

Common Pathology

The UCL is the main stabilizer to valgus stress to the elbow. During the throwing motion, a tremendous amount of valgus stress is applied to the elbow in many cases exceeding the capacity of the UCL resulting in partial or complete disruption of the ligament. This can occur with repetitive microtrauma, a single throw, or a force applied to an outstretched forearm. The patient will complain of medial elbow pain often associated with numbness in the fourth and fifth digits (the ulnar nerve distribution). The numbness is attributed to swelling or edema associated with the UCL injury causing irritation to the ulnar nerve at the cubital tunnel. The common flexor tendon at the medial epicondyle can also be a source of medial elbow pain, making ultrasound a valuable tool in assessing this injury and distinguishing where the pathology is located.

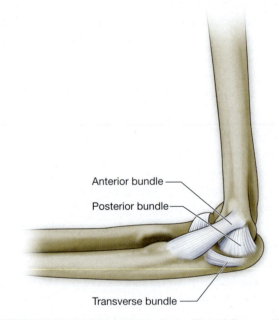

Anterior bundle

Posterior bundle

Transverse bundle

FIGURE 20-1 ■ Anatomy of the ulnar collateral ligament (UCL) demonstrating the three bundles.

Ultrasound Imaging Findings (Figure 20-2)

The UCL is best visualized in the long axis using a high-frequency linear array transducer at a depth between 2 and 3 cm. Common findings include a discontinuous or heterogenous appearing fiber pattern of the ligament with or without hypoechoic swelling associated with the injury. The common flexor tendon can be injured simultaneously, so thorough ultrasound is required to identify other pathology. In addition to static images, dynamic valgus stress testing of the UCL should always be performed during ultrasound evaluation to further assess the competency of the ligament and to help distinguish partial- from full-thickness tears.[1]

Indications for Injections of the Ulnar Collateral Ligament

Injection of regenerative solutions or only needle tenotomy can be performed for patients with recalcitrant pain that is unresponsive to active rest to include physical therapy, no throwing, and possibly antiinflammatories typically lasting 3 months or more. Clinical outcomes of guided versus unguided injection has not been described and the author cannot justify an injection into the UCL without ultrasound guidance.

Equipment

- Needle: 20- to 22-gauge, 1.5-inch needle; may use 25–27 gauge for local anesthesia
- Limited amount of local anesthesia to allow for adequate pain control during needle fenestration
- High-frequency linear array transducer

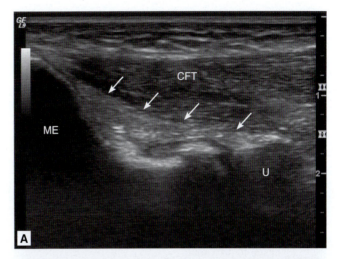

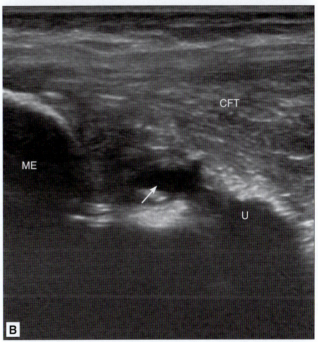

FIGURE 20-2 ■ **A.** Normal appearance of compact fibrillar ulnar collateral ligament (UCL) indicated by *arrows*. Left, proximal; right, distal. **B.** An abnormal proximal UCL with a small anechoic undersurface fluid, indicated with a *small arrow*. CFT, common flexor tendon; ME, medial epicondyle; U, ulna.

Author's Preferred Technique

a. Patient position (Figure 20-3)
    i. Supine with arm abducted at least 45 degrees in 90 degrees of external rotation at the glenohumeral joint
b. Transducer position (see Figure 20-3)
    i. Anatomic sagittal in slight oblique plane on the medial elbow
c. Needle orientation relative to the transducer (see Figure 20-3)
    i. In plane
d. Needle approach (Figure 20-4)
    i. Distal to proximal
e. Target
    i. The entire length of the UCL, though the focus should be on area of pathology
f. Pearls/Pitfalls
    i. Great care must be taken to first identify the ulnar nerve prior to injection.
    ii. Be aware of the patient who has had a previous ulnar nerve transposition or a UCL reconstruction with ulnar nerve transposition as the nerve will be more anterior and superficial overlying the UCL.
    iii. Dynamic evaluation is helpful when interrogating UCL stability. This will often illustrate further abnormal findings.
    iv. The UCL that is injured will often translate or hydrodissect on injection of solution if instability is present.
    v. Consider additional needling of the proximal enthesis to create bleeding from the medial epicondyle.

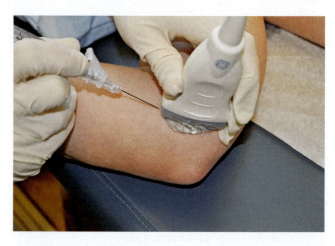

FIGURE 20-3 ▪ Arm abducted greater than 45 degrees with 90 degrees of external rotation at glenohumeral joint demonstrating transducer position and needle entry from distal to proximal.

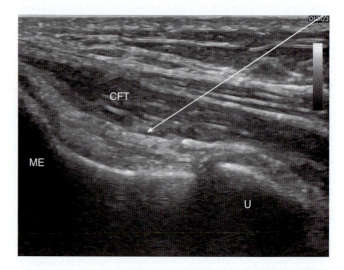

FIGURE 20-4 ▪ Long-axis view of ulnar collateral ligament (UCL) showing needle angle (*white arrow*) from distal to proximal. The needle should track proximal and distal along course of tendon, specifically targeting areas of ligament pathology. Left, proximal; right, distal.

References

1. De Smet, AA, Winter TC, Thomas MB, Bernhardt DT. Dynamic sonography with valgus stress to assess elbow ulnar collateral ligament injury in baseball pitchers. *Skelet Radiol.* 2002;31(11):671–676.
2. Van Holsbeeck MT, Introcaso JH. *Musculoskeletal Ultrasound.* 2nd ed. St. Louis, MO: Mosby; 2001.
3. Jacobson JA: Elbow ultrasound. In: *Fundamentals of Musculoskeletal Ultrasound.* Philadelphia, PA: Saunders; 2007:102–132.
4. Andrews JR, Clancy WG, Whiteside JA. Injuries to the elbow. In: *On-Field Evaluation and Treatment of Common Athletic Injuries.* St Louis, MO: Mosby; 1997;17:225–233.

R. Amadeus Mason, MD

KEY POINTS

- A high-frequency linear array transducer with a large-bore needle (18 gauge) is best for aspiration.
- Be sure to use a large enough gauge needle as fluid is often viscous.
- The olecranon bursa is typically not seen on ultrasound unless distended.

- If unable to withdraw fluid, consider needle fenestration and manual pressure to disperse bursal contents.
- Apply compression sleeve post procedure to reduce recurrence rate.

Pertinent Anatomy

A bursa is a synovial pouch that helps to reduce friction between two adjacent surfaces, typically bone, soft tissues, or skin. Bursa typically contain a very small quantity of fluid, usually no more than a couple of cell layers thick.

The olecranon bursa is the only bursa of the elbow joint. It lies between the skin of the extensor surface of the elbow and the olecranon process of the ulna, but unlike other bursae, it does not communicate with its adjacent joint (Figure 21-1).

Common Pathology

Olecranon bursitis can occur for a number of reasons; trauma (repetitive or acute), infection, and inflammatory medical conditions are the most common.[5,6]

With acute trauma, a hard single blow to the tip of the elbow can cause the bursa to produce excess fluid and swell. Prolonged or repeated pressure such as leaning on the tip of the elbow repeatedly and/or for long periods of time may also cause the bursa to swell. Typically, this type of bursitis develops slowly over several months. Certain occupations (eg, plumbers and heating, ventilation, and air conditioning technicians) are especially vulnerable, as they crawl into tight spaces and repeatedly lean their elbows on hard surfaces. If an injury at the tip of the elbow breaks the skin (eg, an insect bite, scrape, or puncture wound), bacteria may get inside the bursa sac and cause an infection. Occasionally, the bursa may become infected without an obvious injury to the skin; this is usually associated with recurrent or prolonged bursitis. Finally, certain inflammatory medical conditions (eg, rheumatoid arthritis and gout) have been associated with recurrent elbow bursitis.

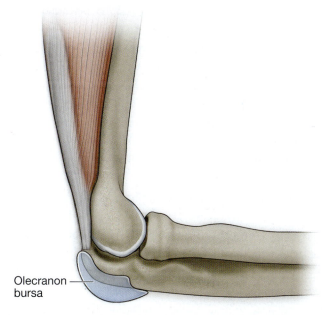

Olecranon bursa

FIGURE 21-1 ■ Lateral view demonstrating the olecranon bursa and its relationship with the triceps tendon and the underlying elbow joint and olecranon.

89

Ultrasound Imaging Findings

The olecranon bursa is best visualized using a high-frequency linear array transducer and depth of less than 3 cm. Initially, scan in the long axis from medial to lateral then switch to the short axis and move from proximal to distal. Common findings include cortical irregularities (bone spurs), calcifications, and loose bodies. The bursal fluid will appear hypoechoic to anechoic depending on whether or not it is complex (with stromal inclusions and loose bodies) or simple (no inclusions) (Figures 21-2 and 21-3).

Indications for Aspiration and Injection of the Olecranon Bursa

Aspiration of the olecranon bursa can be performed for patients with persistent or recurrent swelling that is unresponsive to conservative management with rest/padding/compression, icing, antiinflammatories, and sometimes physical therapy.[5] Aspiration of an inflamed bursa can be performed for relief of discomfort associated with bursitis. If the symptoms of olecranon bursitis are recurrent, corticosteroid injection may be considered. Corticosteroids should not be injected if infection is suspected and the fluid should be sent for Gram stain and culture.[6]

Unguided olecranon bursa aspiration has been well described.[1,2,3] The success rate of these unguided injections is reported between 80% and 100%.[3] Ultrasound-guided bursa injection has not been as well described, but Joines et al. reported a success rate of 90%–100%.[4] In most cases success was measured by lack of recurrence. There have not been any head-to-head studies comparing clinical outcomes of unguided versus ultrasound-guided injection of the olecranon bursa.

Equipment

- Needle: 18-gauge, 1.5-inch needle for aspiration
- Injectate: 1–2 mL of local anesthetic with 25-gauge needle. Following aspiration, consider 0.5–1 mL of local anesthetic and 0.5–1 mL of an injectable corticosteroid
- High-frequency linear array transducer

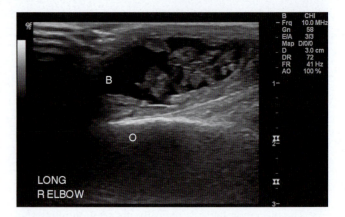

FIGURE 21-2 ■ Long-axis ultrasound image of a fluid-filled olecranon bursa (B). Note the olecranon (O) and hyperechoic debris located inside the bursal collection.

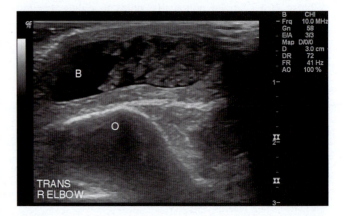

FIGURE 21-3 ■ Short-axis ultrasound image of a fluid-filled olecranon bursa (B). Note the olecranon (O) and hyperechoic debris located inside the bursal collection.

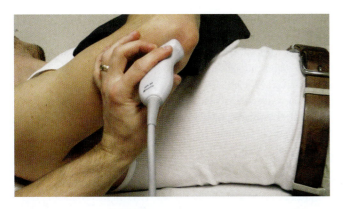

FIGURE 21-4 ▪ Preferred patient positioning for the procedure.

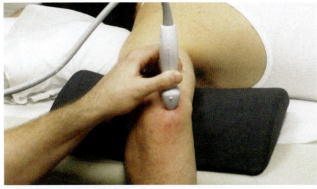

FIGURE 21-5 ▪ Alternate patient positioning for the procedure.

Author's Preferred Technique

a. Patient position
   i. Supine with the shoulder internally rotated and with about 30 degrees of shoulder flexion (Figure 21-4)
b. Alternate patient position
   i. Prone with the shoulder partially abducted and the elbow flexed at the edge of the examination table, allowing for the distal arm to hang off of the side (Figure 21-5)
c. Transducer position (Figures 21-4 and 21-5)
   i. Long axis or short axis to the bursa
d. Needle orientation relative to the transducer
   i. In plane
e. Needle approach (Figure 21-6)
   i. Any approach that directly visualizes cyst is allowed.
f. Target (Figure 21-7)
   i. Middle of bursa
g. Pearls and Pitfalls
   i. Turn the bevel of the needle down to prevent subcutaneous tissue from clogging the opening and impeding flow.
   ii. Use a large enough gauge needle; usually 18 gauge is sufficient.
   iii. Use the transducer to milk fluid to ensure maximal fluid extraction.
   iv. If the patient has a fever, and/or the skin over the bursa is erythematous, warm, and swollen, *do not* inject corticosteroids.
   v. Even though this is a superficial structure, *do not* use a "hockey stick" transducer as your field of view will be too narrow.

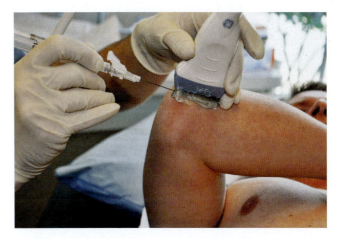

FIGURE 21-6 ▪ Preferred patient positioning with probe and needle showing in-plane approach to the olecranon bursa from proximal to distal. Actual approach may vary.

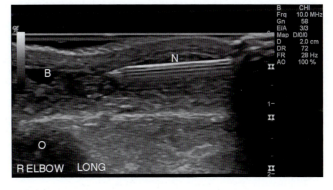

FIGURE 21-7 ▪ This is a long-axis ultrasound image demonstrating needle (N) placement in the fluid-filled olecranon bursa (B). Note the olecranon (O). With ultrasound you can identify any hyperechoic debris that may clog the needle and maneuver the needle to avoid it.

vi. If you are unable to withdraw fluid, consider needle fenestration and manual pressure to disperse bursal contents.

vii. Apply a compression sleeve post procedure as this may help reduce recurrence rate.

References

1. Cardone DA, Tallia AF. Joint and soft tissue injection. *Am Fam Physician*. 2002;66:283–288.

2. Stitik TP, ed. *Injection Procedures: Osteoarthritis and Related Conditions*. New York: Springer; 2011:215–217.

3. Lockman L. Treating nonseptic olecranon bursitis: a 3-step technique. *Can Fam Physician*. 2010 November;56(11):1157.

4. Joines MM, Motamedi K, Seeger LL, DiFiori JP. Musculoskeletal interventional ultrasound. *Semin Musculoskelet Radiol*. 2007;11:192–198.

5. JF Sarwark, ed. *Essentials of Musculoskeletal Care*. 4th ed. Rosemont, IL: American Academy of Orthopaedic Surgeons; 2010.

6. Goddard J, Goddard M. Common musculoskeletal problems. 2010;25–31, DOI:10.1007/978-1-4419-5523-4.

7. Smith DL, McAfee JH, Lucas LM, Kumar KL, Romney DM. Treatment of nonseptic olecranon bursitis. A controlled, blinded prospective trial. *Arch Intern Med*. 1989;149:2527–2530.

Sean W. Mulvaney, MD

KEY POINTS

- A 22- to 25-gauge, 2- to 3.5-inch needle and high-frequency linear array transducer are ideal.
- The deep branch of the radial nerve courses between the deep and superficial heads of the supinator muscle.
- Start procedure in short axis, out-of-plane view but rotate between short and long axis (needle in plane and out of plane) to better visualize nerve during entire procedure.

- It will take significant volume, up to 15 mL, to completely decompress the deep branch of the radial nerve through the supinator musculature.
- A diagnostic nerve block can be performed to help differentiate this syndrome from the nearby lateral epicondylopathy.

Pertinent Anatomy

The deep branch of the radial nerve (DBRN) courses between the deep and superficial heads of the supinator muscle. Once the DBRN exits the supinator muscle it becomes the posterior interosseous nerve (PIN),[1] although some references use PIN to refer to the DBRN.[2,3] The DBRN is vulnerable to entrapment most commonly at the arcade of Frohse (AF),[4,5] although it may become compressed and entrapped as it courses through or exits from the supinator muscle, by a recurrent radial artery (leash of Henry), the medial aspect of the extensor carpi radialis brevis, and the capsule-tendon aponeurosis of the humeroradial joint[6,7] (Figure 22-1).

Common Pathology

Entrapment of the DBRN can present as radial tunnel syndrome (RTS)[8] or as PIN syndrome. PIN syndrome presents with painless wrist extension weakness.[9] RTS presents with pain in the lateral-dorsal proximal forearm area that is exacerbated by forearm pronation and may masquerade as lateral epicondylopathy.[10] RTS is encountered much less frequently than other entrapment neuropathies of the upper limb, such as carpal tunnel syndrome (CTS) or cubital tunnel syndrome. Both RTS and PIN syndrome have been reported in patients with supination/pronation overuse, which has been hypothesized to contribute toward fibrosis of the AF.[11]

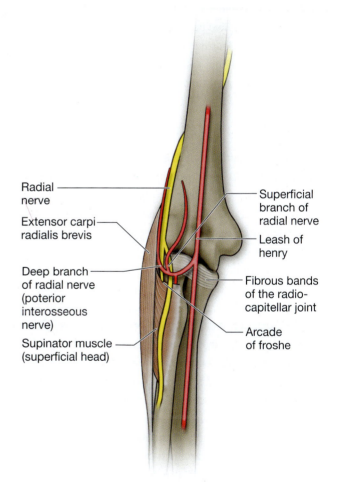

Radial nerve
Extensor carpi radialis brevis
Deep branch of radial nerve (poterior interosseous nerve)
Supinator muscle (superficial head)

Superficial branch of radial nerve
Leash of henry
Fibrous bands of the radio-capitellar joint
Arcade of froshe

FIGURE 22-1 ■ The course of deep branch of the radial nerve (DBRN) and most common sites of entrapment are demonstrated. 1. Arcade of Frohse 2. Fibrous bands anterior to radio-capitellar joint between brachialis and brachioradialis. 3. Leash of Henry. 4. Leading (medial/proximal) edge of the extensor carpi radialis brevis (ECRB). 5. Distal edge of supinator muscle.

Ultrasound Imaging Findings

Ultrasound is ideally suited to structurally assess peripheral nerves and locate areas of peripheral nerve entrapment or injury.[12,13,14] Electromyography (EMG) and nerve conduction studies can indicate conduction within a nerve, but generally not the physical structure of a nerve or the specific location of a nerve injury or entrapment. In addition, electrophysiological studies are imprecise especially when dealing with nerves with a smaller cross-sectional areas or the potential for anastomotic branches.[15,16] EMG studies are normal in the vast majority of patients with RTS and have limited use in diagnosing RTS.[17] The DBRN can be identified with ultrasound imaging.[18] Specific norms for the cross-sectional area of the DBRN at the supinator muscle or at the AF have not been established. In their published study on reference values for nerve cross-sectional area in normal male and female adults, with the largest sample population published, Cartwright and colleagues stated that the mean surface area for the radial nerve at the antecubital fossa was 9.3 mm², with a reference range of 4.5–14.3 mm² (Figures 22-2 and 22-3).

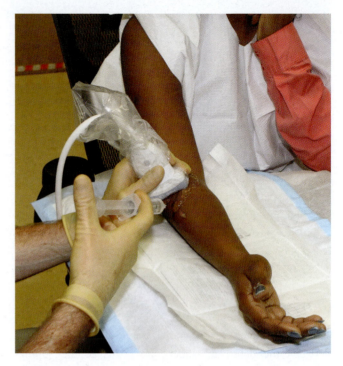

FIGURE 22-2 ■ Patient position for injection of deep branch of the radial nerve (DBRN) around arcade of Frohse (AF).

Indications for Injections of the DBRN

Conservative treatment of RTS can be successful in the minority of patients: rest, activity modification, nonsteroidal antiinflammatory drugs, local corticosteroids, heat, as well as physical therapy involving nerve mobilizations.[19] Most patients with RTS will need further intervention to attempt to relieve their symptoms.[20]

The first mention in the medical literature of using ultrasound-guided percutaneous hydro-neuroplasty, or nerve hydrodissection, was by Mulvaney in the successful treatment of an entrapped lateral femoral cutaneous nerve.[21] Smith and colleagues reported delivering corticosteroid around the median nerve at the carpal tunnel for CTS by ultrasound guidance and "hydrodissecting" around the median nerve with the injectate.[22] According to Smith's article, it appears that their described technique was a means of delivering a corticosteroid in proximity to the median nerve, and did not use hydrodissection as a primary means for the treatment of an entrapped nerve. Clinical outcomes of palpation-guided versus ultrasound-guided injections have not been described.

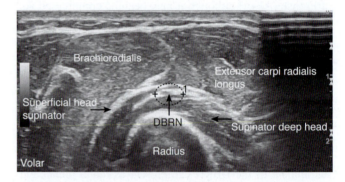

FIGURE 22-3 ■ Deep branch of the radial nerve (DBRN) between the two heads of the supinator in short-axis view.

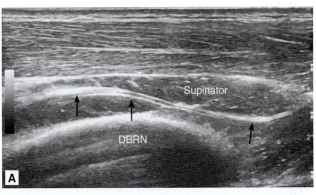

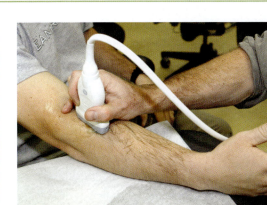

FIGURE 22-4 ▪ **A.** Deep branch of the radial nerve (DBRN) in long-axis view, with probe position shown in **B**.

Equipment

- ▪ Needle: 22- to 25-gauge, 2- to 3.5-inch needle
- ▪ Injectate:
  - • Nerve block: 2 mL of local anesthetic ± injectable corticosteroids
  - • Nerve hydrodissection/decompression: up to 15 mL of total solution (combination of normal saline, local anesthetic, ± dextrose solution) depending on length of nerve entrapment
- ▪ High-frequency linear array transducer

Author's Preferred Injection Technique

a. Patient position (see Figure 22-2)
   i. Seated with arm flexed 20 degrees, arm resting on examination table, thumb pointing toward ceiling
b. Transducer position (see Figure 22-2)
   i. Short axis to the DBRN at the target site (eg, AF)
c. Needle orientation relative to the transducer
   i. Initially out-of-plane, but then switching between in-plane and out-of- plane during procedure
d. Needle approach (Figures 22-4, 22-5, and 22-6)
   i. Distal to proximal
   ii. Once the needle is approximated to the center of the nerve in short axis, switch to long axis.
e. Target (see Figure 22-6)
   i. DBRN mid supinator injecting toward AF

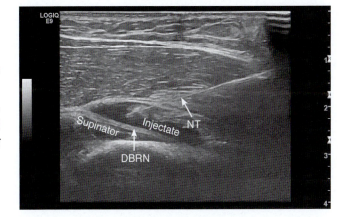

FIGURE 22-5 ▪ Long-axis view of deep branch of the radial nerve (DBRN) during injection procedure.

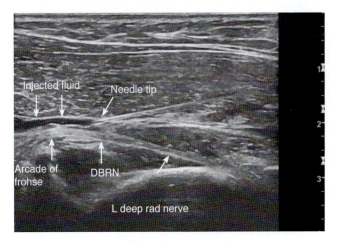

FIGURE 22-6 ▪ Long-axis view of hydroneurolysis of deep branch of the radial nerve (DBRN) approaching the arcade of Frohse (AF) with needle tip and spread of injectate visualized.

f. Pearls/Pitfalls

i. This is an advanced ultrasound-guided technique that requires precise needle and transducer control, constant visualization of the needle tip, and a clear understanding of both the local ultrasound anatomy and the ultrasound anatomy of nerves.

ii. If you are having difficulty identifying the radial nerve, try one of these techniques: in short-axis, identify the radial nerve coming off the spiral groove at the mid-lateral humerus and follow it distally, or while in short-axis, identify the DBRN while performing a short-axis slide in the plane between the superficial and deep heads of the supinator muscle.

iii. To release the entire course of the DBRN, repeat the above procedure in a proximal to distal direction where the nerve exits the supinator muscle and becomes the PIN (Figures 22-7 and 22-8).

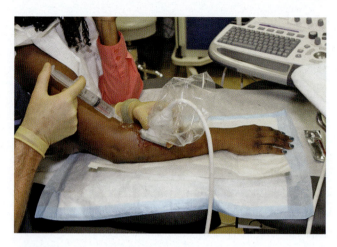

FIGURE 22-7 ■ Patient position for injection/hydroneurolysis of distal edge of supinator.

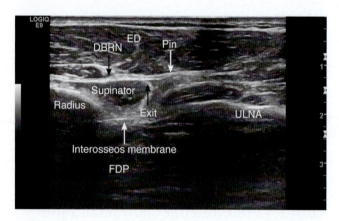

FIGURE 22-8 ■ Long-axis view of deep branch of the radial nerve (DBRN) at distal edge of supinator. PIN, posterior interosseous nerve.

References

1. Ozturk A, Kutlu C, Taskara N, et al. Anatomic and morphometric study of the arcade of Frohse in cadavers. *Surg Radiol Anat.* 2005;27:171–175.
2. Bodner G, Huber B, Schwabeggar A, Lutz M, Waldenberger P. Sonographic detection of radial nerve entrapment within a humerus fracture. *J Ultrasound Med.* 1999;18(10):703–706.
3. Moore KL, Dalley AF. *Clinically Oriented Anatomy.* 4th ed. Philadelphia, PA: Lippincott; 713, 730.
4. Arle JE, Zager EL. Surgical treatment of common entrapment neuropathies in the upper limbs. *Muscle Nerve.* 2000;23:1160–1174.
5. Cravens G, Kline DG. Posterior interosseous nerve palsies. *Neurosurgery.* 1990;27:397–402.
6. Konjengbam M, Elangbam J. Radial nerve in the radial tunnel: anatomic sites of entrapment neuropathy. *Clin Anat.* 2004;17:21–25.
7. Riffaud L, Morandi X, Godey B, et al. Anatomic bases for the compression and neurolysis of the deep branch of the radial nerve in the radial tunnel. *Surg Radiol Anat.* 1999;21:229–233.
8. Roles NC, Maudsley KH. Radial tunnel syndrome: resistant tennis elbow as nerve entrapment. *J Bone Joint Surg Br.* 1972;54:499–508.
9. Vikram K, Craig J, van Holsbeeck M, Ditmars D. Entrapment of the posterior interosseous nerve at the arcade of Frohse with sonographic, magnetic resonance imaging, and intraoperative confirmation. *J Ultrasound Med.* 2009;28:807–812.
10. Lister GD, Belsole RB, Kleinert HE. The radial tunnel syndrome. *J Hand Surg Am.* 1979;4:52–59.
11. Chien AJ, Jamadar DA, Jacobson JA, Hayes CW, Louis DS. Sonography and MR imaging of posterior interosseous nerve syndrome with surgical correlation. *AJR Am J Roentgenol.* 2003;181:219–221.
12. Cartwright MS, Shin HW, Passmore LV. Ultrasound findings of the ulnar nerve in adults. *Arch Phys Med Rehabil.* 2007;88:394–396.

13. Werner RA, Jacobson JA, Jamadar DA. Influence of body mass index on median nerve function, carpal canal pressure and cross-sectional area of the median nerve. *Muscle Nerve.* 2004;30;4:481–485.

14. Yoshii Y, Vilarraga HR, Henderson J, et al. Ultrasound assessment of the displacement and deformation of the median nerve in the human carpal tunnel with active finger motion. *J Bone Joint Surg.* 2009;91:2922–2930.

15. Hsu JC, Paletta GA, Gambardella RA et al. Musculocutaneous nerve injury in major league pitchers: a report of 2 cases. *Am J Sports Med.* 2007;35:1003–1006.

16. Maeda S, Kawai K, Koizumi M et al. Morphological study of the communication between the musculocutaneous and median nerves. *Anat Sci Int.* 2009;84:34–40.

17. Barnum M, Mastey RD, Weiss AP, Akelman E. *Hand Clin.* 1996;12(4):679–689.

18. Kinni V, Craig J, van Holsbeeck M, Ditmars D. Entrapment of the posterior interosseus nerve at the arcade of Frohse with sonographic, magnetic resonance imaging, and intraoperative confirmation. *J Ultrasound Med.* 2009;28:807–812.

19. Thatte MR, Mansukhani KA. Compressive neuropathy in the upper limb. *Indian J Plast Surg.* 2011;44:283–297.

20. Barnum M, Mastey RD, Weiss AP, Akelman E. *Hand Clin.* 1996;12(4):679–689.

21. Mulvaney S. Ultrasound-guided percutaneous neuroplasty of the lateral femoral cutaneous nerve for the treatment of meralgia paresthetica: a case report and description of a new ultrasound-guided technique. *Curr Sports Med Report.* 2011;10:2; 99–104.

22. Smith J, Wisniewski SJ, Finnoff JT, Payne JM. Sonographically guided carpal tunnel injections, the ulnar approach. *J Ultrasound Med.* 2008;27:1485–1490.

Evan Peck, MD / Brian J. Shiple, DO

KEY POINTS

- Use a high-frequency, linear array transducer.
- Use a small-gauge (eg, 25) and relatively short (eg, 1.5-inch) needle.
- Ulnar perineural injection can be used therapeutically, diagnostically, or to obtain regional anesthesia prior

to an invasive procedure for the corresponding ulnar-innervated regions of the fingers, hand, or wrist.
- Avoid injecting directly into the nerve or adjacent vascular structures.

Pertinent Anatomy

The ulnar nerve originates from the C8 and T1 nerve roots, which each contribute to form the medial cord of the brachial plexus. The ulnar nerve forms from the medial cord and descends posteromedially on the humerus. It travels through the cubital tunnel and enters the flexor compartment of the forearm between the two heads of flexor carpi ulnaris muscle. There it innervates the flexor carpi ulnaris as well as the medial half of the flexor digitorum profundus. The nerve then joins with the ulnar artery and travels deep to the flexor carpi ulnaris muscle (Figure 23-1).

Approximately 5 cm proximal to the wrist, the ulnar nerve then divides into dorsal and palmar branches. The dorsal branch supplies cutaneous sensation to the dorsal aspect of the little finger and the ulnar half of the ring finger, except for the nails, and the corresponding aspects of the dorsal hand. The palmar branch passes superficial to the flexor retinaculum (in contrast to the median nerve) and enters the wrist through Guyon's canal, where it supplies cutaneous sensation to the palmar aspect of the little finger and the ulnar half of the ring finger, as well as the nails, and the corresponding aspects of the palm.

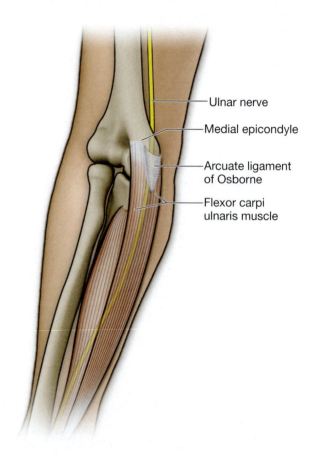

Ulnar nerve

Medial epicondyle

Arcuate ligament of Osborne

Flexor carpi ulnaris muscle

FIGURE 23-1 ■ The ulnar nerve viewed passing posterior to the medial epicondyle.

Common Pathology

The ulnar nerve may be entrapped or injured at the elbow (eg, at the cubital tunnel) or wrist (eg, at Guyon's canal) by several mechanisms, including arterial aneurysms or thrombosis, external compression, fractures, physeal injuries, and repetitive use or improper positioning. More proximal pathology should also be considered when symptoms are in an ulnar nerve distribution, including cervical radiculopathy, thoracic outlet syndrome, or brachial plexus injury. In addition, clinicians should consider the possibility of a more generalized neuropathy, such as that due to alcoholism, diabetes mellitus, drug toxicity, malignancy, rheumatic disease, or thyroid disorders.

Ultrasound Imaging Findings

The ulnar nerve is initially best visualized in its short axis, starting at the elbow where adjacent bony landmarks are easily palpated. A high-frequency linear array transducer is ideal to visualize this superficial structure. The transducer is typically placed such that it spans the medial epicondyle and the olecranon process. The ulnar nerve is normally visible between these two bony landmarks as a round structure containing a fascicular (honeycomb) pattern, which occurs due to alternating areas of hypoechoic nerve fascicles and hyperechoic connective tissue. The ulnar nerve in this position may appear more hypoechoic than a typical nerve, because of the hyperechoic fat that frequently surrounds the nerve near the elbow.

From this position, the ulnar nerve can be traced distally into the cubital tunnel, between the two heads of the flexor carpi ulnaris muscle. The arcuate ligament may be seen superficial to the ulnar nerve in this location. The ulnar nerve can then be followed distally in the forearm, following the aforementioned branches into the wrist and hand. In addition, it may be scanned proximally in the arm to its junction with the medial cord of the brachial plexus. At any point, the transducer may be rotated 90 degrees to visualize the nerve in its long axis.

A cross-sectional area of the ulnar nerve above 7.5 mm^2 at the level of the medial epicondyle is considered abnormal.[1] The nerve should also be evaluated dynamically at the elbow, keeping the transducer in place and visualizing the nerve in its short axis while the patient actively flexes the elbow. The nerve may dislocate medially over the medial epicondyle during elbow flexion. Care should be taken by the sonographer to not apply excessive transducer pressure during this maneuver, which may result in a false negative dislocation sign. Asymptomatic ulnar nerve dislocation occurs in up to 20% of the population, so clinical correlation is advised.[2] Snapping triceps syndrome may also be observed, wherein the medial head of the triceps dislocates medially over the medial epicondyle along with the ulnar nerve upon active flexion of the elbow.

Indications for Ulnar Perineural Injection

Ulnar perineural injection may be considered as a therapeutic maneuver to relieve pain due to ulnar nerve entrapment that is unresponsive to appropriate activity modifications, oral or topical medications, therapeutic modalities, therapeutic exercises, and protection or bracing where indicated. In addition, it may be used for diagnostic purposes if the primary pain generator is uncertain based on history, physical examination, imaging findings, or electrodiagnostic studies.

Ulnar perineural injections may be performed anywhere along the course of the nerve where the entrapment may be occurring or for obtaining regional anesthesia to the ulnar-innervated regions of the fingers, hand, wrist, or forearm.

Equipment

- Needle: 25-gauge, 1.5-inch
- Injectate:
  - Nerve block: 2 mL of local anesthetic ± injectable corticosteroids
  - Nerve hydrodissection/decompression: 5–10 mL of total solution (combination of normal saline, local anesthetic, ± dextrose solution)
- High-frequency linear array transducer

Author's Preferred Technique (below Cubital Tunnel)

a. Patient position

   i. Supine

   ii. Arm abducted to approximately 15–30 degrees in forearm supination

b. Transducer position (Figure 23-2)

   i. Anatomic short-axis plane over the ulnar nerve at the junction of the proximal and middle thirds of the forearm

   ii. If possible, choose a point where the ulnar artery and nerve have not yet become immediately adjacent.

c. Needle orientation relative to the transducer (see Figure 23-2)

   i. In plane

d. Needle approach (Figures 23-2 and 23-3)

   i. Medial to lateral or lateral to medial

e. Target

   i. Area surrounding the ulnar nerve. Create a "halo" of injectate around the nerve.

f. Pearls/Pitfalls

   i. Avoid contact with the ulnar artery. The ulnar artery may lie superficial to the nerve.

   ii. Place the tip of the needle very close to the nerve, but do not touch the nerve. Advise patients to inform you if they feel a sharp pain, which may indicate the needle has touched the nerve. If this occurs, withdraw the needle away from the nerve and redirect it.

   iii. To create the desired "halo" of injectate around the nerve, repositioning of the needle above and below the nerve may be necessary.

   iv. If the ulnar side of the forearm needs to be anesthetized as well, perineural injection may be performed of the ulnar nerve and the medial antebrachial cutaneous nerve at the level of the junction of the metaphysis and diaphysis of the humerus, where the two nerves are in the same plane as the basilic vein, proximal to the medial epicondyle.

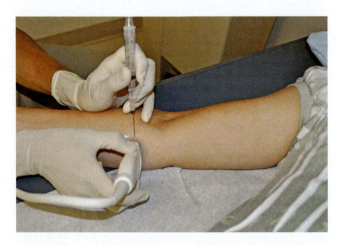

FIGURE 23-2 ■ Transducer position and needle orientation for an anterior, lateral-to-medial approach, transducer short-axis to nerve, needle in-plane ultrasound-guided ulnar perineural injection. Sterile transducer cover not pictured.

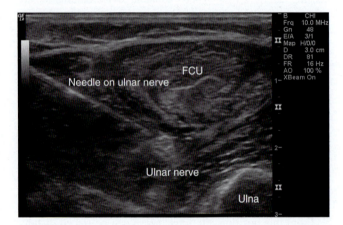

FIGURE 23-3 ■ Ultrasound image for an anterior, lateral-to-medial approach, transducer short-axis to nerve, needle in-plane ultrasound-guided ulnar perineural injection. Needle shown directly adjacent to ulnar nerve.

Author's Preferred Technique (above Cubital Tunnel)

a. Patient position
    i.   Supine
    ii. Arm abducted to approximately 90 degrees in fore-arm supination, placed on a supportive bolster
b. Transducer position (Figure 23-4)
    i.   Anatomic short-axis plane over the ulnar nerve above cubital tunnel
c. Needle orientation relative to the transducer (Figure 23-4)
    i.   In plane
d. Needle approach (Figure 23-5)
    i.   Medial to lateral or lateral to medial
e. Target
    i.   Area surrounding the ulnar nerve. Create a "halo" of injectate around the nerve.
f. Pearls/Pitfalls
    i.   Avoid contact with the ulnar artery. The ulnar artery may lie superficial to the nerve.
    ii. Place the tip of the needle very close to the nerve, but do not touch the nerve. Advise patients to inform you if they feel a sharp pain, which may indicate the needle has touched the nerve. If this occurs, with-draw the needle away from the nerve and redirect it.
    iii. To create the desired "halo" of injectate around the nerve, repositioning of the needle above and below the nerve may be necessary.
    iv. If the ulnar side of the forearm needs to be anesthe-tized as well, perineural injection may be performed of the ulnar nerve and the medial antebrachial cuta-neous nerve at the level of the junction of the me-taphysis and diaphysis of the humerus, where the two nerves are in the same plane as the basilic vein, proximal to the medial epicondyle.

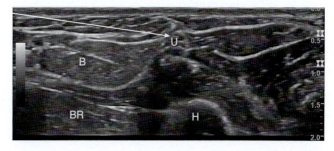

FIGURE 23-4 ■ Transducer position and needle orientation for an anterior, lateral-to-medial approach, transducer short-axis to nerve, needle in-plane ultrasound-guided ulnar perineural injection above the cubital tunnel.

FIGURE 23-5 ■ Ultrasound image for an anterior, medial-to-lateral approach, transducer short-axis to nerve, needle in-plane ultrasound-guided ulnar perineural injection above the cubital tunnel. *Arrow* corresponds to needle position during injection. B, biceps; BR, brachialis; H, humerus; U, ulnar nerve.

References

1. Chiou HJ, Chou YH, Cheng SP, et al. Cubital tunnel syndrome: diagnosis by high-resolution ultrasonography. *J Ultrasound Med.* 1998;17(10):643–648.

2. Okamoto M, Abe M, Shirai H, Ueda N. Morphology and dynam-ics of the ulnar nerve in the cubital tunnel: observation by ultra-sonography. *J Hand Surg Br.* 2000;25(1):85–89.

Victor Ibrahim, MD / Adam D. Weglein, DO, DABMA

KEY POINTS

- Use a high-frequency linear array transducer in short axis to the nerve.
- A 25- to 27-gauge needle, in-plane approach is used.
- Proper identification of local anatomy, including all neurovascular structures, is essential prior to the procedure.
- Injection can be performed for therapeutic or diagnostic value.

Pertinent Anatomy

The median nerve receives nerve fibers from the C5–C7 roots on the lateral brachial cord and C8–T1 roots on the medial cord. The median nerve surfaces from the elbow cubital fossa and passes between the two heads of the pronator teres after passing through the ligament of Struthers and then traveling superficial to the flexor digitorum profundus and beneath flexor digitorum superficial[1] (Figure 24-1). The nerve has several clinically relevant divisions including the anterior interosseous branch, which arises near the pronator teres muscle. The anterior interosseous nerve provides motor innervation to flexor pollicis longus, radial half of the flexor digitorum profundus, and the pronator quadratus.[2]

Common Pathology

Symptoms of median nerve entrapment at the pronator teres muscle may be very similar to carpal tunnel syndrome. Pain is commonly reported over the mid forearm and follows the distal median nerve distribution along with weakness of the muscles innervated by the anterior interosseous nerve. This is most often seen with sports or careers that require extensive amounts of forearm rotational movement, which may lead to pronator muscle hypertrophy.

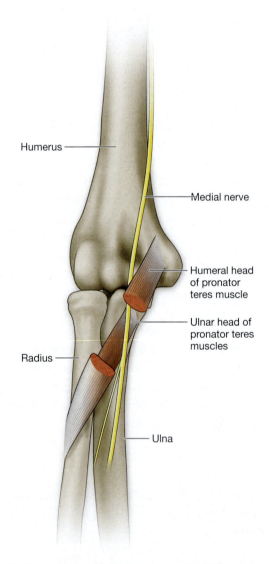

FIGURE 24-1 ■ Illustration demonstrating the median nerve running between the two heads of the pronator teres (humeral head cut to show nerve) where pronator syndrome occurs.

Ultrasound Image Findings

The median nerve may be scanned in a short-axis view along the length of the elbow. In cases of moderate-to-severe compression, enlargement of the nerve may be seen proximal to the site of compression on ultrasound evaluation (Figure 24-2). The median nerve should be followed in short-axis view until it dives posteriorly into the pronator teres (Figure 24-3). The probe is then rotated 90 degrees to create an in-plane view of the median nerve diving between the two heads of the pronator teres muscle (Figure 24-4).

Indications for Injections of Median Nerve

Pain in the distribution of the median nerve with clinical evidence or suspicion of entrapment at the pronator teres is the primary indication for this injection. Patients traditionally undergo conservative management including antiinflammatory medications, bracing, and occupational or physical therapy prior to injection. There are established techniques for nonguided injections of this target, which requires large volumes of anesthetic to approach near 100% rate of nerve palsy.[3] Ultrasound-guided injection technique has been described by Yang Soo Lee with 100% accuracy reported, but no comparative studies have been done to date.[4]

Equipment

■ Needle: 25- to 27-gauge, 1.5- to 2-inch needle
■ Injectate
  • Nerve block: 2 mL of local anesthetic ± injectable corticosteroids
  • Nerve hydrodissection and decompression: 5–10 mL of total solution (combination of normal saline, local anesthetic, ± dextrose solution)
■ High-frequency linear array transducer

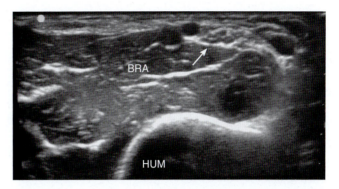

FIGURE 24-2 ■ Short-axis view of the median nerve (*arrow*) proximal to the pronator teres with enlargement in the nerve, but intact axons. This is commonly seen is acute to subacute nerve entrapment proximal to the lesion. BRA, brachialis; HUM, humerus.

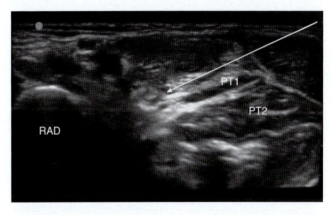

FIGURE 24-3 ■ Short-axis view of the median nerve and pronator teres muscle at the radial head. There is thickening of the perineural sheath evidenced by hyperechoic patterning at the perineural space. The *arrow* represents angle of needle entry around median nerve in plane from medial to lateral. PT1, proximal head of pronator teres; PT2, distal head of pronator teres; RAD, radius.

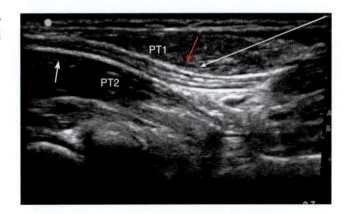

FIGURE 24-4 ■ Long-axis view of the median nerve showing the full length of the entrapment. Note the "bird beak" appearance (*red arrow*) where proximal thickening and then more distal tapering of the nerve occurs. Also note the change in echogenicity of the nerve from proximal (*white arrow*) to distal (*red arrow*). The *arrow* represents angle of needle entry around median nerve, in plane, from distal to proximal.

Author's Preferred Technique

a. Patient position (Figure 24-5)
    i. Seated or supine
    ii. Forearm supinated with the elbow in a neutral position
b. Transducer position (see Figure 24-5)
    i. Long-axis view of the median nerve in the distal antecubital fossa
c. Needle orientation relative to the transducer (see Figures 24-4 and 24-5)
    i. In plane
d. Needle approach (see Figure 24-4)
    i. Distal to proximal
e. Target (see Figure 24-4)
    i. Median nerve between the heads of the pronator teres
f. Pearls and Pitfalls
    i. Intravascular injection is a potential concern. It is recommended that color Doppler ultrasound be used to ensure nonvascular needle position.
    ii. Intraneural injection is also a potential concern and, therefore, caution should be taken to remain in the perineural space.
    iii. The diagnostic and therapeutic value of this injection relies significantly on proper identification of the median nerve. To confirm anatomy, the practitioner should scan proximal to distal in order to identify the proper track of the median nerve. If aberrant anatomy is suspected, revision of the injection approach and application should be considered.
    iv. In-plane injection of this nerve is ideal for hydroneurolysis as the nerve is tortuous and this allows better expansion of the muscle bellies of the pronator.

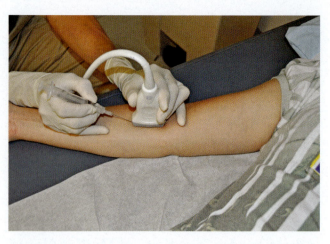

FIGURE 24-5 ■ Patient, transducer, and needle positioning for long-axis, in-plane injection from distal to proximal of the median nerve between heads of the pronator teres.

Alternate Injection Technique

a. Patient position (Figure 24-6)

   i. Seated or supine

   ii. Forearm supinated with the elbow in a neutral position.

b. Transducer position (see Figure 24-6)

   i. Short-axis view of the median nerve in the distal antecubital fossa

c. Needle orientation relative to the transducer (see Figures 24-3 and 24-6)

   i. In plane

d. Needle approach (see Figure 24-3)

   i. Lateral to medial

e. Target

   i. Median nerve between the heads of the pronator teres

f. Pearls and Pitfalls

   i. This technique is appropriate for diagnostic nerve block or regional anesthesia but may not allow for adequate hydroneurolysis of nerve.

   ii. See pearls and pitfalls of Author's Preferred Technique.

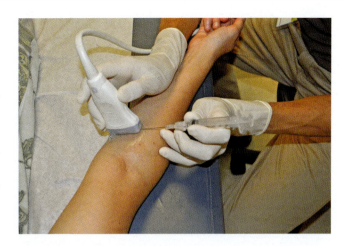

FIGURE 24-6 ▪ Patient, transducer, and needle positioning for short-axis, in-plane injection from lateral to medial of the median nerve between heads of the pronator teres.

References

1. Fuss FK, Wurzl GH. Median nerve entrapment: pronator teres syndrome. *Surg Radiol Anat.* 1990;12(4):267–271.
2. Wertsch JJ, Melvin J. Median nerve anatomy and entrapment syndromes: a review. *Arch Phys Med Rehabil.* 1982;63(12):623–627.
3. Grutter P, Desilva GL, Meehan RE, Desilva SP. The accuracy of distal posterior interosseous and anterior interosseous nerve injection. *J Hand Surg Am.* 2004;29(5):865–870.
4. Lee J, Lee YS. Percutaneous chemical nerve block with ultrasound-guided intraneural injection. *Eur Radiol.* 2008;18(7):1506–1512.

Hand and Wrist

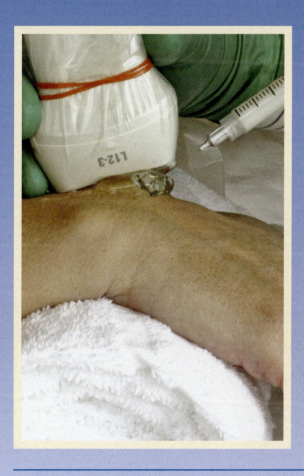

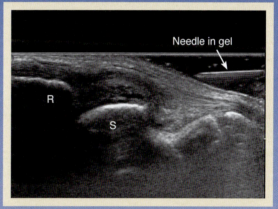

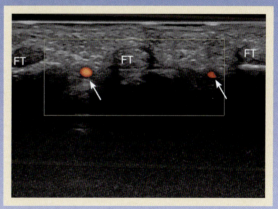

Darryl Eugene Barnes, MD

KEY POINTS

- A 25- to 27-gauge needle is recommended.
- The radiocarpal joint is condyloid type of synovial articulation.
- The radiocarpal joint extends from the radial to the ulnar sides of the wrist.
- There are in- and out-of-plane approaches to ultrasound-guided injection of the radiocarpal joint.

Pertinent Anatomy

The radiocarpal joint is condyloid type of synovial articulation, considered the "wrist joint" proper, which is formed proximally by the concave articular facet surface of the radius, distal surface of the triangular fibrocartilage complex (TFCC), and distally by the convex articular surfaces of the scaphoid, lunate, and triquetrum (often includes the pisotriquetral joint). The radiocarpal joint capsule inserts into the distal radius, ulnar, and the proximal carpal row and is stabilized by extrinsic carpal ligaments (Figure 25-1). This articulation allows for extension, flexion, and ulnar and radial deviation of the wrist.

Important dorsal wrist landmarks to consider when doing an ultrasound-guided injection into the radiocarpal joint are as follows (Figure 25-2A, B):

1. Lister's tubercle
2. Extensor pollicis longus tendon (third wrist extensor compartment)
3. Extensor digitorum tendons (fourth wrist extensor compartment)
4. Scapholunate ligament (see Figure 25-1)

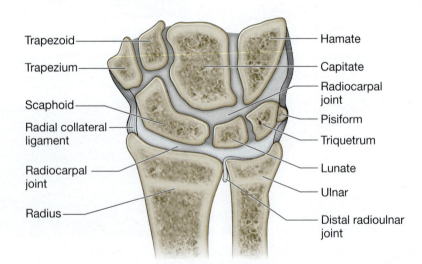

FIGURE 25-1 ■ Depicts the relationship of the radius, triangular fibrocartilage complex (TFCC), and proximal carpal row that forms the radiocarpal joint. Radiocarpal joint (1), TFCC (2), distal radial ulnar joint (3), radius (R), ulna (U), scaphoid (S), lunate (L), triquetrum (T), pisiform (P), scapholunate ligament (4), lunotriquetral ligament (5), joint capsule (6).

Common Pathology

The radiocarpal joint is intimately associated with important soft-tissue stabilizers to the carpus (ie, scapholunate and lunotriquetral ligaments and the TFCC), making this joint subject to injury and disease resulting in wrist pain and dysfunction. Injury can be caused either indirectly by damage to the intercarpal ligaments (ie, scapholunate ligament) creating instability in the wrist joint or directly by traumatic, inflammatory, or degenerative processes affecting the articulations.

Ultrasound Imaging Findings

The radiocarpal joint is best visualized dorsally in the long-axis plane with the wrist in slight flexion using a high-frequency linear array transducer (see Figure 25-2A). Findings may include synovitis (effusion and pannus), cortical irregularities, and cartilage degeneration (except for the central articular surfaces).

Indications for Injection of the Radiocarpal Joint

Injection of the radiocarpal joint should be conducted for diagnostic and/or therapeutic reasons in those patients with wrist pain where disease of the joint is suspected and have not responded to common less invasive treatments (ie, nonsteroidal antiinflammatory drugs, icing, and physical therapy). It is important to note that the scapholunate ligament should be interrogated with ultrasound examination to ensure documentation of the integrity of this structure prior to injection. In addition, this ligament should be avoided when placing the needle into the joint during the procedure. Ultrasound-guided injection into this joint has been described by Lohman et al. with a success rate of 93.5%.[2] Clinical outcomes of guided injection have not been described.

Equipment

■ Needle: 25- to 27-gauge, 1- to 1.5-inch needle
■ Injectate: 1 mL of local anesthetic and 0.5–1.0 mL of an injectable corticosteroid
■ High-frequency linear array transducer

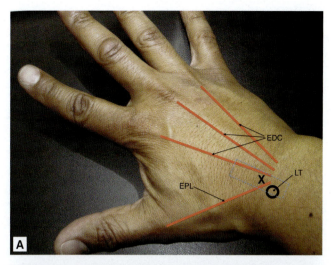

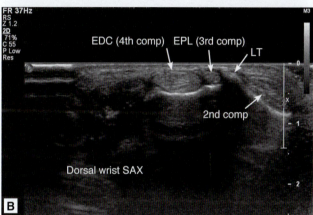

FIGURE 25-2 ■ **A.** Shows surface anatomy of Lister's tubercle (LT), extensor pollicis longus tendon (EPL), extensor digitorum tendons (EDC), and the injection site (X). Transducer placement indicated by *dotted line.* **B.** Dorsal wrist short-axis view demonstrating Lister's tubercle and extensor compartments 2, 3, and 4. EDC, extensor digitorum tendons; EPL, extensor pollicis longus tendon; LT, Lister's tubercle; SAX, short axis.

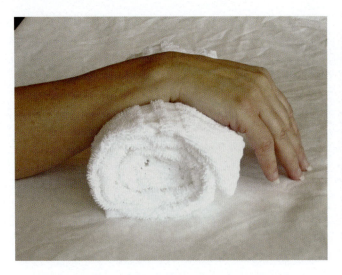

FIGURE 25-3 ■ Shows arm-wrist-hand position for injection.

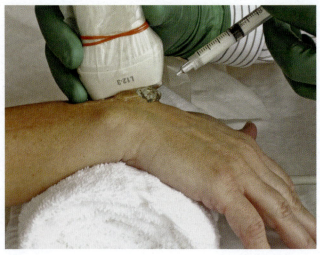

FIGURE 25-4 ■ Demonstrates transducer and needle position for in-plane distal to proximal injection.

Author's Preferred Technique

a. Patient position (Figure 25-3)
   i. Seated or supine
   ii. Arm resting in pronation on table in front of seated patient or in the pronated position in supine patient.
   iii. Wrist slight flexed resting on a bump (ie, rolled towel)
b. Transducer position (Figure 25-4)
   i. Dorsal and long axis to wrist
c. Needle orientation relative to the transducer (see Figure 25-4)
   i. In plane
d. Needle approach
   i. Distal to proximal (Figure 25-5A, B)
e. Target
   i. Radiocarpal joint

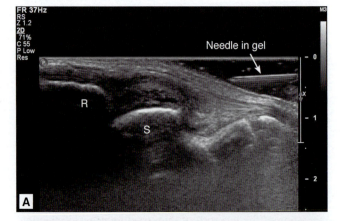

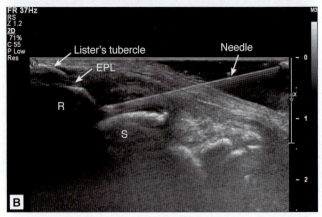

FIGURE 25-5 ■ **A.** Shows ultrasonographic dorsal long-axis view of the wrist. Demonstrates a standoff technique with the needle in sterile gel and in plane with the target (radiocarpal joint). **B.** Demonstrates the needle tip in the radiocarpal joint and Lister's tubercle and part of the extensor pollicis longus (EPL) tendon. R, radius; S, scaphoid.

Alternate Injection Technique

a. Patient position (see Figure 25-3)
    i.   Seated or supine
    ii. Arm resting in pronation on table in front of seated patient or in the pronated position in supine patient.
    iii. Wrist slight flexed resting on a bump (ie, rolled towel)
b. Transducer position (see Figure 25-6)
    i.   Dorsal and long axis to wrist
c. Needle orientation relative to the transducer (Figure 25-6)
    i.   Out of plane
d. Needle approach (Figure 25-7)
    i.   Ulnar to radial or radial to ulnar
    ii. Walk-down technique
e. Target
    i.   Radiocarpal joint

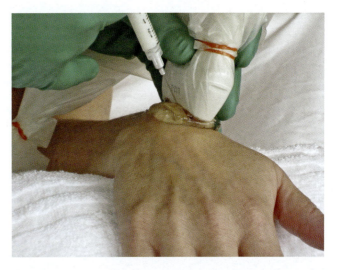

FIGURE 25-6 ▪ Demonstrates transducer and needle position for out-of-plane ulnar to radial injection.

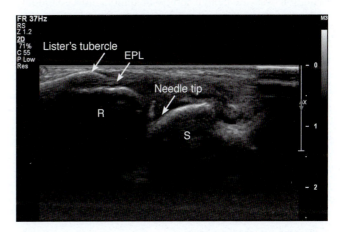

FIGURE 25-7 ▪ Demonstrates the needle tip in the radiocarpal joint and Lister's tubercle and part of the extensor pollicis longus (EPL) tendon. R, radius; S, scaphoid.

References

1. Bianchi S, Martinoli C. Wrist. In: Bianchi S, Martinoli C, Baert AL, Knauth M, Sartor K, eds. *Ultrasound of the Musculoskeletal System*. Berlin: Springer-Verlag; 2007:472.

2. Lohman M, Vasenius J, Nieminen O. Ultrasound guidance for puncture and injection in the radiocarpal joint. *Acta Radiol.* 2007;48:744–747.

B. Elizabeth Delasobera, MD / Garry Wai Keung Ho, MD, CAQSM / Thomas M. Howard, MD, FACSM

KEY POINTS

- Typically an 18-gauge, 1.5-inch needle for aspiration; a 21- to 25-gauge, 1.5-inch needle for trephination, injection, and rupture.
- A high-frequency linear array transducer is used.
- The most common location is in the dorsal wrist in association with the scapholunate joint.

- Surgery and aspiration with injection of cysts have nearly equivalent recurrence rates.
- Preferred initial treatment method is aspiration and injection, followed by trephination and then rupture.

Pertinent Anatomy

Ganglion cysts are benign soft tissue tumors most commonly occurring in the wrist but also occurring in other joints and tendon sheaths. The dorsal aspect of the wrist is the most common location (60–70%) for ganglion cysts to occur, typically involving the scapholunate joint (Figure 26-1). Volar wrist ganglia (15–20%) are usually associated with the radioscaphoid and scaphotrapezial joints. Of note, volar ganglion cysts typically lie in close proximity to the median nerve and its palmar cutaneous branch, as well as the radial artery (see Figure 26-1). The flexor tendon sheaths (10%) also commonly give rise to ganglion cysts.[1–3]

Common Pathology

Ganglion cysts are benign soft-tissue tumors. There are a number of etiological theories as to the origin of these cysts. Commonly held thought includes an evagination of synovium from inflammatory processes afflicting the tenosynovium or intraarticular structures. Another possible cause describes ganglion cysts to be the result of degeneration of connective tissue with attritional cyst formation. Ganglion cysts average 1–2 cm in diameter, may be unilobulated or multiloculated, and are frequently described as firm cystic structures tethered by a pedicle to a nearby joint capsule or tendon sheath. Their lumen is typically filled with viscous gelatinous fluid, surrounded by an outer fibrous coating with its inner proteinaceous walls theoretically lined by synovium.[3] They are more commonly seen in females in the second and third decades of life.[2] Clinically, they often present as a slow-growing, firm swelling in the wrist or hand that may be painless, or can be associated with achy, dull pain, which may radiate proximally. Pain is often exacerbated with activity or direct pressure, and can lead to decreased

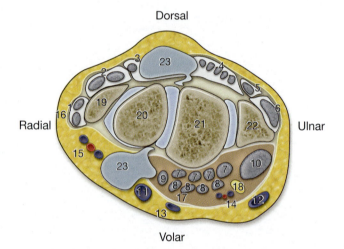

FIGURE 26-1 ■ Anatomical depiction of dorsal and volar wrist ganglion cyst. Axial section of the wrist through scapholunate joint. 1. First dorsal extensor compartment: abductor pollicis longus (APL), extensor pollicis brevis (EPB). 2. Second dorsal extensor compartment: extensor carpi radialis longus (ECRL), extensor carpi radialis brevis (ECRB). 3. Third dorsal extensor compartment: extensor pollicis longus (EPL). 4. Fourth dorsal extensor compartment: extensor digitorum communis (EDC), extensor indicis proprius (EIP). 5. Fifth dorsal extensor compartment: extensor digiti minimi (EDM). 6. Sixth dorsal extensor compartment: extensor carpi ulnaris (ECU). 7. Flexor digitorum profundus (FDP). 8. Flexor digitorum superficialis (FDS). 9. Flexor pollicis longus (FPL). 10. Pisiform recess. 11. Flexor carpi radialis (FCR). 12. Flexor carpi ulnaris (FCU). 13. Palmaris. 14. Ulnar artery. 15. Radial artery. 16. Superficial branch of the radial nerve. 17. Median nerve. 18. Ulnar nerve. 19. Distal radius. 20. Scaphoid. 21. Lunate. 22. Triquetrum. 23. Ganglion (synovial) cyst(s).

range of motion and grip strength. Volar ganglia may cause paresthesias from compression of the ulnar or median nerve.

Indications for Injections of Ganglion Cyst

Treatment of wrist ganglion cysts classically includes three options: watchful waiting, aspiration with injection, or surgery. In patients with minimal pain and unaffected range of motion, watchful waiting may be preferable as 50% of cysts will resolve spontaneously.[1] If the cyst is symptomatic, then aspiration with injection or surgical excision should be considered. In a recent study, 219 patients were randomized to either aspiration with injection or surgical excision of their wrist ganglion cyst. In the nonsurgical group, the cyst was first aspirated and then injected with a separate needle with 2 mL of triamcinolone acetonide 10%. In this study, 8.4% had recurrence rate at 6 months, while there was a 21.5% recurrence rate with surgical excision. The surgical group also had more postoperative pain and stiffness.[2] Other similarly designed studies have shown similar recurrence rates with aspiration and injection compared to surgery in dorsal ganglion cysts.[1] However, a number of studies have shown that volar ganglion cysts are more likely to recur without surgical excision.[1,2] None of these studies were performed with ultrasound guidance, and there are no studies comparing treatment of ganglion cysts with palpation versus ultrasound-guided technique.

Equipment

- Needle
  - 25-gauge, 1.5-inch needle for local anesthetic administration
  - 18- to 22-gauge, 1.5-inch needle for aspiration and fenestration
- Injectate
  - 0.5 mL of local anesthesia and 0.5 mL of injectable corticosteroid
  - For rupture of the cyst, use 2–3 mL of sterile saline
- High-frequency linear array transducer

Author's Preferred Technique

a. Patient position
   i. Seated or supine
   ii. Hand resting comfortably on table, palm down
b. Transducer position (Figure 26-2)
   i. Aligned to get best view of the cyst, can be long axis or short axis to wrist

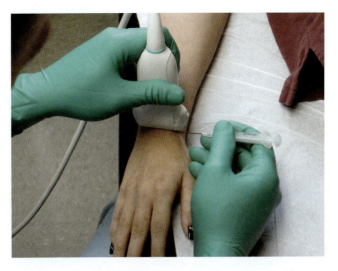

FIGURE 26-2 ■ Probe and needle positioning for dorsal wrist ganglion cyst. Procedure is in plane with transducer placed in long axis to the wrist joint in this photograph.

c. Needle orientation relative to the transducer (see Figure 26-2)
    i. In plane
d. Needle approach
    i. Any angle that the cyst is maximally visualized
e. Target (Figure 26-3)
    i. Middle of the cyst cavity
f. Pearls and Pitfalls
    i. Confirm the cyst in at least two planes and use color Doppler ultrasound to ensure it is not a vascular structure, anisotropic psoas tendon, or solid tumor.
    ii. If attempting, but unable to aspirate the cyst using a 22-gauge needle, try an 18-gauge needle or consider rupturing it with normal saline or fenestrating it to disperse its contents.
    iii. Should the cyst not automatically decompress with rupturing or fenestrating techniques, manual pressure can be applied to assist the process.

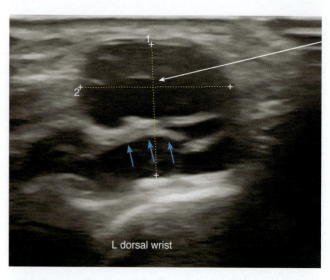

FIGURE 26-3 ■ Ultrasound appearance of dorsal wrist ganglion. Note hyperechoic debris seen within the ganglion cyst (*blue arrows*) and placement of needle (*white arrow*) in the middle of the cyst cavity.

References

1. Gude, W, Morelli, V. Ganglion cysts of the wrist: pathophysiology, clinical picture, and management. *Curr Rev Musculoskelet Med.* 2008 Dec;1(3-4):205–211.
2. Paramhans, D, Nayak, D, Mathur, R, Kushwah K. Double dart technique of instillation of triamcinolone in ganglion over the wrist. *J Cutan Aesthet Surg.* 2010 Jan-Apr;3(1):29–31.
3. Genova, R. Ganglion wrist. Medscape Reference: Emedicine. http://emedicine.medscape.com/article/1243454-overview. Updated August 2009. Accessed November 19, 2011.

Darryl Eugene Barnes, MD

KEY POINTS

- Use a 25- to 27-gauge, 1.5-inch needle.
- Use a high-frequency linear array transducer.
- The distal radial ulnar joint (DRUJ) is an L-shaped joint that is separated from the radiocarpal joint and stabilized by the triangular fibrocartilage complex (TFCC).
- Extensor digiti minimi is located superficial to the dorsal capsule of the DRUJ.
- DRUJ injection approach is dorsal short axis to wrist, in-plane, and ulnar to radial.

Pertinent Anatomy

The distal radial ulnar joint (DRUJ) is an L-shaped joint that is separated from the radiocarpal joint and stabilized by the triangular fibrocartilage complex (TFCC) and formed by the distal epiphysis of the radius (sigmoid notch) and the distal rounded head of the ulna (Figure 27-1). This articulation allows for pronation and supination of the hand.

The extensor digiti minimi tendon is located superficial to the DRUJ and is an important anatomical landmark when performing an ultrasound-guided injection of this joint

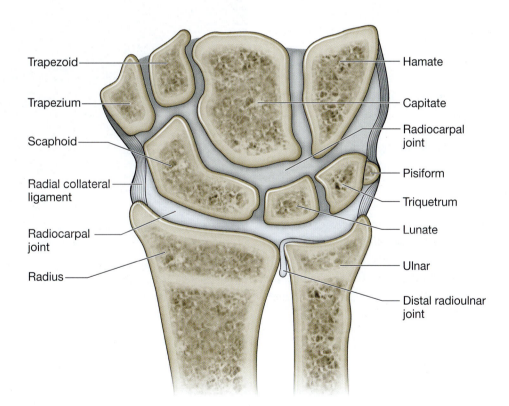

FIGURE 27-1 ■ Depicts the components of the distal radial ulnar joint (DRUJ). Distal radius (sigmoid notch) (1), distal rounded head of the ulna (2), TFCC (3), radiocarpal joint (4).

(Figure 27-2). The distal portion of the dorsal interosseous artery may be seen in this area (with the assistance of the color or power Doppler feature) and should be avoided when performing injections into the DRUJ.

Common Pathology

The DRUJ is minimally congruous and its stability is dependent on soft tissue restraints (ie, TFCC), making this joint subject to injury resulting in ulnar-sided wrist pain. Injury can be caused either indirectly by damage to the TFCC creating instability in the DRUJ or directly by traumatic, inflammatory, or degenerative processes affecting the articulation.

Ultrasound Imaging Findings

The DRUJ is best visualized dorsally in the short-axis plane using a high-frequency linear array transducer (Figure 27-3). Joint effusions are better seen proximal to the joint line where the joint capsule is less compliant. Other findings may include synovitis (effusion and pannus), cortical irregularities, and cartilage degeneration (except for the central articular surface).

Indications for Injection of the Distal Radial Ulnar Joint

Injection of the DRUJ should be conducted for diagnostic and/or therapeutic reasons in those patients with ulnar-sided wrist pain where disease of the DRUJ is suspected and patients have not responded to common less-invasive treatments (ie, nonsteroidal antiinflammatory drugs, icing, and physical therapy). In addition, wrist arthrography or magnetic resonance arthrography are implemented to rule out TFCC tears; this requires injection of the DRUJ. Smith et al. reported 100% success rate with ultrasound-guided injections into the DRUJ.[3] Clinical outcomes of guided injection have not been described.

Equipment

- Needle: 25- to 27-gauge, 1- to 1.5-inch needle
- Injectate: 0.5 mL of local anesthetics and 0.5 mL of an injectable corticosteroid
- High-frequency linear array transducer

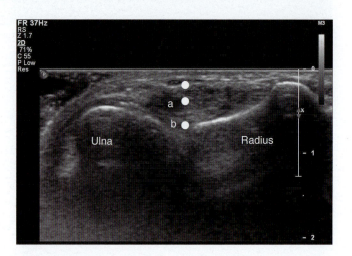

FIGURE 27-2 ■ Demonstrates the relationship of the extensor digiti minimi (a) in short axis (viewed with anisotropy) and the dorsal capsule of the distal radial ulnar joint (DRUJ) (b). *Dots* represent walk-down technique for out-of-plane injection into the joint.

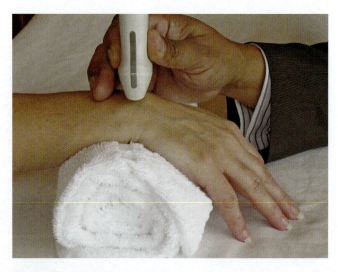

FIGURE 27-3 ■ Depicts the position of the transducer on the dorsum of the wrist and wrist position with a rolled towel to create slight flexion in the resting patient.

Author's Preferred Technique

a. Patient position (see Figure 27-3)
   i. Seated or supine
   ii. Arm resting in pronation on table in front of seated patient or in the pronated position in supine patient.
   iii. Wrist slight flexed resting on a bump (ie, rolled towel)
b. Transducer position (Figure 27-4)
   i. Dorsal and short axis to wrist
c. Needle orientation relative to the transducer (see Figure 27-4)
   i. In plane
d. Needle approach (Figures 27-4 and 27-5)
   i. Ulnar to radial deep to the extensor digiti minimi tendon
   ii. Use standoff oblique technique
e. Target
   i. DRUJ
f. Pearls and Pitfalls
   i. Use anisotropy of the extensor digiti minimi (EDM) tendon to enhance contrast between the joint capsule and the tendon when placing the needle into the DRUJ.
   ii. Avoid placing the needle too far distally, which may result in an injection into the TFCC.
   iii. Avoid placing the needle too far proximally, which may result in an extraarticular injection.

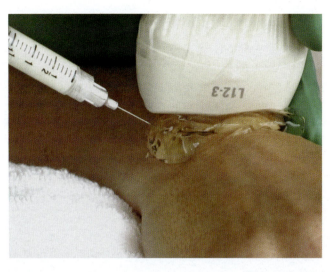

FIGURE 27-4 ■ Short-axis view of wrist with in-plane needle technique visualized (ulnar-to-radial).

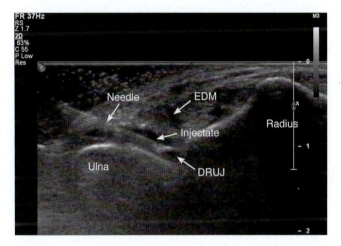

FIGURE 27-5 ■ Demonstrates the ultrasound image of the needle and the injectate in the distal radial ulnar joint (DRUJ) and the relationship of the extensor digiti minimi (EDM).

Alternate Technique

a. Patient position (see Figure 27-3)
   i. Seated or supine
   ii. Arm resting in pronation on table in front of seated patient or in the pronated position in supine patient
   iii. Wrist slight flexed resting on a bump (ie, rolled towel)
b. Transducer position (Figure 27-6)
   i. Dorsal and short axis to wrist
c. Needle orientation relative to the transducer (see Figure 27-6)
   i. Out of plane
d. Needle approach (Figures 27-2 and 27-6)
   i. Distal to proximal, deep to the extensor digiti minimi tendon
   ii. Use walk-down technique
e. Target
   i. DRUJ
f. Pearls and Pitfalls
   i. Place the needle just ulnar to the EDM tendon to avoid piercing the tendon.
   ii. Avoid placing the needle through the TFCC.
      1. To avoid piercing the TFCC, employ the distal to proximal method and not the proximal-to-distal method when using the out-of-plane approach.
      2. Another way to avoid this is to mark the skin over the TFCC (ultrasound assisted) and avoid placing the needle through the skin at this level as you take the distal to proximal out-of-plane approach.

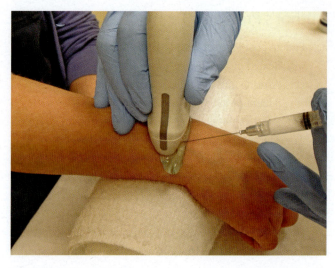

FIGURE 27-6 ■ Short-axis view of wrist with out-of-plane needle technique visualized.

References

1. Buck FM, Nico MAC, Gheno R, Trudell DJ, Resnick D. Ultrasonographic evaluation of degenerative changes in the distal radioulnar joint: correlation of findings with gross anatomy and MR arthrography in cadavers. *Eur J Radiol.* 2011;77:215–221.
2. Bianchi S, Martinoli C. Wrist. In: Bianchi S, Martinoli C, Baert AL, Knauth M, Sartor K, eds. *Ultrasound of the Musculoskeletal System.* Berlin: Springer-Verlag; 2007:472.
3. Smith J, Rizzo M, Sayeed YA, Finnoff JT. Sonographically guided distal radioulnar joint injection: technique and validation in a cadaveric model. *J Ultrasound Med.* 2011;30(11):1587–1592.

Joseph J. Ruane, DO / Paul A. Cook, MD / Jeffrey A. Strakowski, MD

KEY POINTS

- A 25-gauge, 1.5-inch needle is ideal for injection.
- Use a high-frequency linear array transducer.
- An out-of-plane, distal to proximal approach to scapholunate (SL) joint is recommended.
- Ultrasound of SL joint has high specificity, but low sensitivity for dynamic instability evaluation.

Pertinent Anatomy

The wrist is a biaxial ellipsoid joint comprised of eight carpal bones with multiple independent synovial articulations. The carpals form a proximal and distal row, with the proximal row being the more mobile and commonly referred to as an *intercalated segment*. The proximal carpal row consists of the scaphoid, lunate, and triquetrum, and the distal carpal row consists of the trapezium, trapezoid, capitate, and hamate. To maintain mobility without sacrificing stability, a complex interplay of ligaments interconnects the carpals with each other, and with the adjacent metacarpals, ulna, and radius (Figure 28-1). The scapholunate (SL) ligament is the most crucial as the scaphoid bone provides structural support to the rest of the midcarpal joint.

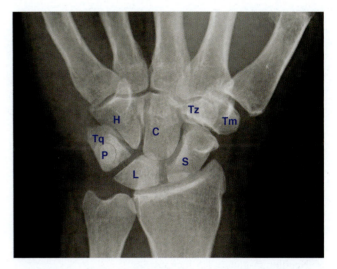

FIGURE 28-1 ■ Bony anatomy of the wrist. C, capitate; H, hamate; L, lunate; P, pisiform; S, scaphoid; Tm, trapezium; Tq, triquetrum; Tz, trapezoid. (Reproduced with permission from Tintinalli JE, Stapczynski JS, Cline DM, et al. *Tintinalli's Emergency Medicine: A Comprehensive Study Guide*. 7th ed. New York: McGraw-Hill; 2011: figure 266-1.)

Common Pathology

Degenerative arthritis is among the most frequently encountered conditions requiring wrist injection, and the most common form is found between the scaphoid, lunate, and radius and is termed the *scapholunate advanced collapse* (SLAC) pattern. This pattern can develop as posttraumatic arthritis following an injury to the joint cartilage, or with carpal instability occurring as a result of injury to the intercarpal ligaments. Provocative maneuvers assist in diagnosis. For example, pain with forced radial deviation implies radiocarpal pathology, such as radioscaphoid impaction secondary to arthritis or chronic SL ligament injury. Additionally, pain with forced radial wrist extension implies pathology at the midcarpal joint. A fall onto an outstretched hand is among the most common mechanisms of a SL injury and could lead to the arthritic patterns described above.

Ultrasound Imaging Findings

The SL joint is best visualized in long axis using a high-frequency linear array transducer and a depth of less than 2 cm. Common findings include the typical cortical irregularities and calcifications seen in osteoarthritis. The SL ligament can be evaluated for thickening or hypoechogenic signal associated with partial tear, or an anechoic void if completely torn.[1] Dynamic imaging can also demonstrate abnormal gapping between these bones in cases of instability, although this has been shown to not be very sensitive, despite good specificity.[2]

Indications

Injection of the SL joint can be performed for patients with recalcitrant pain that is unresponsive to rest, splinting, icing, and antiinflammatory drugs. Injection can also be done for diagnostic purposes to help decide future treatments. In addition, one may wish to inject proliferative agents around the SL joint to attempt to strengthen the ligamentous structures in the region. There is little research comparing placement success or outcomes in palpation-guided versus ultrasound-guided injections of the SL joint.

Equipment

- Needle: 25-gauge, 1.5-inch needle
- Injectate: 0.5–1 mL of local anesthesia and 0.5–1 mL of injectable corticosteroid
- High-frequency linear array transducer

Author's Preferred Technique

a. Patient position
   i. Supine or seated
   ii. Arm adducted to side and palm of hand resting directly on table or folded towel.
b. Transducer position (Figure 28-2)
   i. Begin in short-axis plane over Lister's tubercle and advance distally until the scaphoid, lunate, and SL ligament are in view.
c. Needle orientation relative to the transducer (see Figure 28-2)
   i. Out of plane
d. Needle approach (Figure 28-3)
   i. Distal to proximal
   ii. Needle tilted 30 degrees in the sagittal plane
   iii. Walk-down technique

e. Target
   i. Advance needle toward radius into the SL joint capsule
f. Pearls and Pitfalls
   i. This is a great technique for easy access to SL joint without having to travel as far with needle as in-plane approach.

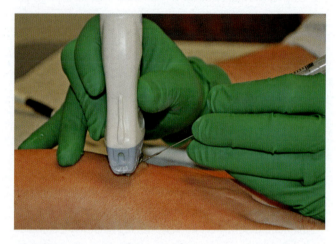

FIGURE 28-2 ■ Transducer and needle position for out-of-plane injection of the scapholunate joint.

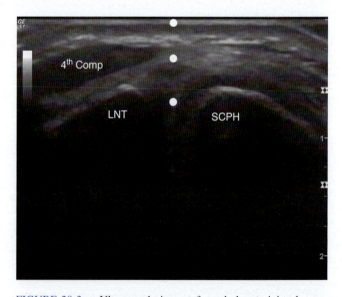

FIGURE 28-3 ■ Ultrasound picture of scapholunate joint demonstrating out-of-plane walk-down technique (*dots*). 4th Comp, fourth extensor compartment; LNT, lunate; SCPH, scaphoid.

Alternate Technique

a. Patient position
   i. Supine or seated
   ii. Arm adducted to side and palm of hand resting directly on table or folded towel
b. Transducer position (Figure 28-4)
   i. Begin in short-axis plane over Lister's tubercle and advance distally until the scaphoid, lunate and SL ligament are in view.
c. Needle orientation relative to the transducer (see Figure 28-4)
   i. In plane
d. Needle approach (Figure 28-5)
   i. Radial to ulnar
   ii. Stand-off oblique technique
e. Target
   i. Advance needle toward radius into the SL joint capsule.
f. Pearls and Pitfalls
   i. This technique is best if attempting proliferation of ligaments with biologics.
   ii. Steep access to joint will necessitate standoff approach for this injection.

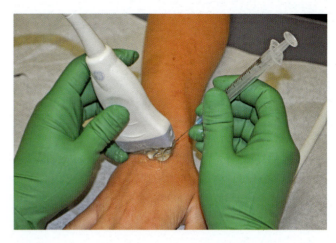

FIGURE 28-4 ▪ Transducer and needle position for in-plane approach to the scapholunate joint.

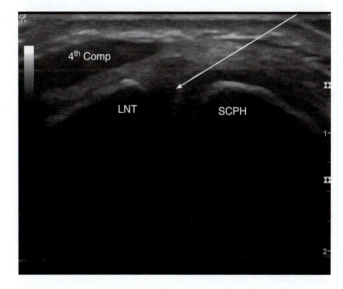

FIGURE 28-5 ▪ Ultrasound picture of scapholunate joint demonstrating in-plane radial to ulnar technique. *Arrow* shows needle angle into joint capsule. 4th Comp, fourth extensor compartment; LNT, lunate; SCPH, scaphoid.

References

1. Jacobson JA. Wrist and hand ultrasound. In: Jacobson JA, ed. *Fundamentals of Musculoskeletal Ultrasound.* Philadelphia, PA: Saunders Elsevier; 2007:144–147.

2. Dao KD, Solomon DJ, Shin AY, Puckett ML. The efficacy of ultrasound in the evaluation of dynamic scapholunate ligamentous instability. *J Bone Joint Surg Am.* 2004;86(7):1473–1478.

John FitzGerald, MD

KEY POINTS

- A 25-gauge, 1.5-inch needle is ideal.
- Use a high-frequency linear array transducer or "hockey stick" transducer.
- The carpal-metacarpal joint (CMC) joint is most accessible from a dorsal approach.
- Use caution to avoid the neurovascular bundle.
- The "seagull" sign indicates joint space on the dorsal approach.

Pertinent Anatomy

The carpal-metacarpal (CMC) joint is key articulation for mobility of the thumb and therefore is susceptible to degenerative arthritis. The trapezium bone articulates with the first metacarpal bone. The radial artery branches near the CMC joint to form the deep and superficial palmar arteries and can therefore envelope the joint. The radial nerve runs along the radial artery. The abductor pollicis longus (APL) and extensor pollicis brevis (EPB) tendons are on the radial side of the joint. The anatomic snuff box is bound by APL and EPB (radial side), and extensor carpi radialis and extensor pollicis longus (dorsal aspect); the carpal trapezium bone comprises the floor with the base of first metacarpal forming the anterior wall of the box. The radial artery can be found at the base of the snuff box (Figure 29-1).

Common Pathology

The CMC joint is susceptible to degenerative arthritis. Patients may complain of pain gripping or holding items. On examination, there may be "squaring" of the joint and crepitus with circumlocution.

Ultrasound Imaging Findings

The CMC joint can be visualized using a high-frequency linear array transducer and shallow depths of less than 1 cm. Common findings may include an enlarged triangular joint space,[1] irregular cortices, sometimes with erosions (eg, with inflammatory osteoarthritis), and effusion.

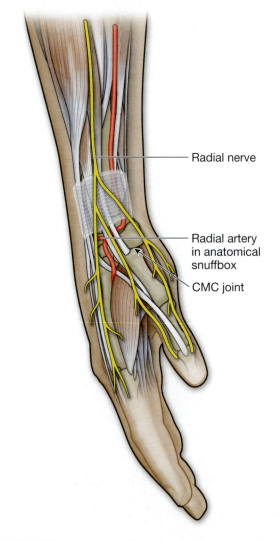

Radial nerve

Radial artery in anatomical snuffbox

CMC joint

FIGURE 29-1 ■ Anatomy of carpal-metacarpal joint region.

Indications for Injections of the Carpal-Metacarpal Joint

Injection of the CMC joint is indicated for patients with pain of the CMC joint that is refractory to conservative therapy, which may include analgesics or antiinflammatories, topical treatments (antiinflammatories, analgesics or counterirritants), splinting, and/or occupational therapy.

Equipment

- Needle: 25-gauge, 1.5-inch needle
- Injectate: 0.5–1 mL of local anesthetic and 0.5–1 mL of injectable corticosteroid
- High-frequency linear array transducer or "hockey stick" transducer

Author's Preferred Technique

a. Patient position (Figure 29-2)
   i. Seated or supine
   ii. Hand placed on stable surface with medial hand on table
b. Transducer position (see Figure 29-2)
   i. Over the anatomic snuff box and aligned along the long axis of the carpal-metacarpal joint
c. Needle orientation relative to the transducer (Figures 29-3 and 29-4)
   i. In plane
   ii. Standoff oblique technique
d. Target: (Figure 29-5)
   i. CMC joint space
e. Pearls and Pitfalls
   i. Care is taken to avoid the neurovascular bundle.
   ii. The joint space is identified by the "seagull" appearance of the carpal and metacarpal hyperechoic reflection.

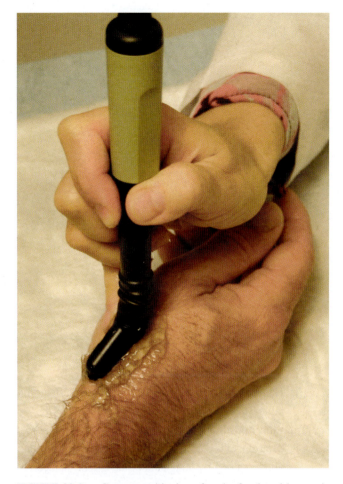

FIGURE 29-2 ▪ Correct positioning of probe for dorsal long-axis view of carpal-metacarpal joint.

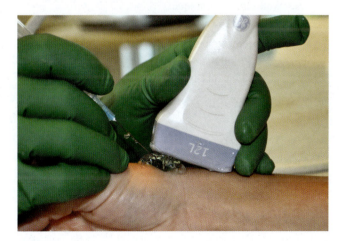

FIGURE 29-3 ▪ Close-up view of dorsal long-axis view of carpal-metacarpal joint with in-plane, standoff technique to joint.

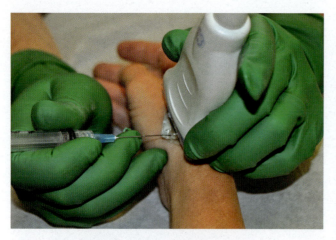

FIGURE 29-4 ■ Close-up view of dorsal long-axis view of carpal-metacarpal joint with out-of-plane technique.

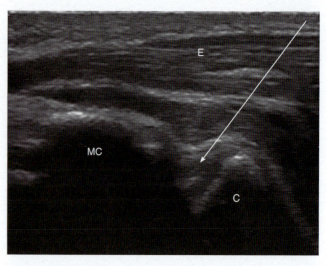

FIGURE 29-5 ■ Dorsal long-axis view of the carpal-metacarpal joint. Note needle angle of entry for in-plane technique. A standoff oblique technique would allow a less steep angle of entry. C, carpal bone; E, extensor tendons; MC, metacarpal bone.

Alternate Technique

a. Patient position
   i. Seated or supine
   ii. Hand placed on stable surface with medial hand on table
b. Transducer position (see Figure 29-2)
   i. Transducer is placed over the anatomic snuff box and aligned along the long axis of the carpal-metacarpal joint.
c. Needle orientation relative to the transducer
   i. Out of plane
   ii. Walk-down technique
d. Target (Figure 29-6)
   i. CMC joint space
e. Pearls and Pitfalls
   i. See "Pearls and Pitfalls" in the "Author's Preferred Technique."

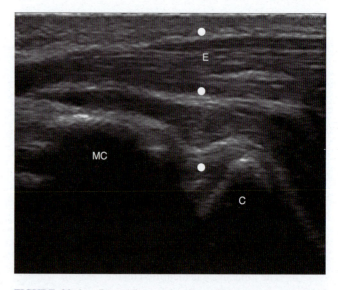

FIGURE 29-6 ■ Dorsal long-axis view of the carpal-metacarpal joint. *Dots* represent walk-down technique to CMC joint. C, carpal bone; E, extensor tendons; MC, metacarpal bone.

Reference

1. Iagnocco A. Usefulness of high resolution US in the evaluation of effusion in osteoarthritic first carpometacarpal joint. *Scand J Rheumatol.* 2000;29:170–173.

Kevin B. Dunn, MD, MS

KEY POINTS

- A 25-gauge, 1.5-inch needle is ideal.
- Use a high-frequency linear array transducer.
- The scaphotrapeziotrapezoidal (STT) joint is the second most common site of osteoarthritis (OA) in the wrist.

- The preferred technique is volar, long axis with the thumb, out of plane.
- The literature reports 100% accuracy with this technique.

Pertinent Anatomy

The scaphotrapeziotrapezoidal (STT) joint is a dome-shaped joint on the radial side of the wrist, primarily involved in movement of the thumb.[1] The scaphoid bridges the proximal and distal carpal rows on the radial side. The scaphoid has articulations with the distal radius, lunate, capitate, trapezium, and trapezoid.[2] Superior and lateral to the scaphoid, the trapezium articulates with the scaphoid and the base of the first metacarpal. Medially, the trapezoid articulates with the trapezium and the scaphoid, as well as the capitate and the base of the second metacarpal[2] (Figure 30-1).

Common Pathology

The STT joint is the second most common site of osteoarthritis (OA) in the wrist.[3] Although the true prevalence is not known, studies have shown a range in STT-joint OA from 15% in radiographic studies, up to 83.3% in cadaveric studies.[1,3,4,5] The incidence of clinical OA of the STT joint is estimated to be 11%.[5,6] Isolated STT-joint OA more commonly affects women after the age of 50, compared to men.[7] Isolating STT-joint pain is complicated by commonly affected surrounding structures, including the first carpal-metacarpal (CMC) joint. The clinical presentation is described as deep aching pain, medially within the thenar imminence, not necessarily associated with thumb motion.[2]

Nonoperative treatment for STT-joint OA includes activity modification, rest, splinting, and injections. Operative treatments include arthrodesis, trapeziectomy, soft tissue interposition, and implant replacement.[2]

Ultrasound Imaging Findings

The STT joint is visualized using high-frequency linear array transducer at shallow depth. The patient is positioned seated or supine with the palm up. To view using a palmar approach,

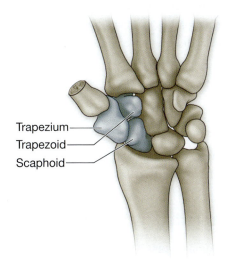

Trapezium
Trapezoid
Scaphoid

FIGURE 30-1 ■ Bony anatomy that comprises the scaphotrapeziotrapezoidal (STT) joint.

the transducer is placed in long axis with the thumb metacarpal. The transducer is translated proximally as the first CMC joint is identified. As the transducer continues to be translated proximally, the palmar aspect of the STT joint is visualized. The joint space is visualized between the adjacent bony acoustic landmarks of the scaphoid and trapezium. The transducer is then moved to center the joint on the display screen.

Indications for Injections of the Scaphotrapeziotrapezoidal Joint

Injection of the STT joint can be performed for patients with recalcitrant pain that is unresponsive to rest, icing, antiinflammatories, and splinting. There is also a diagnostic role in differentiating first CMC-joint pain from STT-joint pain.

Injection of the STT joint based on palpation has not been described. Smith et al. demonstrated that sonographically guided STT joint injections performed via a palmar approach are significantly more accurate than palpation-guided injections performed via a dorsal approach.[8] In this study, the ultrasound-guided injections had an accuracy rate of 100%, whereas the palpation-guided injections had an accuracy rate of 80%.[8] Clinical outcomes have not been described.

Equipment

- Needle: 25-gauge, 1.5-inch needle
- Injectate: 0.5–1.0 mL of local anesthetic and 0.5–1.0 mL of an injectable corticosteroid
- High-frequency linear array transducer

Author's Preferred Technique

a. Patient position (Figure 30-2)
   i. Seated or supine
   ii. Palm up
b. Transducer position (see Figure 30-2)
   i. In long axis with thumb metacarpal
c. Needle orientation relative to the transducer (see Figure 30-2)
   i. Out of plane
d. Needle approach (Figure 30-3)
   i. Radial to ulnar
   ii. Use walk-down technique
e. Target (Figure 30-3)
   i. Palmar aspect of STT joint
f. Pearls and Pitfalls
   i. An injection in the location disperses throughout the other midcarpal joints.[5]
   ii. The superficial palmar branch of the radial artery courses within the subcutaneous tissue over the scaphoid tubercle.
   iii. Once the joint space is visualized, radial-ulnar deviation can be used to palmarflex and dorsiflex the scaphoid, until joint and capsuloligamentous visualization is optimal.[6]

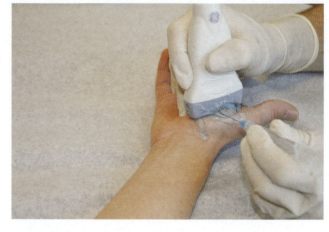

FIGURE 30-2 ■ Transducer, needle, and wrist position for volar, long-axis, out-of-plane technique to the scaphotrapeziotrapezoidal (STT) joint.

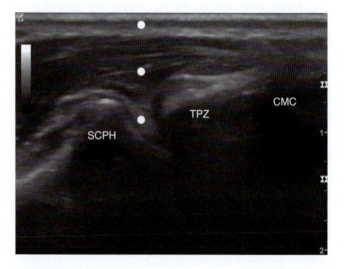

FIGURE 30-3 ■ Ultrasound picture of volar, scaphotrapeziotrapezoidal (STT) joint demonstrating out-of-plane walk-down technique (*dots*). Right side of screen is proximal; left side is distal. CMC, carpal-metacarpal joint; SCPH, scaphoid; TPZ, trapezium.

Alternate Technique

a. Patient position (Figure 30-4)
   i. Seated or supine
   ii. Palm down
b. Transducer position (see Figure 30-4)
   i. Just radial to the extensor pollicis longus tendon in the anatomic snuffbox, in long axis with thumb metacarpal
c. Needle orientation relative to the transducer (see Figure 30-4)
   i. Out of plane
d. Needle approach (Figure 30-5)
   i. Radial to ulnar
   ii. Use walk-down technique
e. Target (see Figure 30-5)
   i. Dorsal aspect of STT joint
f. Pearls and Pitfalls
   i. Pulsation of the dorsal carpal arch (a branch of the radial artery) should be visible and the vessel should be clearly identified prior to injection.
   ii. Be aware of the superficial branch of the radial nerve and take care to avoid it.

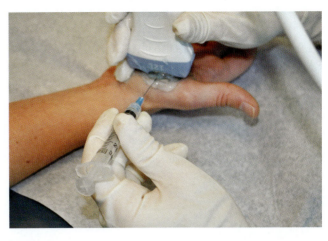

FIGURE 30-4 ■ Transducer, needle, and wrist position for dorsal, long-axis, out-of-plane technique to the scaphotrapeziotrapezoidal (STT) joint.

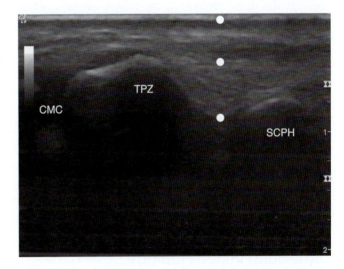

FIGURE 30-5 ■ Ultrasound picture of dorsal, scaphotrapeziotrapezoidal (STT) joint demonstrating out-of-plane walk-down technique (*dots*). Right side of screen is proximal; left side is distal. CMC, carpal-metacarpal joint; SCPH, scaphoid; TPZ, trapezium.

References

1. White L, Clavijo J, Gilula LA, Wollstein R. Classification system for isolated arthritis of the scaphotrapeziotrapezoidal joint. *Scand J Plast Reconstr Surg Hand Surg.* 2010;44:112–117.
2. Wolf JM. Treatment of scaphotrapezio-trapezoid arthritis. *Hand Clin.* 2008;24(3):301–306.
3. Watson HK, Ballet FL. The SLAC wrist: scapholunate advanced collapse pattern of degenerative arthritis. *J Hand Surg Am.* 1984;9(3):358–365.
4. Crosby EB, Linscheid RL, Dobyns JK. Scaphotrapezial trapezoidal arthrosis. *J Hand Surg Am.* 1978;3(3):223–234.
5. Bhatia A, Pisoh T, Touam C, Oberlin C. Incidence and distribution of scaphotrapeziotrapezoidal arthritis in 73 fresh cadaveric wrists. *Ann Chir Main Memb Super.* 1996;15(4):220–225.
6. Wollstein R, Watson HK. Scaphotrapeziotrapezoid arthrodesis for arthritis. *Hand Clin.* 2005;21(4):539–543.
7. Low AK, Edmunds IA. Isolated scaphotrapeziotrapezoidal osteoarthritis: preliminary results of treatment using a pyrocarbon implant. *Hand Surg.* 2007;12(2):73–77.
8. Smith J, Brault JS, Rizzo M, Sayeed YA, Finnoff JT. Accuracy of sonographically guided and palpation guided scaphotrapeziotrapezoid joint injections. *J Ultrasound Med.* 2011;30(11):1509–1515.

Mark-Friedrich Berthold Hurdle, MD

KEY POINTS

- A 25- to 30-gauge needle is ideal.
- A high-frequency linear array transducer or "hockey stick" is required.

- The interphalangeal joint injections are difficult to access in patient with advanced osteoarthritis.
- The dorsal approach with the joint flexed provides better access.

Pertinent Anatomy

The interphalangeal (IP) joints are the two most distal hinge joints of the fingers. The distal interphalangeal (DIP) joint connects the distal phalanx to the middle phalanx, while the proximal interphalangeal joint connects the middle and proximal phalanx. The (IP) joints are stabilized by collateral ligaments as well as the volar and extensor ligament complex (Figure 31-1).

Common Pathology

A host of disorders including degenerative changes, joint infections, and inflammatory disorders can affect the IP joints. Typically, osteoarthritis involves the DIP joints, whereas rheumatoid arthritis prefers the metacarpophalangeal joints.

Ultrasound Image Findings

The IP joins can be assessed for synovitis and are best visualized in the long axis using a high-frequency linear array transducer initially placed directly over the IP joint of interest. These joints can also be scanned in the short axis.

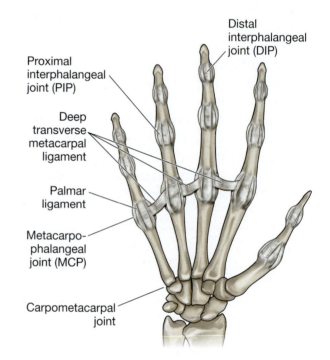

FIGURE 31-1 ■ Illustration of the location of the distal interphalangeal (DIP), proximal interphalangeal (PIP), and metacarpophalangeal (MCP) joints in the hand. (Reproduced with permission from Morton DA, Foreman KB, Albertine KH, eds. *The Big Picture: Gross Anatomy*. New York: McGraw-Hill; 2011: figure 33-5C.)

Indications for Injections of the Interphalangeal Joints

Injection of the IP joints can be performed on patients with IP joint pain that does not respond to conservative interventions including physical therapy, relative rest, antiinflammatories, and modalities. Injection of the IP joints has been described based on palpation or guidance. The rate of periarticular finger joint injections without guidance varies from 15% to 32% in one European study.[1] Ultrasound guidance allows for more accurate needle placement (59% vs. 96%) and aspiration (0% vs. 63%) based on a study by Raza et al.[2]

Equipment

- Needle: 25- to 30-gauge, 0.5- to 1-inch needle for injection
- Injectate: 0.5–1 mL of local anesthetic and 0.5 mL of an injectable corticosteroid
- High-frequency linear array transducer or "hockey stick"

Author's Preferred Technique

a. Patient position (Figure 31-2)
   i. Supine or sitting position
   ii. Wrist pronated
   iii. Cylindrical object or rolled surgical towel placed in the palm for the patient to grip loosely
b. Transducer position (see Figure 31-2)
   i. Parallel to the long bones of the phalanges
c. Needle orientation relative to the transducer (Figure 31-3)
   i. Out of plane
d. Needle approach (see Figure 31-3)
   i. Lateral to medial or medial to lateral
e. Target
   i. Deep to IP joint capsule
f. Pearls and Pitfalls
   i. Once the needle is in place, color Doppler can be used to visualize the digital arteries with the working knowledge that the digital nerves are adjacent to the blood vessels.

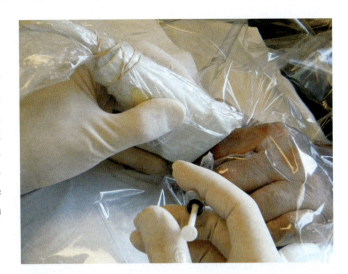

FIGURE 31-2 ■ Short-axis, out-of-plane view of an injection into the proximal interphalangeal (PIP) joint of the second digit. Note transducer position and angle of needle entry directly midline under the transducer.

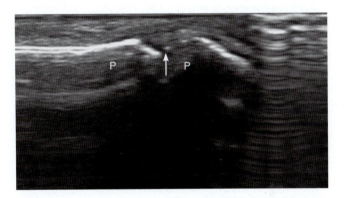

FIGURE 31-3 ■ Ultrasound image demonstrating the final needle position (*arrow* points to needle tip) deep to the joint capsule. P, phalanx.

Alternate Technique

a. Patient position (Figure 31-4)
   i. Supine or sitting position
   ii Wrist pronated
   iii. Cylindrical object or rolled up surgical towel placed in the palm for the patient to grip loosely
b. Transducer position (see Figure 31-4)
   i. Parallel to the long bones of the phalanges
c. Needle orientation relative to the transducer (Figure 31-4)
   i. In plane
d. Needle approach (Figure 31-5)
   i. Proximal to distal
   ii. Standoff oblique technique
e. Target
   i. Deep to IP joint capsule
f. Pearls and Pitfalls
   i. Once the needle is in place, color Doppler can be used to visualize the digital arteries with the working knowledge that the digital nerves are adjacent to the blood vessels.

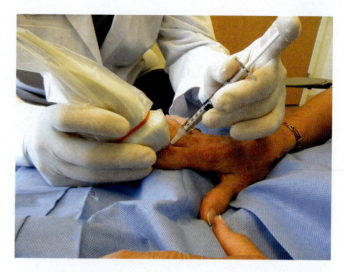

FIGURE 31-4 ■ Long-axis, in-plane view of an injection into the proximal interphalangeal (PIP) joint of the second digit. Note the standoff oblique technique and steep angle of entry.

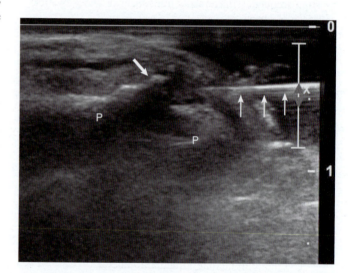

FIGURE 31-5 ■ Ultrasound image demonstrating the needle tip (*thin arrows* highlighting needle tip and shaft) entering the proximal interphalangeal (PIP) joint. Note the hypertrophic dorsal spur (*wide arrow*), which made this technique preferred in this case. P, phalanx.

References

1. Pichler W, Grechenig W, Grechenig S, et al. Frequency of successful intra-articular puncture of finger joints: influence of puncture position and physician experience. *Rheumatology.* 2008;47: 1503–1505.

2. Raza K, Lee CY, Pilling D, et al. Ultrasound guidance allows accurate needle placement and aspiration from small joints in patients with early inflammatory arthritis. *Rheumatology.* (Oxford) 2003;42:976–979.

Ricardo J. Vasquez-Duarte, MD / Jackson Cohen, MD

KEY POINTS

- Use a small gauge (eg, 25) and relatively short (eg, 1.5 inch) needle.
- Use a high-frequency linear array transducer in short-axis view.

- Subcompartmentalization of the extensor pollicis brevis (EPB) tendon occurs in 33% of tendons.
- Short-axis, in-plane approach is the preferred injection technique.

Pertinent Anatomy

The first extensor (dorsal) compartment of the wrist is located just lateral to the radial styloid process and contains the tendons of the extensor pollicis brevis (EPB) and abductor pollicis longus (APL) (Figure 32-1). Important anatomical variations to recognize include the sub-compartmentalization of the EPB tendon in approximately 33% of patients as well as the fact that the APL tendon usually has multiple slips within itself appearing multilamellar.[1]

Common Pathology

The tendons of the first extensor compartment can be injured by shear and repetitive microtrauma resulting in a stenosing tenosynovitis referred to as de Quervain syndrome. De Quervain syndrome is the most common tendonitis of the wrist and is most frequently seen in patients who perform activities requiring forceful grasping coupled with ulnar deviation or repetitive use of the thumb such as golf, racquet sports, or fly-fishing.[2] Patients normally present with

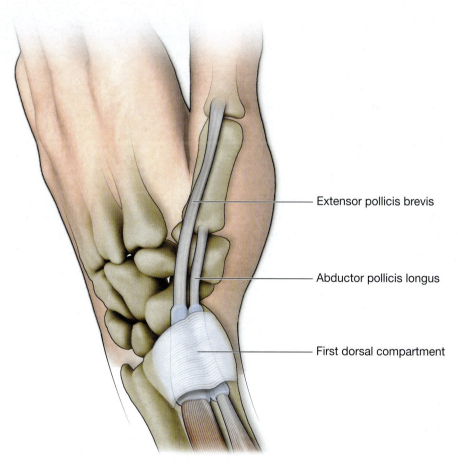

Extensor pollicis brevis

Abductor pollicis longus

First dorsal compartment

FIGURE 32-1 ■ Normal anatomy of the first extensor compartment.

radial wrist pain radiating to the hand, forearm, or thumb in addition to moderate swelling and tenderness over the first dorsal compartment. Finkelstein's test is pathognomonic for diagnosing de Quervain syndrome and is performed by flexing the patient's thumb into the palm while the examiner ulnarly deviates the wrist reproducing the patient's symptoms (Figure. 32-2).

Ultrasound Imaging Findings

The first extensor compartment is best visualized in the short axis using a high-frequency linear array transducer and a depth of less than 3 cm (Figure 32-3).[3] Common findings include anechoic fluid surrounding the tendon, tendon thickening, and intrasubstance tears. Normal variations include a multilamellar APL tendon, which may erroneously be viewed as a split or tear under ultrasound. Also, a septum within the compartment may be present in some patients producing a hypoechoic shadow between the APL and EPB tendons.[4]

Indications for Injections of the First Extensor Compartment

Injection of the first dorsal compartment can be performed for patients with de Quervain syndrome that is unresponsive to rest, ice, bracing, antiinflammatories, and physical therapy. Injection of the first dorsal compartment has been described based on palpation of anatomical landmarks of the wrist by Hazani et al. (ie, unguided).[5] In the majority of patients, the distal aspect of the radial styloid can be easily palpated and used for preinjection marking. However, if the radial styloid process is not palpable, the junction where the APL tendon crosses an imaginary line between Lister's tubercle and the scaphoid tubercle represents the distal edge of the first dorsal compartment. The success rate of these unguided injections varies from 58% to 93% according to multiple studies.[6–14] The presence of two separate compartments divided by a septum contributes to the wide margin of success rates. Ultrasound-guided injections have been described by Jeyapalan et al. with a success rate of 93.75%.[3] Ultrasound guidance ensures correct needle placement, avoids intratendinous injection, and allows imaging of any septum in the first dorsal compartment. The visualization of each tendon through ultrasound imaging also helps identify the exact location of the tenosynovitis, which may involve one or both of the tendons. Thus, the injection can

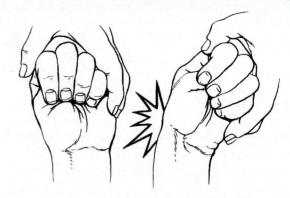

FIGURE 32-2 ■ Finkelstein test. (Reproduced with permission from Skinner HB. *Current Diagnosis and Treatment in Orthopedics.* 4th ed. New York: McGraw-Hill; 2000: figure 10-20.)

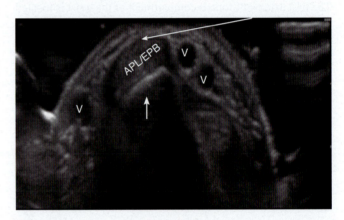

FIGURE 32-3 ■ Ultrasound demonstrating normal appearance of short-axis view of first dorsal compartment (APL/EPB tendons) with *arrow* representing in-plane, lateral-to-medial approach for injection and *small arrow* represents bony landmark on distal radius. Left of screen is medial, right is lateral. APL/EPB, abductor pollicis longus and extensor pollicis brevis; V, vessels.

be performed at the point of maximal inflammation. Moreover, the incidence of reported complications for unguided injections was 36% by Sawaizumi et al.[15] These included atrophy of subcutaneous fat tissue and/or depigmentation around the needle insertion site. In contrast, Jeyapalan et al. reported no complications when injections were performed under ultrasound guidance.[3]

Equipment

- ■ Needle: 25-gauge, 1.5-inch needle
- ■ Injectate: 1 mL of local anesthetic and 0.5 mL of an injectable corticosteroid
- ■ High-frequency linear array transducer

Author's Preferred Technique

a. Patient position
   i. Seated with arm at patient's side in neutral rotation
   ii. Ulnar aspect of forearm positioned on table with wrist in neutral position
b. Transducer position (Figure 32-4)
   i. Anatomic cross-section view of the first extensor wrist compartment
c. Needle orientation relative to the transducer (see Figure 32-4)
   i. In plane
d. Needle approach (see Figure 32-3)
   i. Lateral to medial.
   ii. The bevel of the needle should be turned away from the tendon to avoid intratendinous injection.
e. Target (see Figure 32-3)
   i. APL and EPB tendon sheath(s) in the first extensor compartment
f. Pearls and Pitfalls
   i. Identify exact location of tenosynovitis for more precise needle placement.
   ii. Be wary of misdiagnosing multilamellar APL tendon slip as tendon pathology.
   iii. View the spread of injectate to assure that it courses through the entire compartment of tendon.
   iv. Be sure to locate and avoid the radial artery.

Alternate Technique

a. Patient position
   i. Seated
   ii. Arm at patient's side in neutral rotation
   iii. Ulnar aspect of forearm positioned on table with wrist in neutral position
b. Transducer position (Figure 32-5)
   i. Anatomic cross-section view of the first extensor wrist compartment
c. Needle orientation relative to the transducer (Figure 32-5)
   i. Out of plane
d. Needle approach (Figure 32-6)
   i. Distal to proximal or proximal to distal
   ii. The bevel of the needle should be turned away from the tendon to avoid intratendinous injection

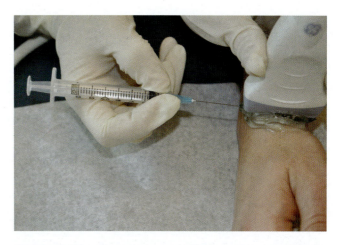

FIGURE 32-4 ■ Positioning and needle entry for short-axis, in-plane approach from lateral to medial for injection of first dorsal compartment.

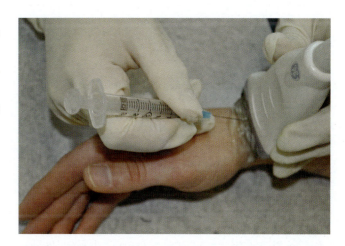

FIGURE 32-5 ■ Positioning and needle entry for short-axis, out-of-plane approach from proximal to distal for injection of first dorsal compartment.

e. Target (Figure 32-6)
    i. APL and EPB tendon sheath(s) in the first extensor compartment
f. Pearls and Pitfalls
    i. See "Pearls and Pitfalls" under "Author's Preferred Technique"

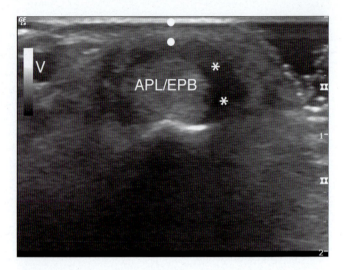

FIGURE 32-6 ■ Ultrasound image showing short-axis view of first dorsal compartment (APL/EPB tendons) with *dots* representing out-of-plane walk-down technique. Left of screen is medial; right is lateral. *Asterisk* represent fluid surrounding the first dorsal compartment consistent with de Quervain syndrome. APL/EPB, abductor pollicis longus and extensor pollicis brevis; V, vessels.

References

1. Motoura H, Shiozaki K, Kawasaki K. Anatomical variations in the tendon sheath of the first compartment. *Anat Sci Int.* 2010 Sep;85(3):145–151. Epub December 29, 2009.
2. Rettig AC. Athletic injuries of the wrist and hand: part II: overuse injuries of the wrist and traumatic injuries to the hand [Review]. *Am J Sports Med.* 2004 Jan-Feb;32(1):262–273.
3. Jeyapalan K, Choudhary S. Ultrasound-guided injection of triamcinolone and bupivacaine in the management of De Quervain's disease. *Skeletal Radiol.* 2009 Nov;38(11):1099–1103. Epub June 1, 2009.
4. Choi SJ, Ahn JH, Lee YJ, et al. de Quervain disease: US identification of anatomic variations in the first extensor compartment with an emphasis on subcompartmentalization. *Radiology.* 2011 Aug;260(2):480–486. Epub May 25, 2011.
5. Hazani R, Engineer NJ, Cooney D, Wilhelmi BJ. Anatomic landmarks for the first dorsal compartment. *Eplasty.* 2008;8:e53. Epub November 18, 2008.
6. Anderson BC, Manthey R, Brouns MC. Treatment of De Quervain's tenosynovitis with corticosteroids. A prospective study of the response to local injection. *Arthritis Rheum.* 1991;34:793–798.
7. Harvey FJ, Harvey PM, Horsley MW. De Quervain's disease: surgical or nonsurgical treatment. *J Hand Surg Am.* 1990;15:83–87.
8. Jirarattanaphochai K, Saengnipanthkul S, Vipulakorn K, Jianmongkol S, Chatuparisute P, Jung S. Treatment of de Quervain disease with triamcinolone injection with or without nimesulide. A randomized, double-blind, placebocontrolled trial. *J Bone Joint Surg Am.* 2004;86:2700–2706.
9. Lane LB, Boretz RS, Stuchin SA. Treatment of de Quervain's disease: role of conservative management. *J Hand Surg Br.* 2001;26:258–260.
10. McKenzie JM. Conservative treatment of de Quervain's disease. *Br Med J.* 1972;4:659–660.
11. Weiss AP, Akelman E, Tabatabai M. Treatment of de Quervain's disease. *J Hand Surg Am.* 1994;19:595–598.
12. Zingas C, Failla JM, Van Holsbeeck M. Injection accuracy and clinical relief of de Quervain's tendinitis. *J Hand Surg Am.* 1998;23:89–96.
13. Sawaizumi T, Nanno M, Ito H. De Quervain's disease: efficacy of intra-sheath triamcinolone injection. *Int Orthop.* 2007;31:265–268.
14. Mirzanli C, Ozturk K, Esenyel CZ, et al. Accuracy of intra-sheath injection techniques for de Quervain's disease: a cadaveric study. *J Hand Surg Eur Vol.* Epub May 18, 2011.
15. Sawaizumi T, Nanno M, Ito H. De Quervain's disease: efficacy of intra-sheath triamcinolone injection. *Int Orthop.* 2007 Apr;31(2):265–268. Epub June 8, 2006.

Ricardo J. Vasquez-Duarte, MD / Jackson Cohen, MD

KEY POINTS

- Use a small-gauge (eg, 25) and relatively short (eg, 1.5-inch) needle.
- Use a high-frequency linear array transducer.

- The second dorsal compartment of wrist is anatomically located on the radial side of Lister's tubercle.
- A short-axis, in-plane approach is the preferred injection technique.

Pertinent Anatomy

The second extensor (dorsal) compartment of the wrist is located on the radial side of Lister's tubercle, with the extensor carpi radialis longus (ECRL) and extensor carpi radialis brevis (ECRB) tendons passing over the radial styloid process and inserting on the second and third metacarpal bases, respectively (Figure 33-1A and B).[1]

Common Pathology

At the present time, no pathology of the second extensor compartment distal to the intersection of the tendons has been described in the literature. However, overuse of the ECRB and ECRL tendons in the distal second extensor compartment with repetitive wrist extension motions such as racquet sports and weightlifting among other similar activities can lead to inflammation, creating a tenosynovitis within the compartment. Patients may present with dorsoradial distal wrist pain radiating down the thumb or up the radial aspect of the forearm coupled with moderate swelling and tenderness just radial to Lister's tubercle.

Ultrasound Imaging Findings

The second extensor compartment is best visualized in the short axis using a high-frequency linear array transducer and a depth of less than 3 cm. Common findings include fluid around the tendon, tendon thickening, and intrasubstance tears.

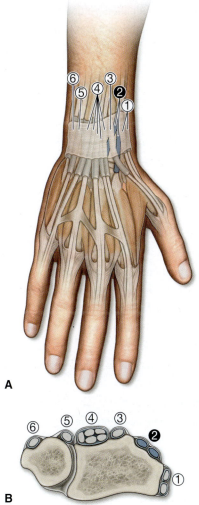

A

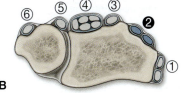

B

FIGURE 33-1 ■ **A.** Anatomy of the dorsal compartments of the wrist. **B.** Short axis view of the dorsal wrist. ❷ ECRL, extensor carpi radialis longus; ECRB, extensor carpi radialis brevis.

Indications for Injections of the Second Extensor Compartment

Injection of the second dorsal compartment can be performed for patients with tenosynovitis of the ECRB or ECRL that is unresponsive to rest, icing, antiinflammatories, and physical therapy. Injection of the second dorsal compartment for the treatment of tenosynovitis distal to the intersection of the tendons of the first and second extensor compartments has not been described in literature up to the present time. Because of the paucity of literature regarding the effectiveness of steroid injections for this condition, it is difficult to quantify the success rate of palpation-guided injections. In addition, no studies exist comparing palpation-guided to ultrasound-guided injections into the second dorsal compartment.

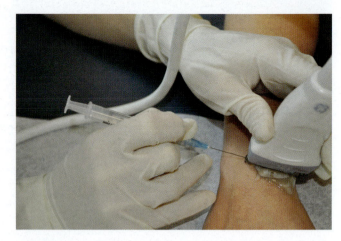

FIGURE 33-2 ■ Linear array transducer is transverse to the compartment, and the needle approach is ulnar to radial, in plane.

Equipment

- Needle: 25-gauge, 1.5-inch needle
- Injectate: 0.5 mL of local anesthetic and 0.5 mL of an injectable corticosteroid
- High-frequency linear array transducer

Author's Preferred Technique

a. Patient position (Figure 33-2)
   i. Seated
   ii. Arm at patient's side in pronation
   iii. Forearm positioned on table with wrist in pronation
b. Transducer position (see Figure 33-2)
   i. Anatomic short-axis view to the second extensor wrist compartment
c. Needle orientation relative to the transducer (Figures 33-2 and 33-3)
   i. In plane
d. Needle approach (see Figure 33-3)
   i. Ulnar to radial or radial to ulnar
   ii. Bevel of needle turned away from the tendon to avoid intratendinous injection
e. Target
   i. Tendon sheath of the ECRL and ECRB tendons
f. Pearls and Pitfalls
   i. Identify the exact location of tenosynovitis.
   ii. The course of the needle tip can be visualized continuously as it moves toward the tendon sheath.
   iii. Be sure to assess for vessels in a pre-scan of area prior to injection.

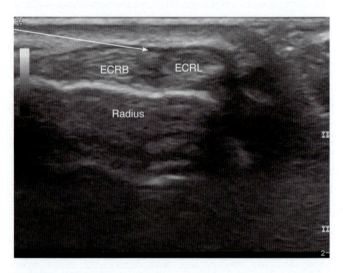

FIGURE 33-3 ■ Transverse view of second dorsal compartment with *arrow* representing needle entry from ulnar to radial, in plane. ECRB, extensor carpi radialis brevis; ECRL, extensor carpi radialis longus.

Alternate Technique

a. Patient position (Figure 33-4)
   i. Seated
   ii. Arm at patient's side in pronated position
   iii. Forearm positioned on table with wrist in pronated position
b. Transducer position (Figure 33-4)
   i. Anatomic short-axis view to the second extensor wrist compartment
c. Needle orientation relative to the transducer (Figures 33-4 and 33-5)
   i. Out of plane
d. Needle approach
   i. Distal to proximal
   ii. Bevel of the needle turned away from the tendon to avoid intratendinous injection
e. Target
   i. Tendon sheath of the ECRL and ECRB tendons
f. Pearls and Pitfalls
   i. Identify the exact location of tenosynovitis.
   ii. There is poorer visualization of needle tip with this technique.

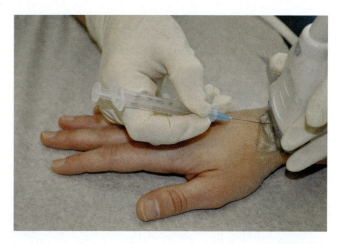

FIGURE 33-4 ■ Linear array transducer is transverse to the compartment, and the needle technique is out of plane, distal to proximal.

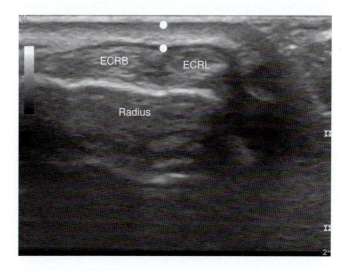

FIGURE 33-5 ■ Transverse view of second dorsal compartment with *dots* representing the walk-down technique to target area from distal to proximal, out of plane. ECRB, extensor carpi radialis brevis; ECRL, extensor carpi radialis longus.

References

1. Lee JC, Healy JC. Normal sonographic anatomy of the wrist and hand. *Radiographics.* 2005 Nov-Dec;25(6):1577–1590.

2. Rettig AC. Athletic injuries of the wrist and hand: part II: overuse injuries of the wrist and traumatic injuries to the hand [Review]. *Am J Sports Med.* 2004 Jan-Feb;32(1):262–273.

CHAPTER 34

Intersection Syndrome of the First and Second Dorsal Compartments Injection

Bradly S. Goodman, MD / Prasanth Nuthakki, MD / Matthew Thomas Smith, MD / Srinivas Mallempati, MD

KEY POINTS

- A 25-gauge, 1.5-inch needle is preferred.
- A high-frequency linear array transducer is used for injection.
- Localize the injection site by visualizing the second compartment in short-axis view and then slide the probe proximal until the tendons of the second compartment

intersect under the musculotendinous junction of the first compartment.
- It is preferable to inject with the transducer in short axis and in plane.
- Aim for the space in between the intersecting tendon compartments.

Pertinent Anatomy

There are six compartments located at the dorsal wrist, wherein various tendons pass that aid in the extension of the wrist and fingers, and extension and abduction of the thumb. The first dorsal compartment crosses the wrist at the lateral aspect of the distal radius and has the largest anatomic variability among individuals.[1] It contains, from radial to ulnar, the tendons of the abductor pollicis longus (APL) and extensor pollicis brevis (EPB). The second compartment crosses the wrist at the dorsal aspect of the radius and contains the tendons of the extensor carpi radialis longus (ECRL) and

extensor carpi radialis brevis (ECRB). The APL and EPB myotendons cross obliquely and superficially over the ECRL and ECRB tendons at an approximately 60-degree angle in the distal forearm. This is approximately 4–6 cm proximal to Lister's tubercle (Figure 34-1).[2,3]

Common Pathology

Intersection syndrome is classically a result of inflammation and subsequent tenosynovitis where the first and second compartments cross in the distal forearm. Symptoms are characterized by pain and swelling at the site of compartment

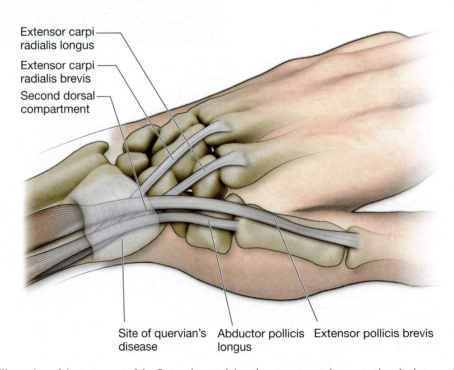

Extensor carpi radialis longus

Extensor carpi radialis brevis

Second dorsal compartment

Site of quervian's disease

Abductor pollicis longus

Extensor pollicis brevis

FIGURE 34-1 ■ Illustration of the crossover of the first and second dorsal compartment demonstrating the intersection area.

intersection. The purported cause is overuse of the wrist, particularly with movements involving repetitive wrist flexion and extension. Examples include weightlifting or occupational work such as carpentry.

Ultrasound Imaging Findings

The tendons are best visualized under short axis with a high-frequency linear array transducer.

Under ultrasound, intersection syndrome appears as a hypoechoic area between the intersection of the two compartments. This is likely due to local edema in the surrounding soft tissues and thickening of the tendon sheaths. There is often hyperemia seen at this intersection when power Doppler is used.

Indications for Injection in Intersection Syndrome

Injection of the intersecting tendons is appropriate in patients for whom pain is refractory to conservative measures, including rest, splinting, ice, nonsteroidal antiinflammatory drugs, and physical therapy.[4]

Equipment

- Needle: 25-gauge, 1.5-inch needle dependent on patient anatomy and operator preference
- Injectate: 1 mL of local anesthetic and 1 mL of injectable corticosteroid
- High-frequency linear array transducer

Author's Preferred Technique

a. Patient position (Figure 34-2)
   i. Seated or supine
   ii. Forearm in neutral position with the radial aspect of the forearm facing the ultrasonographer
b. Transducer position (see Figure 34-2)
   i. Transverse plane short axis to the intersecting compartments (ECRB and ECRL)
c. Needle orientation relative to the transducer (see Figure 34-2)
   i. Out of plane
d. Needle approach (Figure 34-3)
   i. Distal to proximal or proximal to distal
   ii. Use a walk-down technique

e. Target (see Figure 34-3)
   i. Where the APL and EPB musculotendinous junction crosses over the ECRL and ECRB tendons
f. Pearls and Pitfalls
   i. Once the needle is in the desired position, the ultrasonographer may consider rotating the transducer 90 degrees to confirm the needle position in the long-axis, in-plane view.
   ii. The muscles of the first compartment will often appear relatively hypoechoic in this region and should not be confused with inflammatory fluid.

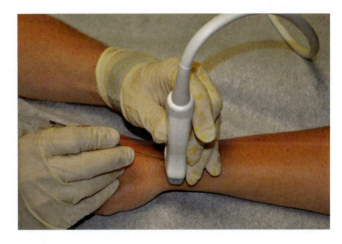

FIGURE 34-2 ■ Shows both the patient and transducer positioning for a short-axis, out-of plane injection technique.

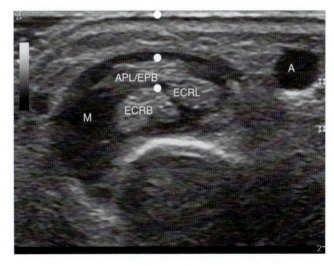

FIGURE 34-3 ■ Ultrasound image of short axis of intersection region demonstrating walk-down technique for out-of plane injection. *Dots* represent needle walk down. A, artery; APL/EPB, abductor pollicis longus, extensor pollicis brevis; ECRB, extensor carpi radialis brevis; ECRL, extensor carpi radialis longus; M, muscle.

Alternate Technique

a. Patient position (Figure 34-4)
   i. Seated or supine
   ii. Forearm in neutral position with the radial aspect of the forearm facing the ultrasonographer
b. Transducer position (see Figure 34-4)
   i. Transverse plane short axis to the intersecting compartments (ECRB and ECRL)
c. Needle orientation relative to the transducer (see Figure 34-4)
   i. In plane
d. Needle (Figure 34-5)
   i. Radial to ulnar or ulnar to radial
e. Target (see Figure 34-5)
   i. Where the APL and EPB musculotendinous junction crosses over the ECRL and ECRB tendons
f. Pearls and Pitfalls
   i. The needle may have further tissue to traverse to get to the desired target with this technique.
   ii. A standoff technique may also be helpful because of the curvature of the wrist. A smaller transducer would be less cumbersome.

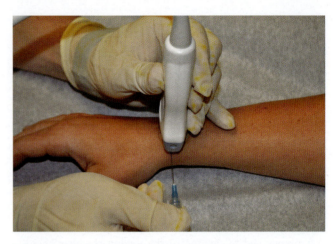

FIGURE 34-4 ■ Shows both the patient and transducer positioning for a short-axis, in-plane injection technique.

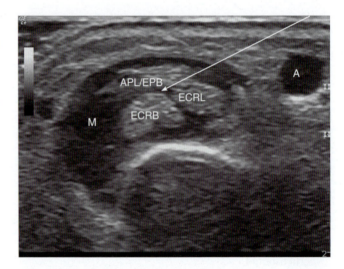

FIGURE 34-5 ■ Ultrasound image of short axis of intersection region. *Arrow* represents needle positioning for in-plane, radial to ulnar approach to injection. A, artery; APL/EPB, abductor pollicis longus, extensor pollicis brevis; ECRB, extensor carpi radialis brevi; ECRL, extensor carpi radialis longus; M, muscle.

References

1. Hazani R, Engineer NJ, Cooney D, Wilhelmi BJ. Anatomic landmarks for the first dorsal compartment. *Eplasty.* 2008;8:e53. Epub November 18, 2008.
2. Lee RP, Hatem SF, Recht MP. Extended MRI findings of intersection syndrome. *Skeletal Radiol.* 2009;38(2):157–163.
3. Bodor M, Fullerton B. Ultrasonography of the hand, wrist, and elbow. *Phys Med Rehabil Clin N Am.* 2010;21(3):509–531.
4. Browne J, Helms CA. Intersection syndrome of the forearm. *Arthritis Rheum.* Jun 2006;54(6):2038.
5. O'Neill, J. *Musculoskeletal Ultrasound: Anatomy and Technique.* New York: Springer; 2008:137–139.

Sean N. Martin, DO

KEY POINTS

- Use a 23- to 25-gauge, 1.5-inch needle, distal to proximal, in plane.
- Use a high-frequency linear array transducer.

- Lister's tubercle should serve as major landmark for identifying this compartment.
- Extensor pollicis longus tendon rupture is a known complication following corticosteroid injection.

Pertinent Anatomy

Located just ulnar (medial) to Lister's tubercle, the third dorsal compartment of the wrist contains the extensor pollicis longus (EPL) exclusively (Figure 35-1A and B). This tendon contributes extension of the thumb and is accentuated during sonography by actively resisting the patient while he or she performs this motion.

Common Pathology

Pathology of the EPL tendon is often that of localized tenosynovitis. This is most prominent as the thin tendon courses next to Lister's tubercle. Often, fluid is seen within the tendon sheath just proximal to the tubercle. Patients typically describe pain localized to this location and, potentially, crepitus with movement of their thumb. Less commonly, the EPL tendon can become irritated immediately after its intersection with the extensor carpi radialis longus tendon.[1] Isolated partial tears of the EPL tendon, either related to or independent from tenosynovitis, can be seen on ultrasound imaging. One predisposing factor to a tear is a previous distal radius fracture adjacent to a particularly thin portion of the tendon.[1] It should be noted, as well, that complete EPL rupture is a known complication of distal radius fractures. Presence of rheumatoid arthritis and use of corticosteroids (both locally and systemically) are also known risk factors for tendon rupture.[2]

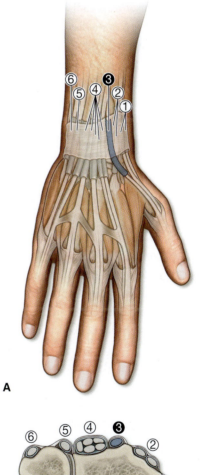

A

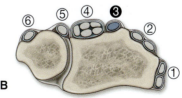

B

FIGURE 35-1 ■ **A.** Anatomy of the dorsal compartments of the wrist. **B.** Short axis view of the dorsal wrist. ❸ EPL, extensor pollicis longus.

Ultrasound Imaging Findings

The third compartment is most easily visualized in long and short axis using a high-frequency linear array transducer at a depth of less than 2 cm. Often it is helpful to float the transducer using a thick layer of ultrasound gel. This compartment is most easily identified by first locating the prominent Lister's tubercle, which separates the third (ulnar aspect of the tubercle) and second compartments (radial aspect of the tubercle). This tubercle is seen as a hyperechoic prominence of the dorsal radius. Correct identification of the EPL is most reliably accomplished by visualization of the tendon at this location as the tendon crosses the tendons of the second dorsal compartment (extensor carpi radialis longus and extensor carpi radialis brevis) as it courses distally. The tendon is most easily tracked using a short-axis view while remembering that the tendon courses obliquely from medial to lateral. Imprecise scanning through anisotropy may provide the false appearance of a pathologic tendon, so it is imperative to not scan this tendon obliquely. Distally, the EPL tendon becomes closely approximated to the tendon of the extensor pollicis brevis just prior to its insertion on the distal phalanx of the thumb.

Indications for Injections of the Third Dorsal Compartment

Ultrasound-guided corticosteroid injection of the third dorsal compartment is typically reserved for localized tenosynovitis that is unresponsive to more conservative measures. At the time of publication, there is a void of studies on the efficacy of this procedure through either palpation- or ultrasound-guided technique.

Equipment

- Needle: 23- to 25-gauge, 1.5-inch needle
- Injectate: 0.5 mL of local anesthetic and 0.5 mL of an injectable corticosteroid
- High-frequency linear array transducer

Author's Preferred Injection Technique

a. Patient position (Figure 35-2)
    i. Seated with hand resting prone on a flat surface
b. Transducer position (see Figure 35-2)
    i. Short axis to EPL tendon
c. Needle orientation relative to the transducer (Figures 35-2 and 35-3)
    i. In plane
d. Needle approach (see Figure 35-3)
    i. Ulnar to radial or radial to ulnar
e. Target (see Figure 35-3)
    i. Space between tendon sheath and tendon
f. Pearls and Pitfalls
    i. Be sure to scan the area prior to injecting and use power Doppler to avoid any nerves or vessels in the area.
    ii. Active patients should be counseled on reports of rupture of the EPL tendon following corticosteroid injection.[3]

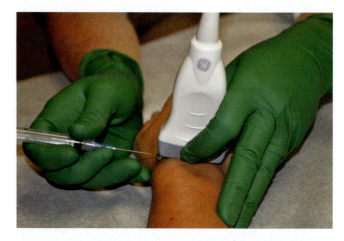

FIGURE 35-2 ■ High-frequency linear array transducer is transverse to the compartment and needle approach is in plane.

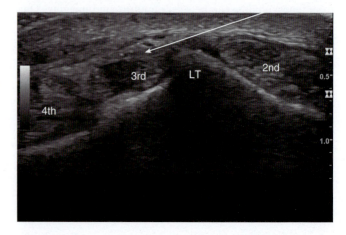

FIGURE 35-3 ■ Transverse view of EPL tendon with "hockey stick" probe. *Arrow* represents needle entry from radial to ulnar, in plane. 2nd, second dorsal compartment; 3rd, third dorsal compartment; 4th, fourth dorsal compartment; LT, Lister's tubercle.

Alternate Technique

a. Patient position (Figure 35-4)

   i. Seated with hand resting prone on a flat surface

b. Transducer position (see Figure 35-4)

   i. Long axis over EPL tendon

c. Needle orientation relative to the transducer (Figures 35-4 and 35-5)

   i. In plane

d. Needle approach (see Figure 35-5)

   i. Distal to proximal

e. Target (see Figure 35-5)

   i. Space between tendon sheath and tendon

f. Pearls and Pitfalls

   i. Short-axis scanning should also be used to confirm both orientation of the needle toward the desired tendon and placement of the needle between the sheath and the tendon.

   ii. Active patients should be counseled on reports of rupture of the EPL tendon following corticosteroid injection.[3]

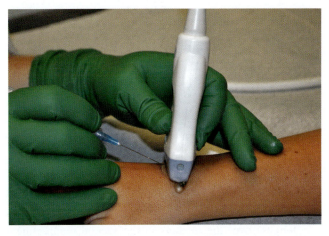

FIGURE 35-4 ■ High-frequency linear array transducer longitudinal to compartment; needle approach is in plane.

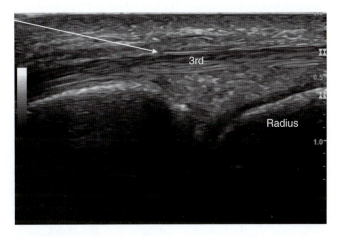

FIGURE 35-5 ■ Long-axis view of extensor pollicis longus (EPL) tendon with "hockey stick" probe. *Arrow* represents needle entry into tendon sheath from distal to proximal. 3rd, third dorsal compartment.

References

1. Bianchi S, Martinoli C. *Ultrasound of the Musculoskeletal System.* New York: Springer; 2007.

2. Björkman A, Jörgsholm P. Rupture of the extensor pollicis longus tendon: a study of aetiological factors. *Scand J Plast Reconstr Surg Hand Surg.* 2004;38(1):32–35.

3. Mills SP, Charalambous CP, Hayton MJ. Bilateral rupture of the extensor pollicis longus tendon in a professional goalkeeper following steroid injections for extensor tenosynovitis. *Hand Surg.* 1009;14(2-3):135–137.

Bradly S. Goodman, MD / Matthew Thomas Smith, MD / Prasanth Nuthakki, MD / Srinivas Mallempati, MD

KEY POINTS

- A 22- to 30-gauge, 1- to 1.5-inch needle is used.
- A high-frequency linear array transducer is used.
- Pathologically, distal intersection syndrome is a tenosynovitis caused by friction of the tendon of the third dorsal compartment of the wrist (extensor pollicis longus) over the tendons in the second compartment (extensor carpi radialis longus, and extensor carpi radialis brevis).
- Symptoms are characterized by pain and swelling in the dorsal radial forearm around the area of Lister's tubercle.
- It occurs much less commonly than proximal intersection syndrome.

Pertinent Anatomy

The extensor pollicis longus (EPL) originates from the dorsal ulna and interosseous membrane and represents the third dorsal wrist compartment. On its course to its insertion into the base of the distal phalanx of the thumb, it uses Lister's tubercle as a pulley, then crosses superficially to the tendons of the extensor carpi radialis longus (ECRL) and extensor carpi radialis brevis (ECRB), the second dorsal compartment (Figure 36-1).

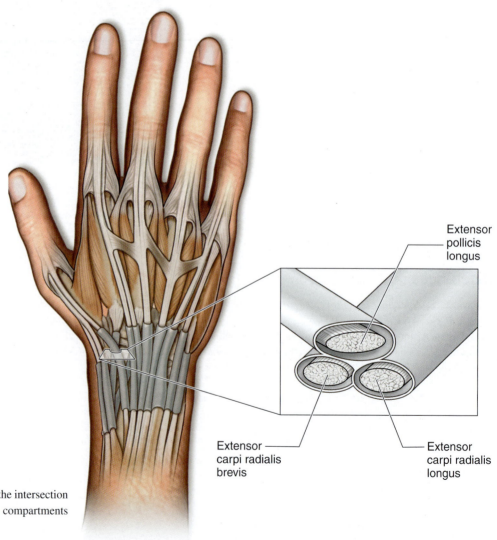

Extensor pollicis longus

Extensor carpi radialis brevis

Extensor carpi radialis longus

FIGURE 36-1 ■ Illustration of the intersection between second and third dorsal compartments distal to Lister's tubercle.

Common Pathology

The unique anatomic arrangement of the EPL to Lister's tubercle and the underlying ECRL and ECRB has been implicated as a predisposing factor to tenosynovitis and spontaneous ruptures of the EPL (Figure 36-2). Furthermore, recent studies have shown that this anatomic arrangement may potentially lead to tenosynovitis and tendinosis in potentially any of the tendons in these two compartments proximal or distal to Lister's tubercle. Cvitanic et al. have recently described communicating foramina between the tendinous sheaths of the second and third compartments.[1] The spread of synovial fluid containing inflammatory mediators by way of these foramina may also contribute to this finding. Distal intersection syndrome may be clinically mistaken for proximal intersection syndrome, de Quervain tenosynovitis, carpal-metacarpal arthritis of the thumb, wrist osteoarthritis, or superficial radial nerve pathology (Wartenberg syndrome).[2] Many of these conditions are commonly seen and can occur in conjunction with distal intersection syndrome. Because of their similarity in clinical presentation, ultrasound of this region may be clinically useful to discriminate between these pathologies.

Ultrasound Imaging Findings

The tendons are best visualized under short axis with high-frequency linear array transducer.

Ultrasound findings may show pathology at any of the three tendons involved in distal intersection syndrome. Commonly, tendon or synovial sheath thickening may be present, as well as peritendinous edema. This may be located just proximal or distal to Lister's tubercle, or at the extensor retinaculum. In addition, power Doppler should be used to assess for hyperemia in the region.

Indications for Injection in Intersection Syndrome

Injection of the intersecting tendons is appropriate in patients for whom pain is refractory to conservative measures, including rest, splinting, ice, removal of offending agent, nonsteroidal antiinflammatory drugs, and occupational therapy.

Equipment

- Needle: 22- to 30-gauge needle, 0.5- to 1.5-inch long
- Injectate: 0.5–1 mL of local anesthetic and 0.5–1.0 mL of an injectable corticosteroid
- High-frequency linear array transducer

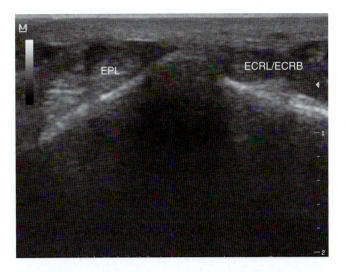

FIGURE 36-2 ■ Ultrasound image of relationship between second and third dorsal compartments at level of Lister's tubercle. EPL, extensor pollicis longus; ECRL/ECRB, extensor carpi radialis longus and extensor carpi radialis brevis.

Author's Preferred Technique

a. Patient position (Figure 36-3)
    i. Seated or supine
    ii. Forearm in neutral position with radial aspect of the forearm facing the ultrasonographer
b. Transducer position (see Figure 36-3)
    i. Short axis to intersecting tendons
c. Needle orientation relative to the transducer (see Figure 36-3)
    i. Out of plane
d. Needle approach (Figure 36-4)
    i. Distal to proximal or proximal to distal
e. Target (see Figure 36-4)
    i. The target space is where the EPL tendon crosses superficially to the ECRL and ECRB tendons.
f. Pearls and Pitfalls
    i. In the short-axis, out-of-plane approach, advancement of the needle should be stopped as soon as the tip is visible on the ultrasound monitor. After the needle tip is visualized, the needle tip may be stepped down to the desired position.
    ii. Once the needle is in the desired position, the ultrasonographer can rotate the transducer 90 degrees to confirm the needle position with an in-plane view.

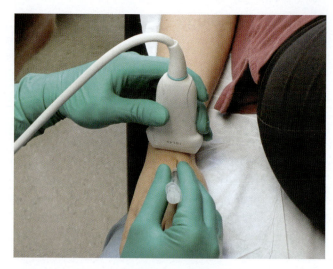

FIGURE 36-3 ■ Transducer and needle entry for out-of plane, distal-to-proximal technique to distal intersection area.

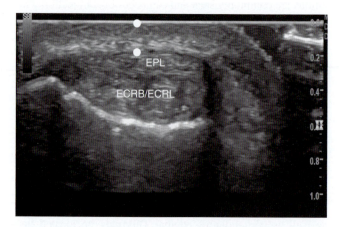

FIGURE 36-4 ■ Ultrasound image of distal intersection syndrome taken with "hockey stick" probe at 18 MHz. *Dots* represent walkdown, out-of-plane technique, from distal to proximal. EPL, extensor pollicis longus; ECRL/ECRB, extensor carpi radialis longus and extensor carpi radialis brevis.

Alternate Technique

a. Patient position (Figure 36-5)
   i. Seated or supine
   ii. Forearm in neutral position with radial aspect of the forearm facing the ultrasonographer
b. Transducer position (see Figure 36-5)
   i. Short axis to intersecting tendons
c. Needle orientation relative to the transducer (see Figure 36-5)
   i. In plane
d. Needle approach (Figure 36-6)
   i. Radial to ulnar or ulnar to radial
e. Target (see Figure 36-6)
   i. The target space is where the EPL tendon crosses superficially to the ECRL and ECRB tendons.
f. Pearls and Pitfalls
   i. The operator should be positioned on the side of patient adjacent to the forearm being injected. The needle should be visualized while advancing to the target.
   ii. The technique requires further tissue to traverse to get to the desired target. An oblique standoff technique may also be helpful.
   iii. A smaller transducer would be less cumbersome.

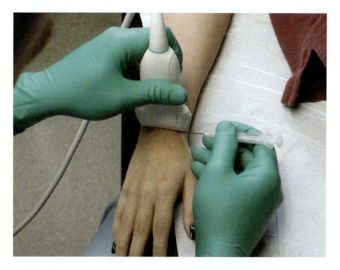

FIGURE 36-5 ■ Transducer and needle entry for in-plane, radial-to-ulnar technique to distal intersection area.

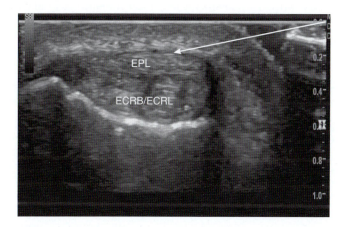

FIGURE 36-6 ■ Ultrasound image of distal intersection syndrome taken with "hockey stick" probe at 18 MHz. *Arrow* represents in-plane technique from radial to ulnar. APL, abductor pollicis longus; ECRL/ECRB, extensor carpi radialis longus and extensor carpi radialis brevis.

References

1. Cvitanic OA, Henzie GM, Adham M. Communicating foramen between the tendon sheaths of the extensor carpi radialis brevis and extensor pollicis longus muscles: imaging of cadavers and patients. *AJR Am J Roentgenol.* 2007;189(5):1190–1197.
2. Parelada AJ, Gopez AG, Morrison WB, et al. Distal intersection tenosynovitis of the wrist: a lesser-known extensor tendinopathy with characteristic MR imaging features. *Skeletal Radiol.* 2007;36(3):203–208.
3. Narouze SN. *Atlas of Ultrasound-Guided Procedures in Interventional Pain Management.* New York: Springer; 2011; 316.

Sean N. Martin, DO

KEY POINTS

- Use a 23- or 25-gauge, 1.5-inch needle, distal to proximal.
- Use a high-frequency linear array transducer.
- Identification of individual tendons is only accomplished by dynamic scanning while the patient alternatively flexes and extends the fingers.
- Use the long-axis view to guide the needle to the appropriate depth, but short axis to confirm appropriate placement within sheath.

Pertinent Anatomy

The extensor digitorum communis (EDC) and extensor indicis proprius (EIP) tendons of the wrist share a common synovial sheath, making up the fourth dorsal compartment of the wrist. This compartment is located immediately ulnar (medial) to the extensor pollicis longus and Lister's tubercle. This compartment is easily identified grossly during resisted wrist extension. The tendons within this compartment are closely spaced and impossible to differentiate without dynamic scanning during selective finger flexion and extension (Figure 37-1A and B).

Common Pathology

Pathology of the fourth dorsal compartment typically arises from overuse injuries causing tenosynovitis or secondary to muscular hypertrophy resulting in localized irritation. EIP syndrome is a rare entity that presents as pain and swelling over the middle aspect of the dorsal wrist. Patients will endorse worsening of pain when their index finger is extended against resistance with their wrist is the extended position. Aside from overuse injuries, rarely a patient will suffer a traumatic dislocation of the EDC tendon. If the hand is forcibly flexed by an external object while the patient is actively extending the digits, the sagittal bands can rupture, displacing the EDC tendon into the metacarpal space.

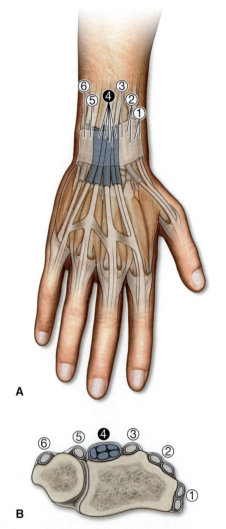

FIGURE 37-1 ■ **A.** Anatomy of the dorsal compartments of the wrist. **B.** Short axis view of the dorsal wrist. ❹ EDC, extensor digitorum comminus; EIP, extensor indices proprius.

Ultrasound Imaging Findings

The tendons of the fourth compartment are easily visualized in long and short axes using a high-frequency linear array transducer at a depth of less than 2 cm. Depth and focal zones should be adjusted to account for the relative superficial location of this compartment. Often it is helpful to float the transducer using a thick layer of ultrasound gel. By placing Lister's tubercle on one side of the screen, often the entire compartment can be visualized in short axis at the wrist. Identification of individual tendons within this compartment is only possible by having the patient alternate between flexion and extension of individual digits while scanning the tendons in cross section (see Figure 37-1). The hyperechoic signal of the tendons becomes more pronounced as they course distally. At the wrist, the extensor retinaculum can be seen coursing in a transverse-oblique direction. This structure typically appears hyperechoic, but can be falsely displayed as hypoechoic secondary to anisotropy.[1] From the wrist, the tendons can be traced as they exit their common synovial sheath. Ultrasound imaging becomes easier as the tendons diverge. Thin sagittal bands can be identified at the level of the metacarpal heads and connecting the interdigitating extensor tendons. At the phalanges, the tendons flatten and broadly cover the majority of the dorsal surface. The tendons then divide into a central slip, inserting onto the base of the middle phalanx and two lateral slips, which insert on the base of the distal phalanx. Once the central slip is identified, the lateral slips can be seen by performing a short-axis slide. Throughout the examination, long- and short-axis views should be used to assess for swelling of the tendon sheath, evaluate for tears, and dynamically assess sliding of the tendon within the compartment.[2] Power Doppler should also be used to assess for hyperemia associated with acute tenosynovitis (Figure 37-2).

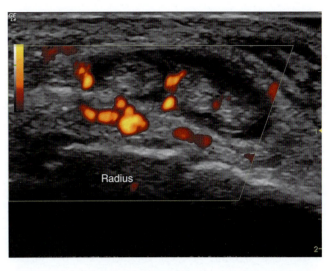

FIGURE 37-2 ■ Short-axis view of the fourth dorsal compartment with hyperemia seen with power Doppler.

Indications for Injections of the Fourth Dorsal Compartment

Ultrasound-guided corticosteroid injection of the fourth dorsal compartment is indicated in recalcitrant cases of tendinopathy and tenosynovitis that is unresponsive to more conservative measures. At the time of publication, there is a void of studies on the efficacy of this procedure by either palpation or ultrasound guidance.

Equipment

- ▪ Needle: 23- to 25-gauge, 1.5-inch needle
- ▪ Injectate: 0.5 mL of local anesthetic and 0.5 mL of an injectable corticosteroid
- ▪ High-frequency linear array transducer

Author's Preferred Technique

a. Patient position (Figure 37-3)
   i. Seated with hand resting prone on a flat surface
b. Transducer position (see Figure 37-3)
   i. Short axis to tendons of the fourth dorsal compartment
c. Needle orientation relative to the transducer (see Figure 37-3)
   i. In plane
d. Needle approach (Figures 37-3 and 37-4)
   i. Ulnar to radial or radial to ulnar
e. Target (Figure 37-4)
   i. Space between tendon sheath and tendon
f. Pearls and Pitfalls
   i. Be sure to scan the area prior to injecting and use power Doppler to avoid any nerves or vessels in the area.

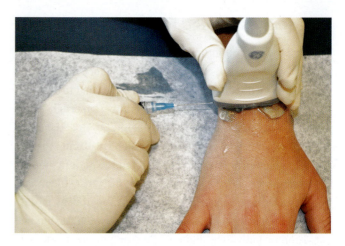

FIGURE 37-3 ▪ Linear array transducer is transverse to the compartment and needle approach is in plane.

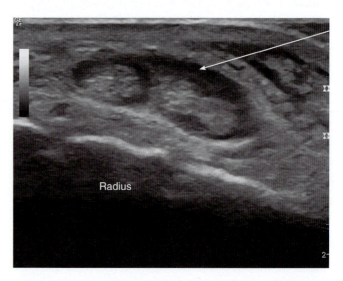

FIGURE 37-4 ▪ Transverse view of fourth dorsal compartment with *arrow* representing needle entry from ulnar to radial, in plane.

Alternate Technique

a. Patient position (Figure 37-5)

   i. Seated with hand resting prone on a flat surface

b. Transducer position (see Figure 37-5)

   i. Short axis to tendons of the fourth dorsal compartment

c. Needle orientation relative to the transducer (see Figure 37-5)

   i. Out of plane

   ii. Use walk-down technique

d. Needle approach (Figures 37-5 and 37-6)

   i. Distal to proximal

e. Target (Figure 37-6)

   i. Space between tendon sheath and tendon

f. Pearls and Pitfalls

   i. Superficial nature of this tendon sheath allows ease of out-of-plane approach to tendon sheath with less soft tissue to traverse to get to the target area.

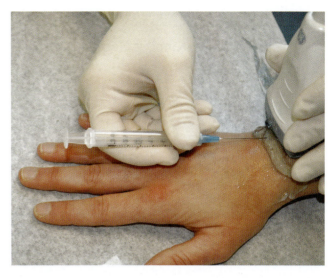

FIGURE 37-5 ■ Linear array transducer is transverse to the compartment and needle approach is out of plane.

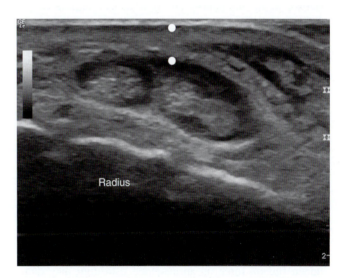

FIGURE 37-6 ■ Short-axis view of fourth dorsal compartment with *dots* representing walk-down technique to target area from distal to proximal, out of plane.

References

1. Jacobson J. *Fundamentals of Musculoskeletal Ultrasound.* St. Louis: Elsevier; 2007.
2. Bianchi S, Martinoli C. *Ultrasound of the Musculoskeletal System.* New York: Springer; 2007.
3. Cooney W, Linscheid R. *Wrist: Diagnostic and Operative Treatment.* Philadelphia, PA: Lippincott Williams and Wilkins; 1998.

Todd P. Stitik, MD / Kambiz Nooryani, MD / Prathap Jayaram, MD / Asal Sepassi, MD

KEY POINTS

- Use a 25- to 30-gauge, 1- to 1.5-inch needle.
- Use a high-frequency linear array transducer in the short axis, in plane.
- The fifth compartment overlies the distal ends of the radioulnar joint on the dorsal aspect of the wrist, and it contains the extensor digiti minimi (EDM) tendon.

- Avoid the ulnar styloid when injecting.
- An oblique standoff technique may be needed.

Pertinent Anatomy

The extensor digiti minimi (EDM) muscle, also known as extensor digiti quinti proprius, is a slender muscle of the forearm, located on the ulnar side of the extensor digitorum communis (EDC). Its tendon is located within the fifth dorsal wrist compartment.

The EDM's origin is at the lateral epicondyle of the humerus, and it inserts at the extensor expansion of the fifth digit. The EDM extends the fifth digit at the metacarpal and interphalangeal joints. The posterior interosseous nerve (C7, C8), the continuation of the deep branch of the radial nerve, innervates the EDM. The interosseous artery is the arterial supply of the EDM (Figure 38-1A and B).

Common Pathology

Sudden flexion force on an extended fifth digit may damage the EDM tendon and/or muscle. Strain of EDM tendon is relatively common in sports that are prone to wrist tendinitis including tennis, basketball, golf, weightlifting, and rock climbing.[1] Systemic illnesses associated with tendinitis, including diabetes, rheumatoid arthritis, crystal arthropathy, and connective tissue disorders, can also affect the EDM.[1] In addition, Vaughan-Jackson syndrome is characterized by the disruption of the digital extensor tendons, beginning on the ulnar side with the EDM and EDC tendon of the small finger. It is most commonly associated with rheumatoid arthritis.[2] A chronic indolent infection and/or mass lesion of the dorsal aspect of the wrist can also damage or cause tenosynovitis of the EDM. Longstanding Kienböck disease can cause partial damage to EDM, because of continuous friction of EDM tendon against the osteonecrotic lunate bone fragments.[3]

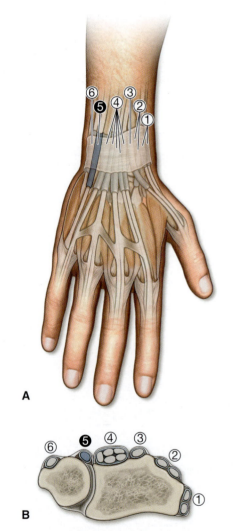

A

B

FIGURE 38-1 ■ **A.** Anatomy of the dorsal compartments of the wrist. **B.** Short axis view of the dorsal wrist. ❺ EDM, extensor digiti minimi.

Ultrasound Imaging Findings

The fifth compartment is palpable by applying slight pressure just lateral to the ulnar styloid process. To palpate the EDM, the patient should rest his or her palm upon a surface and then he or she should extend the little finger. The EDM tendon is best identified in the short-axis plane using a high-frequency linear array transducer at a depth of less than 3 cm. Once the tendon has been identified in this plane, a long-axis probe orientation can then be used to further study the tendon.

Indications for Injections of the Fifth Compartment

Injection of the fifth compartment can be performed for diagnostic and/or therapeutic purposes in patients with recalcitrant pain from tenosynovitis, tendinosis, and a partially torn tendon that is unresponsive to conservative measures, which generally include a splint, nonsteroidal antiinflammatory drugs and/or other analgesics, and activity limitation.

Equipment

- Needle: 25- to 30-gauge, 1- to 1.5-inch needle
- Injectate: 0.5–1.0 mL of local anesthetic and 0.5–1.0 mL of an injectable corticosteroid
- High-frequency linear array transducer

Author's Preferred Technique

a. Patient position (Figure 38-2)
   i. Supine (preferably) or seated
   ii. Extensor side up, wrist partially flexed on towel
b. Transducer position (see Figure 38-2)
   i. Anatomically transverse to the EDM tendon
c. Needle orientation relative to the transducer (see Figure 38-2)
   i. In plane
d. Needle approach (Figure 38-3)
   i. Ulnar to radial direction
   ii. May require oblique standoff technique
e. Target (see Figure 38-3)
   i. EDM tendon sheath
f. Pearls and Pitfalls
   i. It is always best to use the short-axis view initially, to correctly identify the fifth dorsal compartment.
   ii. The needle may need to be bent at the hub to enter the skin at an optimal angle.

iii. Inadvertent blood vessel penetration can be become problematic during the injection, especially the more distal the injection is.
iv. The curvilinear surface of the distal ulna can represent an obstacle to the injection.
v. Injecting too proximally can increase the risk of injecting the wrong compartment because the fourth and the fifth compartments are closer to one another the more proximal the location.

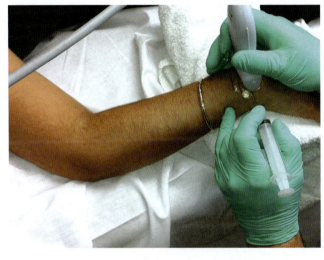

FIGURE 38-2 ■ High-frequency linear array probe transverse to the compartment, and needle approach is in plane.

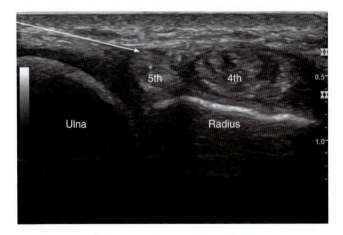

FIGURE 38-3 ■ Transverse view of extensor digiti minimi (EDM) tendon with "hockey stick" probe. *Arrow* represents needle entry from ulnar to radial, in plane. 4th, fourth dorsal compartment; 5th, fifth dorsal compartment.

Alternate Technique

a. Patient position (Figure 38-4)
   i. Supine (preferably) or seated
   ii. Extensor side up, wrist partially flexed on towel
b. Transducer position (see Figure 38-4)
   i. Long axis to the EDM tendon
c. Needle orientation relative to the transducer (see Figure 38-4)
   i. In plane
d. Needle approach (Figure 38-5)
   i. Distal to proximal
e. Target (see Figure 38-5)
   i. EDM tendon sheath

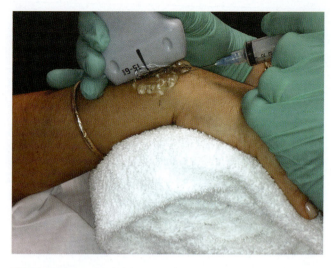

FIGURE 38-4 ■ High-frequency linear array transducer longitudinal to compartment, and needle approach is in plane.

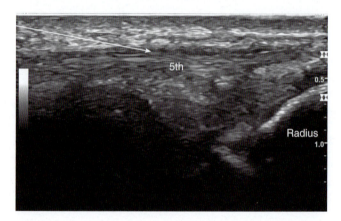

FIGURE 38-5 ■ Long-axis view of extensor carpi ulnaris (ECU) tendon with "hockey stick" probe. *Arrow* represents needle entry into tendon sheath from distal to proximal. 5th, fifth dorsal compartment.

References

1. Youngman J. Wrist tendinitis and wrist injuries: what is wrist tendinitis, how is it caused, and how about wrist tendinitis treatment. http://www.sportsinjurybulletin.com/archive/wrist-tendinitis-treatment.html. Accessed January 15, 2012.

2. McAuliffe JA. Vaughan-Jackson syndrome. *Medscape*. http://emedicine.medscape.com/article/1244987-overview. Access date: July, 2011 through January, 2012.

3. Mazhar T, Rambani R. Vaughan-Jackson-like syndrome as an unusual presentation of Kienböck's disease: a case report. *J Med Case Rep.* 2011;5:325.

Todd P. Stitik, MD / Asal Sepassi, MD / Prathap Jayaram, MD / Kambiz Nooryani, MD

KEY POINTS

- A 25-gauge, 1.5-inch needle is ideal.
- A high-frequency linear array transducer is best.
- The sixth compartment is best seen with the transducer oriented short axis to the wrist.

- Avoid ulnar styloid when injecting.
- The oblique standoff technique may need to be used.

Pertinent Anatomy

The sixth dorsal compartment of the wrist is the most ulnar dorsal compartment of the wrist and is bordered by the extensor retinaculum dorsally and the ulna volarly. It contains the extensor carpi ulnaris (ECU) tendon and sheath. There is a the bandlike subsheath that serves to stabilize ECU tendon within its groove at the distal ulna (Figure 39-1A and B). The ECU muscle has two origins, one at the lateral epicondyle of the humerus and one at the posterior border of the ulna. From its origin, the muscle passes through the ulnar–radial groove, then inserts at the base of the fifth metacarpal. There are no neurovascular structures contained within the sheath.

Common Pathology

After first compartment injuries, the sixth is the most commonly injured dorsal compartment of the wrist.[1] The sixth compartment is most commonly affected by pathology in one of three ways. Acute injuries occur particularly in the case of tennis players who are likely to go from extreme pronation to extreme supination of the wrist. Trauma can occur to both the tendon and the overlying subsheath of the retinaculum. Chronic repetitive injuries to the tendon are typically associated with rowing, racquet sports, and golf. This chronic stress likely first results in tenosynovitis leading to a progressive tendinopathy over time. Lastly, systemic and inflammatory conditions cause the tendon and its synovial lining to become inflamed most commonly as part of rheumatoid synovitis or other systemic inflammatory conditions.

Ultrasound Imaging Findings

The ECU tendon is best identified in the short-axis plane using a high-frequency linear array transducer. Prior to injection, the sixth compartment is palpable by applying slight

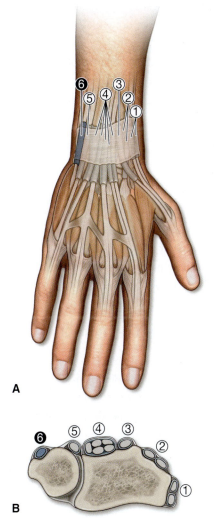

FIGURE 39-1 ■ **A.** Anatomy of the dorsal compartments of the wrist. **B.** Short axis view of the dorsal wrist. ❻ ECU, extensor carpi ulnaris.

pressure just lateral to the ulnar styloid process. To palpate the ECU tendon, have the patient hyperpronate with the wrist slightly flexed. Once the tendon has been identified in this plane, a long-axis probe orientation can then be used to further study the tendon.

Indications for Injections of the Sixth Compartment

Injection of the sixth compartment can be performed for patients with recalcitrant pain from tenosynovitis, tendinosis, and a partially torn ECU tendon that is unresponsive to conservative measures, which generally include a splint, nonsteroidal antiinflammatory drugs and/or other analgesics, and activity limitation.

Injection of the sixth compartment has been described based on palpation of the wrist and hand.[2] However, clinical outcomes of palpation-guided versus ultrasound-guided injection of the sixth compartment of the wrist have not been reported.

Equipment

■ Needle: 25- to 30-gauge, 1- to 1.5-inch needle
■ Injectate: 1 mL of local anesthetic and 1 mL of an injectable corticosteroid
■ High-frequency linear array transducer or "hockey stick" probe

Author's Preferred Technique

a. Patient position (Figure 39-2)
   i. Supine (preferably) or seated
   ii. Extensor side of wrist facing up, wrist on a rolled up towel placed beneath the ventral wrist, slightly flexed and pronated
b. Transducer position (see Figure 39-2)
   i. Anatomic short-axis plane over the dorsal aspect of the wrist
c. Needle orientation relative to the transducer (Figures 39-2 and 39-3)
   i. In plane
d. Needle approach (see Figures 39-2 and 39-3)
   i. Ulnar to radial
e. Target (see Figure 39-3)
   i. ECU tendon sheath

f. Pearls and Pitfalls
   i. Because physiological ECU displacement from its groove is maximal in supination, keep wrist pronated or even hyperpronated if necessary to visualize.
   ii. If necessary, bend the hub of needle to the degree needed for parallel entry point.
   iii. Not taking the ulnar styloid into consideration when positioning the needle can lead to an obstacle for needle advancement.

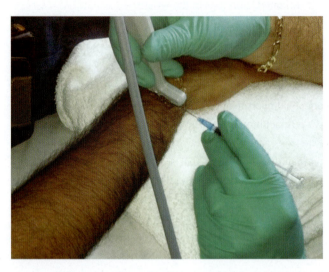

FIGURE 39-2 ■ Compact linear array transducer is transverse to the compartment, and needle approach is in plane.

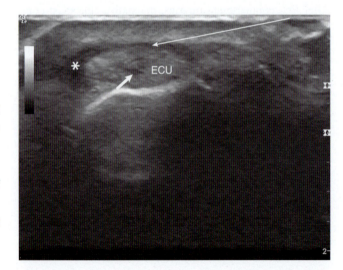

FIGURE 39-3 ■ Transverse view of ECU tendon with *arrow* representing needle entry from ulnar to radial, in plane. Asterisk, fluid surrounding tendon sheath; ECU, extensor carpi ulnaris; wide arrow, hypoechoic cleft in tendon representing longitudinal tear.

Alternate Technique

a. Patient position (Figure 39-4)
    i. Supine (preferably) or seated
    ii. Extensor side of wrist facing up, wrist on a rolled up towel placed beneath the ventral wrist, slightly flexed and pronated
b. Transducer position (see Figure 39-4)
    i. Long axis to the tendon
c. Needle orientation relative to transducer (Figures 39-4 and 39-5)
    i. In plane
d. Needle approach (see Figures 39-4 and 39-5)
    i. Distal to proximal direction
e. Target (see Figure 39-5)
    i. ECU tendon sheath
f. Pearls and Pitfalls
    i. If needle approach from the ulnar to radial direction is not possible because of a lesion or scar tissue over the targeted area, this technique may be applied at the discretion of the treating clinician.
    ii. Because of the possibility of volume averaging, there is an increased risk of injecting the wrong compartment; therefore, this is not a preferred technique.

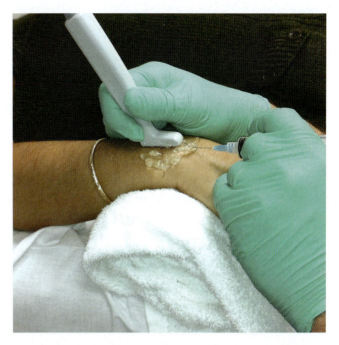

FIGURE 39-4 ■ Compact linear array transducer is long axis to the compartment, and needle approach is in plane.

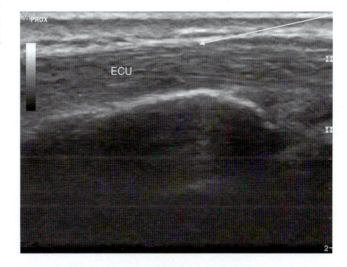

FIGURE 39-5 ■ Long-axis view of extensor carpi ulnaris (ECU) tendon. *Arrow* represents needle entry into tendon sheath.

References

1. Wood MB, Dobyns JH. Sports-related extraarticular wrist syndromes. *Clin Orthop.* 1986;202:93–102.
2. Gilliland CA, Salazar LD, Borchers JR. Ultrasound versus anatomic guidance for intra-articular and periarticular injection: a systematic review. *Phys Sportsmed.* 2011 Oct;39(3):121–131.
3. Duke Orthopaedics. Extensor carpi ulnaris. In: *Wheeless' Textbook of Orthopaedics.* http://www.wheelessonline.com/ortho/extensor_carpi_ulnaris. Accessed November 1, 2011.
4. Lee KS, Ablove RH, Singh S, et al. Ultrasound imaging of normal displacement of the extensor carpi ulnaris tendon within the ulnar groove in 12 forearm-wrist positions. *AJR Am J Roentgenol.* 2009 Sep;193(3):651–655.

CHAPTER 40

Jeffrey A. Strakowski, MD

KEY POINTS

- A 25- to 30-gauge, 1.5-inch needle is ideal.
- A high-frequency linear array transducer is appropriate.
- An in-plane or out-of-plane approach is appropriate.
- Care should be taken to locate and avoid interdigital nerves and arteries.

- A more experienced practitioner can consider a stretch or release of the first annular (A1) pulley.

Anatomy of the Flexor Tendons at the First Annular Pulley

The first annular (A1) pulley arises from the volar plate of the metacarpal phalangeal (MCP) joint (Figure 40-1). It is located approximately 5 mm proximal to the joint and extends to the base of the proximal phalanx with an average length of 1 cm. The proximal finger crease can be used as a surface marker for the A1 pulley. The proximal edge of the A1 pulley lies approximately 2 cm from the proximal finger crease. The distal edge of the pulley lies approximately 1 cm from the proximal finger crease.[1] The flexor digitorum sublimis (FDS) and flexor digitorum profundus (FDP) tendons slide underneath the annular pulleys. At the level of the A1 pulley, the FDS splits and the FDP becomes more superficial.

Common Pathology

Stenosing tenosynovitis at the A1 pulley (aka "trigger finger") can occur with associated conditions such as diabetes mellitus, rheumatoid arthritis, and gout. It also can develop after localized trauma to the base of the digit; however, it more frequently occurs without any established predisposing factor.[2] The patient feels pain, catching, or locking in the finger with flexion and extension as a result of the flexor tendons, or the pulley becoming too thick at the level in which the tendons

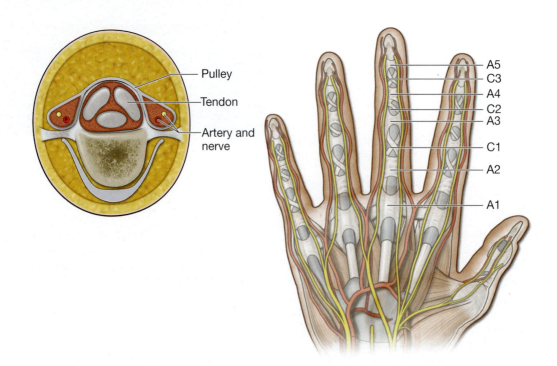

Pulley

Tendon

Artery and nerve

A5
C3
A4
C2
A3
C1
A2
A1

FIGURE 40-1 ■ Illustration of long-axis and short-axis views of the digital flexor tendons and first annular (A1) pulley.

must pass through the pulley. In some circumstances, flexor tendons can develop a palpable nodule from the increased thickness of the synovial sheath at that location. Despite the location of catching at the A1 pulley, the patient often feels as though the problem is at the level of the proximal interphalangeal joint because of the snapping of the flexor tendons. In severe cases, the finger can become locked in flexion.

Ultrasound Imaging Findings

The flexor tendons and A1 pulley are best visualized using a high-frequency linear array transducer. Tenosynovitis can be identified by a hypoechoic layer around the flexor tendons and enlargement of the tendons and sheath just distal to the A1 pulley. The pulley itself is identified as a thin hypoechoic line volar to the flexor tendons at and just proximal to the MCP joint (Figures 40-2 and 40-3).[3] Dynamic imaging can be used to view the bunching and catching of the tendons with flexion and extension. The nearby digital nerves and vessels, located lateral and medial to the flexor tendons, are identified in order to plan an appropriate placement of the needle (Figure 40-4).[4] Use of ultrasound guidance can improve needle placement accuracy, enhancing both safety in avoidance of neurovascular structures, and potential efficacy by more precise placement of steroid to the desired target.[5]

Indications

Steroid injection at the A1 pulley for stenosing tenosynovitis can be helpful for alleviating symptoms of pain, locking, and catching with flexion and extension of the involved digit.[6] Injections should be applied with caution or avoided in circumstances of uncontrolled diabetes mellitus, immunosuppression, active systemic or localized infection, compromised skin over the region, or a history of prior adverse reaction to injection of steroid or local anesthetic.

Equipment

- Needle: 25- to 30-gauge, 1- to 1.5-inch needle
- Injectate: 0.5 mL of local anesthetic and 0.5 mL of an injectable corticosteroid
- High-frequency linear array transducer

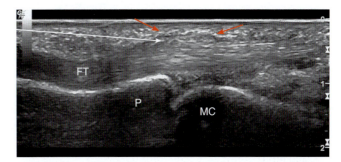

FIGURE 40-2 ■ Sonogram of the flexor tendons and first annular (A1) pulley in long axis. Note the relative thickening of the A1 pulley above the flexor tendons. *Red arrows* demonstrate A1 pulley. *White arrow* represents needle angle for long axis, in-plane technique from distal to proximal. FT, flexor tendons; MC, metacarpal; P, phalanx.

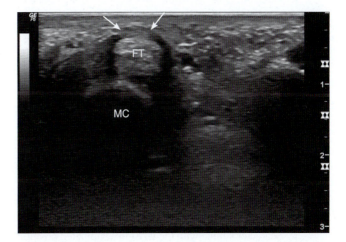

FIGURE 40-3 ■ Sonogram of the flexor tendons and first annular (A1) pulley in short axis. Note the relative thickening of the A1 pulley above the flexor tendons. *Arrow* represents needle angle for long-axis, in-plane approach from distal to proximal. FT, flexor tendons; MC, metacarpal; P, phalanx.

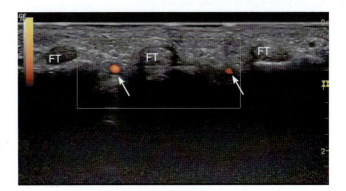

FIGURE 40-4 ■ Sonogram demonstrating the digital nerves and vessels adjacent to the flexors tendons as seen with Doppler flow. *Arrows* point to interdigital arteries.

Author's Preferred Technique

a. Patient position (Figure 40-5)
   i. Seated or supine with the wrist in a supinated position
b. Transducer position (see Figure 40-5)
   i. Long axis to flexor tendons and A1 pulley at level of MCP joint
c. Needle orientation relative to the transducer (Figures 40-2 and 40-5)
   i. In plane
d. Needle approach (see Figure 40-2)
   i. Distal to proximal or proximal to distal
e. Target (see Figure 40-2)
   i. Just inferior to A1 pulley, superficial to flexor tendons
f. Pearls and Pitfalls
   i. Once in good position for the injection, consider switching to short-axis view to establish position of interdigital nerves prior to injection.
   ii. The experienced practitioner may consider stretch or release procedure of the A1 pulley (discussed in Chapter 104).
   iii. Procedure is same for A1 pulley of the thumb. For this pulley, it is only the flexor pollicis longus that is entrapped.

Alternate Technique 1

a. Patient position (Figure 40-6)
   i. Seated or supine with the wrist in a supinated position
b. Transducer position (Figures 40-6 and 40-7)
   i. Short axis to flexor tendons and A1 pulley at level of MCP joint
c. Needle orientation relative to the transducer (see Figure 40-7)
   i. In plane
d. Needle approach (see Figure 40-7)
   i. Ulnar to radial or radial to ulnar
e. Target (see Figure 40-7)
   i. Just inferior to A1 pulley, superficial to flexor tendons
f. Pearls and Pitfalls
   i. Pre-scan the area to locate interdigital nerves so they can be avoided for procedure.
   ii. The procedure is the same for the A1 pulley of the thumb. For this pulley, it is only the flexor pollicis longus tendon that is entrapped.

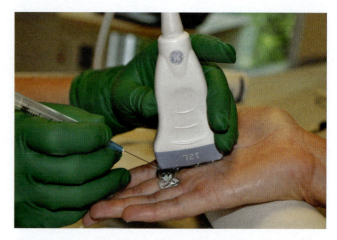

FIGURE 40-5 ■ Transducer and needle placement for long-axis, in-plane approach from distal to proximal.

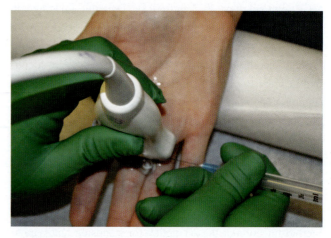

FIGURE 40-6 ■ Transducer and needle placement for short-axis, in-plane approach from ulnar to radial.

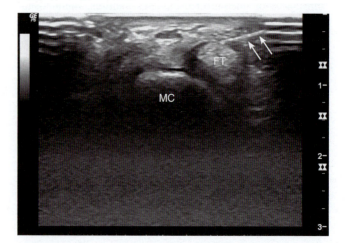

FIGURE 40-7 ■ Demonstration of the needle in-plane technique to the first annular (A1) pulley injection with the target in short-axis view. *Arrows* highlight the needle path deep to the pulley.

Alternate Technique 2

a. Patient position (Figure 40-8)
    i. Seated or supine with the wrist in a supinated position
b. Transducer position (see Figure 40-8)
    i. Short axis to flexor tendons and A1 pulley at level of MCP joint
c. Needle orientation relative to the transducer (see Figure 40-8)
    i. Out of plane
d. Needle approach (Figure 40-9)
    i. Distal to proximal
    ii. Use walk-down technique
e. Target (see Figure 40-9)
    i. Lateral to tendon, within flexor tendon sheath
f. Pearls and Pitfalls
    i. This technique does not directly target the pulley, but lateral placement of medicine is easier and avoids intratendinous needle placement.
    ii. The procedure is the same for the A1 pulley of the thumb. For this pulley, it is only the flexor pollicis longus tendon that is entrapped.

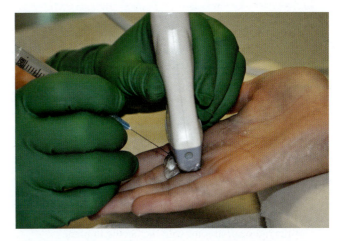

FIGURE 40-8 ■ Transducer and needle placement for short-axis, out-of-plane approach.

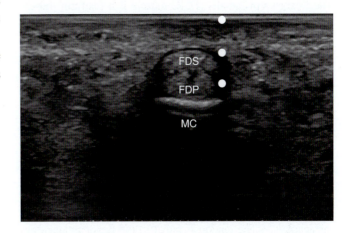

FIGURE 40-9 ■ Sonogram demonstrating the first annular (A1) pulley in short-axis view. *Dots* represent the walk-down technique. FDP, flexor digitorum profundus; FDS, flexor digitorum superficialis; MC, metacarpal.

References

1. Florini HJ, Santos JBG, Kirakaw CK, et al. Anatomical study of the a1 pulley: length and location by means of cutaneous landmarks on the palmar surface. *J Hand Surg.* March 2011;36(3):464–468.
2. Chambers RG Jr. Corticosteroid injections for trigger finger. *Am Fam Physician.* 2009 Sep 1;80(5):454.
3. Bodor M, Flossman T. Ultrasound-guided first annular pulley injection for trigger finger. *J Ultrasound Med.* 2009 Jun;28(6):737–743.
4. Smith J, Rizzo M, Lai JK. Sonographically guided percutaneous first annular pulley release: cadaveric safety study of needle and knife techniques. *J Ultrasound Med.* 2010 Nov;29(11):1531–1542.
5. Lee DH, Han SB, Park JW, et al. Sonographically guided tendon sheath injections are more accurate than blind injections: implications for trigger finger treatment. *J Ultrasound Med.* 2011 Feb;30(2):197–203.
6. Marks MR, Gunther SF. Efficacy of cortisone injection in treatment of trigger fingers and thumbs. *J Hand Surg.* 1989;14-A:722–727.

Rebecca Ann Myers, MD / Jennifer K. Malcolm, DO / Mark Edward Lavallee, MD, CSCS, FACSM

KEY POINTS

- Use a high-frequency linear array transducer to perform procedure.
- The flexor carpi radialis tendon may develop a tenosynovitis.
- The ultrasound transducer should be long axis at the level of the radiocarpal joint with the needle in plane.

- Color Doppler imaging aids in avoiding puncture of the radial artery.
- Ganglion cysts may occur adjacent to the distal flexor carpi radialis tendon sheath.

Pertinent Anatomy (Figure 41-1A, B)

The flexor carpi radialis (FCR) muscle is a fusiform muscle that originates at the medial epicondyle of the humerus medial to the pronator teres muscle.[1] The FCR tendon originates approximately 15 cm proximal to the radiocarpal joint, and becomes completely tendinous approximately 8 cm proximal to this joint.[2] The tendon then travels distally crossing over the scaphoid and trapezius. It travels through a fibro-osseus tunnel consisting of the trapezial crest palmarly, trapezial body radially, trapezoid dorsally, and retinacular septum ulnarly.[2] The tendon angles approximately 30–45 degrees and divides into two sections distal to the trapezium.[2] The distal attachments are on the volar surface of the base of the second and third metacarpals.[1,2] The tendon is radial to the flexor retinaculum and therefore does not pass through the carpal tunnel. Distally the radial artery courses lateral to the tendon. Ulnar and deep to the FCR tendon is the flexor pollicis longus and median nerve.

Common Pathology

Pain along the radial aspect of the wrist may be common, but the FCR is an uncommon cause of radiovolar wrist pain and is often overlooked. Because of the limited space within the fibro-osseus tunnel, small boney abnormalities such as osteophytes may predispose the tendon to injury. A reactive tenosynovitis has been reported with characteristics similar to de Quervain syndrome.[3] Flexor carpi radialis tendon rupture is a rare cause of wrist pain associated with rheumatologic disease or pantrapezial osteoarthritis.[4]

In addition, ganglion cysts may occur adjacent to the distal FCR tendon sheath. Twenty percent of wrist ganglia are found over the volar wrist, with the most common site between the FCR and abductor pollicis longus at the scapho-trapezoid joint.[5]

Aspiration of these cysts will be covered in another chapter.

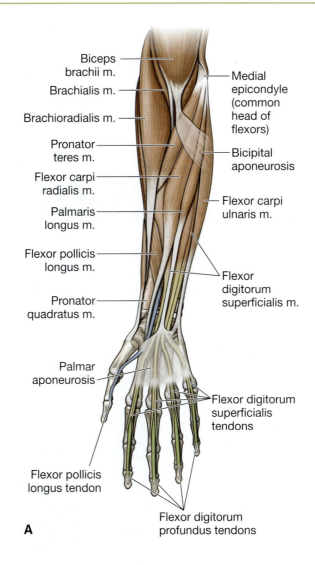

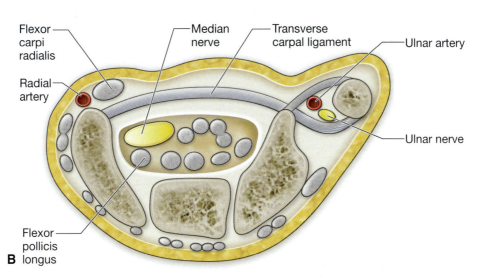

FIGURE 41-1 ■ **A.** (Reproduced with permission from Morton DA, Foreman KB, Albertine KH, eds. *The Big Picture: Gross Anatomy*. New York: McGraw-Hill; 2011: figure 32-1B.) **B.** Cross-sectional view of wrist demonstrating the flexor carpi radialis (FCR) tendon. Note the relationship between FCR and radial artery as well as transverse carpal ligament (TCL).

Ultrasound Imaging

The FCR tendon is best visualized in long axis using a high-frequency linear array transducer at a depth of 2.0 cm (Figure 41-2). Ultrasound identification of the radial artery in short axis should be noted given its close proximity to the FCR tendon (Figure 41-3).

Indications for Injection of the Flexor Carpi Radialis

Anesthetic injection with or without steroid can aid in the diagnosis and treatment of patients with pain at the radiovolar aspect of the wrist (suspicious for tenosynovitis). If a ganglion cyst is identified, aspiration should be attempted prior to injection.

Equipment

- Needle: 25-gauge, 1.5-inch needle
- Injectate: 0.5 mL of local anesthetic and 0.5 mL of injectable corticosteroid
- High-frequency linear array transducer

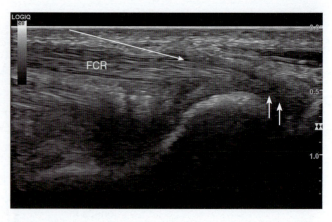

FIGURE 41-2 ▪ Ultrasound image long axis to the FCR tendon with "hockey stick" transducer. Note the steep angle of the FCR tendon as it attaches distally and the anisotropy in this region (*small arrows*). *Long arrow* is angle of needle entry for in-plane approach to tendon sheath. FCR, flexor carpi radialis.

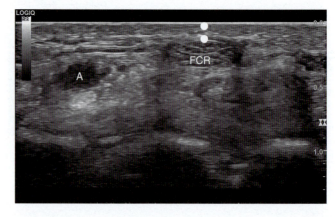

FIGURE 41-3 ▪ Ultrasound image short axis to flexor carpi radialis (FCR) tendon with high-frequency linear array transducer. Note the location of the radial artery (A) in relationship to the FCR tendon. *Dots* represent out-of-plane walk-down technique to tendon sheath.

Author's Preferred Technique

a. Patient position
   i. Seated or supine
   ii. Patient's hand palm side up with forearm and hand supported on a firm surface
b. Transducer position (Figure 41-4)
   i. Long axis to the FCR tendon at the level of the radio-carpal joint
c. Needle orientation relative to the transducer (Figures 41-2 and 41-4)
   i. In plane
d. Needle approach (see Figures 41-2 and 41-4)
   i. Proximal to distal
e. Target (see Figure 41-2)
   i. FCR tendon sheath
f. Pearls and Pitfalls
   i. Consider color Doppler imaging during injections to avoid puncture of the radial artery during the injection and to visualize injectate in sheath versus surrounding tissue.
   ii. If resistance is met while injecting, slightly retract the needle until the bolus easily flows within the tendinous sheath.
   iii. Gentle active wrist flexion may help to identify the tendon and confirm needle location within the tendinous sheath.
   iv. The FCR tendon may be differentiated from the flexor pollicis longus tendon by dynamic testing, that is, having the patient independently flex the wrist and thumb.

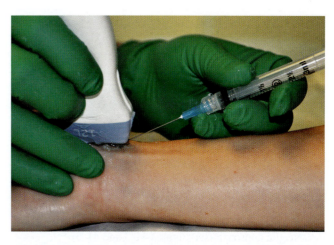

FIGURE 41-4 ▪ Setup for long-axis, in-plane approach to flexor carpi radialis (FCR) tendon sheath.

Alternate Technique

a. Patient position
  i. Seated or supine
  ii. Patient's hand palm side up with forearm and hand supported on a firm surface
b. Transducer position (Figure 41-5)
  i. Short axis to the forearm at the level of the radiocarpal joint
c. Needle orientation relative to the transducer (Figures 41-3 and 41-5)
  i. Out of plane
d. Needle approach (see Figures 41-3 and 41-5)
  i. Proximal to distal
  ii. Use walk-down technique
e. Target (see Figure 41-3)
  i. FCR tendon sheath
f. Pearls and Pitfalls
  i. See "Pearls and Pitfalls" under "Author's Preferred Technique."

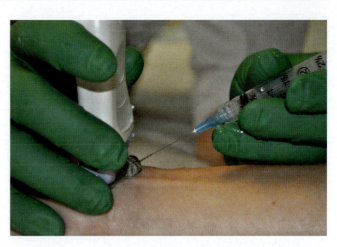

FIGURE 41-5 ■ Setup for short-axis out-of plane approach to the flexor carpi radialis (FCR) tendon sheath.

References

1. Moore KL, Dalley AF. *Clinically Oriented Anatomy*. 4th ed. New York: Lippincott Williams and Wilkins; 1999:736–737.
2. Bishop AT, Gabel G, Carmichael SW. Flexor carpi radialis tendonitis part I: operative anatomy. *J Bone Joint Surg Am.* 1994;74(7):1009–1014.
3. Fitton JM, Shea FW, Goldie W. Lesions of the flexor carpi radialis tendon and sheath causing pain at the wrist. *J Bone Joint Surg Am.* 1968;50(2):359–363.
4. Tonkin MA, Ster HS. Spontaneous rupture of the flexor carpi radialis tendon. *J Hand Surg.* 1991;16B(1):72–74.
5. Gude W, Morelli V. Ganglion cysts of the wrist: pathophysiology, clinical picture, and management. *Curr Rev Musculoskelet Med.* 2008;1(3-4):205–211.

Luis Baerga-Varela, MD

KEY POINTS

- Use a high-frequency linear array transducer in short axis view.
- Use a 25- to 27-gauge, 1.25- to 1.5-inch needle, in-plane approach.
- Avoid injecting intratendon; avoid median and ulnar nerves and ulnar artery.
- Check for and avoid persistent median artery.

Pertinent Anatomy

The flexor digitorum profundus (FDP) muscle originates from the proximal ulna and the interosseous membrane and divides distally into four slips that pass superficial to the pronator quadratus and insert into the distal phalanx of the second through fifth fingers. The flexor digitorum superficialis (FDS) muscle consists of three heads originating in the medial epicondyle, proximal ulna, and proximal radius, which merge at the forearm. The FDS splits distally into four slips, passing superficial to the tendons of the FDP and inserting into the middle phalanx of second through fifth digits.[1]

The FDP and superficialis tendons pass through the carpal tunnel at the wrist. They are enveloped by a common synovial sheath, while a separate sheath envelops the smaller flexor pollicis longus (FPL) tendon. Within the carpal tunnel, the median nerve is located superficial to the FDS on the radial side[2] (Figure 42-1). Occasionally, a bifid median nerve may be found and/or a persistent median artery of the forearm. The persistent median artery of the forearm when present is located between the two bundles of a bifid median nerve or on the ulnar side of a normal median nerve.[3]

Common Pathology

Pathology of the FDS and FDP tendons at the wrist is not common. In fact, besides traumatic ruptures, there is hardly any literature describing pathology of these tendons at the wrist. Occasionally, FDS and FDP tenosynovitis, secondary to rheumatologic conditions such as rheumatoid arthritis,[4] systemic lupus erythematosus, and spondyloarthropathies among others, can be seen.

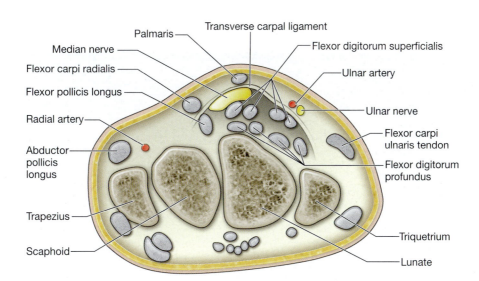

FIGURE 42-1 ■ Cross-section of the wrist at the proximal border of first carpal row (wrist crease).

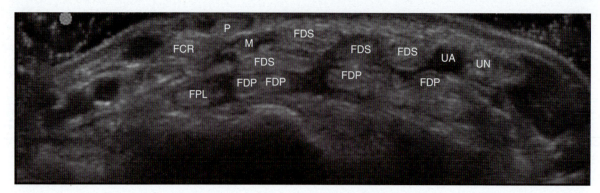

FIGURE 42-2 ■ Normal sonographic view of the flexor digitorum tendons at the level of the wrist crease: FCR, flexor carpi radialis; FDP, flexor digitorum profundus; FDS, flexor digitorum superficialis; FPL, flexor pollicis longus; M, median nerve; P, palmaris; UA, ulnar artery; and UN, ulnar nerve.

Ultrasound Imaging Findings

The FDS and FDP tendons are best visualized in short axis using a high-frequency linear array transducer at a depth of 1–2 cm. Scanning should start at the proximal carpal tunnel, where the four tendons of the FDS are seen superior to the four tendons of the FDP. Just radial to these tendons, the smaller FPL tendon will be noted. The median nerve will be noted superficial and slightly radial with its usual relatively hypoechoic honeycomb appearance. By tilting the probe back and forth, the tendon's anisotropy can be used to distinguish the tendons from the median nerve. The convex band of the transverse carpal ligament is noted overlying the tendons and medial nerve. Because of the transverse carpal ligament's convex shape and anisotropy, the ligament appears hypoechoic in areas. The ulnar artery and nerve should be identified in Guyon's canal. The FDS and FDP tendons should be assessed in this short-axis view by scanning both distally in the distal carpal tunnel and more proximally into the forearm until the musculotendinous junction is reached. The probe can then be turned into a long-axis view, where each tendon can be assessed individually (Figure 42-2).

Common pathologic findings of tendinopathy would include increased interfibrillar distance (hypoechoic tendon appearance) and tendon thickening. Tenosynovitis findings would include fluid within the common tendon sheath (Figure 42-3).

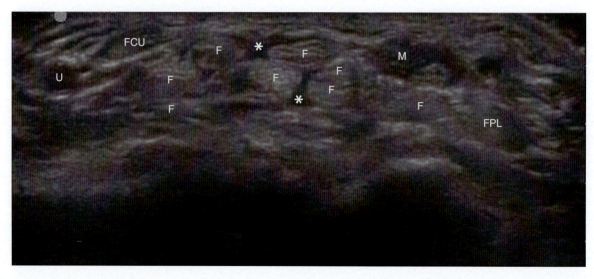

FIGURE 42-3 ■ Flexor digitorum tenosynovitis (*asterisks*), F, flexor tendons; FCU, flexor carpi ulnaris; FPL, flexor pollicis longus; M, median nerve; and U, ulnar artery.

Indications for Injections of the Flexor Digitorum Profundus and Superficialis Tendon Sheath

There is no literature describing the indications for injection of the FDS and FDP at the wrist. Nevertheless, one may choose to inject the common tendon sheath in patients with symptomatic tenosynovitis.

Equipment

- Needle: 27-gauge, 1.25-inch needle or 25-gauge, 1.5-inch needle
- Injectate: 0.5–1 mL of local anesthetic and 0.25–0.5 mL of an injectable corticosteroid
- High-frequency linear array transducer

Author's Preferred Technique

a. Patient position (Figure 42-4)
    i. Wrist supinated and relaxed in slight extension
b. Transducer position (see Figure 42-4)
    i. Anatomic transverse plane over proximal carpal tunnel
    ii. Probe placed at level of wrist crease
c. Needle orientation relative to transducer (see Figure 42-4)
    i. In plane
d. Needle approach (see Figure 42-4)
    i. Ulnar to radial
    ii. Oblique standoff technique

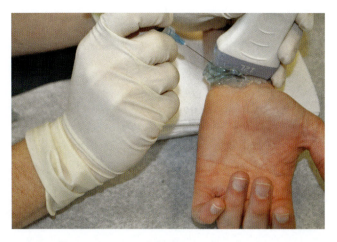

FIGURE 42-4 ▪ Patient positioning, transducer positioning and needle orientation: Wrist supinated and relaxed in slight extension, transducer in anatomical short-axis plane, and needle in plane with transducer from ulnar to radial.

e. Target (Figure 42-5)
    i. Common synovial sheath of FDS and FDP.
    ii. More specifically, one can target between the FDS tendons to the third and fourth digits, to avoid the ulnar artery and median nerve. There is a small gap between these two tendons, which helps identify them.
f. Pearls and Pitfalls
    i. Avoid the ulnar artery and nerve on ulnar side. These should be identified prior to injection.
    ii. Avoid the median nerve and, if present, persistent median artery of the forearm. Doppler should be used to identify the presence of a persistent median artery just ulnar to the median nerve.
    iii. An oblique standoff technique may be used to better visualize the needle, due to the steeper needle angle of entry (see Figure 42-4).

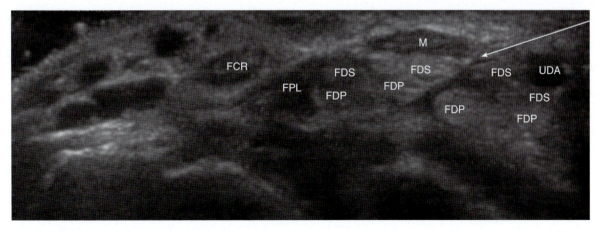

FIGURE 42-5 ▪ Flexor digitorum tendon sheath injection target. *Arrow* indicates path of needle to target space. Notice the gap between third and fourth FDS tendons, a good target to deposit medication. FCR, flexor carpi radialis; FDP, flexor digitorum profundus; FDS, flexor digitorum superficialis; FPL, flexor pollicis longus; M, median nerve.

References

1. Martinolli C, Bianchi S. Forearm. In: Bianchi S, Martinolli C, eds. *Ultrasound of the Musculoskeletal System.* 1st ed. Berlin: Springer; 2007:409–423.

2. Bianchi S, Martinolli C. Wrist. In: Bianchi S, Martinolli C, eds. *Ultrasound of the Musculoskeletal System.* 1st ed. Berlin: Springer; 2007:425–494.

3. Iannicelli E, Chianta GA, Salvini V, et al. Evaluation of bifid median nerve with sonography and MR imaging. *J Ultrasound Med.* 2000 Jul;19(7):481–485.

4. Filippucci E, Gabba A, Di Geso L, et al. Hand tendon involvement in rheumatoid arthritis: an ultrasound study. *Semin Arthritis Rheum.* 2011 Nov 3. [Epub ahead of print]

Jeffrey A. Strakowski, MD

KEY POINTS

- A 22- to 25-gauge needle with high-frequency linear array transducer is ideal.
- Caution should be used to avoid injection into the median nerve.
- The in-plane view of the needle allows more reliable tracking of the needle tip.

- The ulnar side of the carpal tunnel allows better space for injection approach in most people.
- Attention to surface anatomic landmarks can assist with reliable needle placement in conjunction with ultrasound guidance.

Anatomy of the Carpal Tunnel

The carpal tunnel space is bordered by the carpal bones on its radial, ulnar, and dorsal sides, as well as the carpal ligament on its volar aspect. This space contains the median nerve as well as the four tendons of the flexor digitorum superficialis, four tendons of the flexor digitorum profundus, and the flexor pollicis longus (Figure 43-1). The median nerve is typically superficial to the flexor tendons and lies in the middle of the carpal tunnel space relative to the radial

and ulnar sides. It usually lies between the more superficial flexor carpi radialis tendon on the radial side, and palmaris longus on the ulnar side. There are two bursa in the carpal tunnel space. The radial bursa contains the flexor pollicis longus tendon, and the ulnar bursa contains the flexor digitorum superficialis and profundus tendons. With the wrist in the supinated position, the median nerve lies on top of the ulnar bursa but below the transverse carpal ligament (see Figure 43-1).

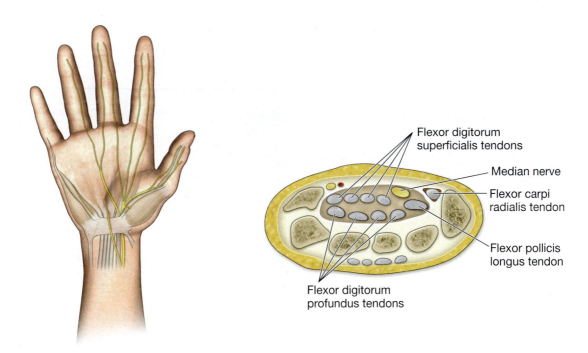

FIGURE 43-1 ■ Illustration of the carpal tunnel space in both long-axis (*left*) and short-axis (*right*) views of the median nerve. The short-axis view displays the structures in and around the carpal tunnel space and includes: flexor digitorum superficialis tendons; flexor digitorum profundus tendons; flexor carpi radialis tendon; flexor pollicis longus tendon; median nerve.

Common Pathology

The walls of the carpal tunnel are relatively unyielding to expansion, and increasing pressure can result in median nerve compromise, which results in the most commonly occurring mono-neuropathy in the human body. This can create paresthesias and pain in the hand and, in some cases, weakness of the median innervated hand intrinsic muscles. Electrodiagnostic techniques including electromyography and nerve conduction studies are highly sensitive for identifying median mononeuropathy at the carpal tunnel.

Ultrasound Imaging Findings

The carpal tunnel space is best visualized using a high-frequency linear array transducer. Median neuropathy at the carpal tunnel can be identified by proximal swelling of the nerve seen in short-axis view of the more proximal aspect of the carpal tunnel. Most studies suggest abnormality if the cross-sectional area is greater than 11 mm (Figure 43-2). Long-axis view of the nerve can further display the proximal swelling as well as a "notch sign" at the site of compression.[2] Ultrasound can be used to assess for potential predisposing factors for median neuropathy, such as arthritic narrowing of the space, tenosynovitis, masses, postsurgical scarring, and encroaching lumbrical or flexor digitorum muscles. The presence of anatomic variants, such as a bifid median nerve, persistent median artery, or an ulnar-lying position of the median palmar sensory branch, should be noted, as these could lead to altering the desired position of the needle.[3]

Indications

Carpal tunnel injection for steroid can be helpful for alleviating symptoms from median neuropathy at the carpal tunnel that have been refractory to other conservative measures such as activity modification and splinting.[1] It is particularly useful in more acute or subacute cases as well as neuropathy that is identified as mild to moderate with electrodiagnostic techniques.

Patient Positioning

Different Techniques

With all of the techniques described here, the surface anatomy of the flexor carpi radialis and palmaris longus (when present) is identified (Figure 43-3). The level of the proximal and distal wrist creases is also noted for the injection position.[4]

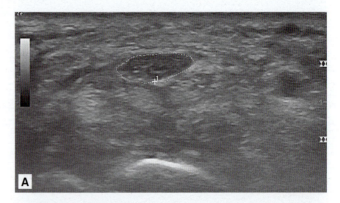

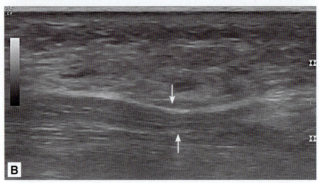

FIGURE 43-2 ■ **A.** Ultrasound scan demonstrating an abnormal enlargement of the median nerve in the proximal carpal tunnel in short-axis view. **B.** Long-axis view of the median nerve in the carpal tunnel space demonstrating a notch sign at the site of compression (*arrows*) and proximal swelling of the nerve.

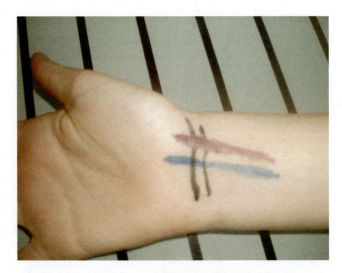

FIGURE 43-3 ■ Photograph illustrating the surface landmarks of the palmaris longus tendon (*blue*), flexor carpi radialis tendon (*red*), and proximal and distal palmar creases (*black*).

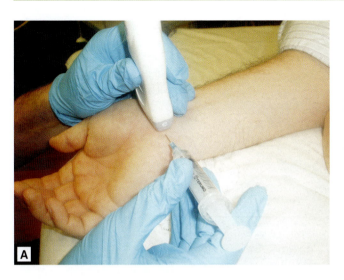

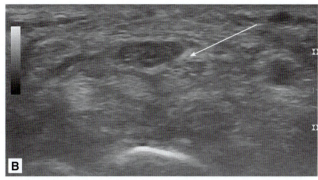

FIGURE 43-4 ■ (**A**) Surface and (**B**) ultrasound view of needle injection with the ulnar to radial in-plane approach.

Equipment

■ Needle: 22- to 25-gauge, 1- to 1.5-inch needle
■ Injectate: 1 mL of local anesthetic and 0.5–1.0 mL of injectable corticosteroids
■ High-frequency linear array transducer

Author's Preferred Technique[5]

a. Patient position
   i. Seated or supine with the wrist in a supinated position and the wrist in slight dorsiflexion over a small rolled towel
b. Transducer position (Figure 43-4A)
   i. Short axis to the median nerve and carpal tunnel at the distal palmar crease
c. Needle orientation relative to the transducer
   i. In plane
d. Needle approach (Figure 43-4B)
   i. Ulnar to radial

e. Target (Figures 43-5 and 43-6)
   i. Deep and superficial to the median nerve along the ulnar and radial bursa
f. Pearls and Pitfalls
   i. Be sure to visualize the ulnar nerve and artery and to confirm that the needle passes superficial to these structures.
   ii. Make sure you see the needle tip during the entire procedure to avoid inadvertent intraneural placement of needle.
   iii. If you are new to this procedure, it is safest to dispense the medicine at a further distance from the nerve and not to approach the radial and ulnar bursa. Successful treatment does not necessitate including these bursa.

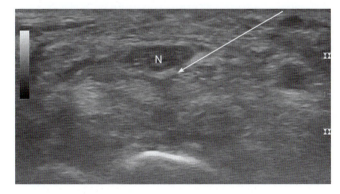

FIGURE 43-5 ■ Needle injection into the ulnar bursa. *Arrow* represents path of needle to target. N, median nerve.

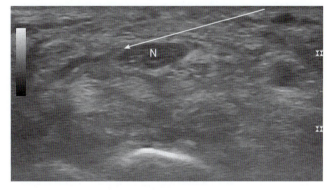

FIGURE 43-6 ■ Needle injection into the radial bursa. *Arrow* represents path of needle to target. N, median nerve.

Alternate Technique 1

a. Patient position
    i. Seated or supine with the wrist in a supinated position and the wrist in slight dorsiflexion over a small rolled towel
b. Transducer position (Figure 43-7A)
    i. Short axis to the median nerve and carpal tunnel at the distal palmar crease
c. Needle orientation relative to the transducer
    i. Out of plane
d. Needle approach (Figure 43-7B)
    i. Proximal to distal
e. Target (see Figure 43-7B)
    i. Ulnar side of median nerve
f. Pearls and Pitfalls
    i. When using this technique, be careful when advancing the needle as the needle tip cannot be visualized past the transducer.

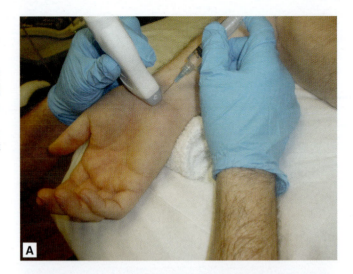

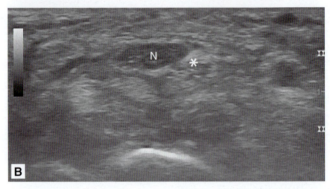

FIGURE 43-7 ■ **(A)** Surface and **(B)** ultrasound view of injection with *asterisk* representing target for out-of-plane approach. N, median nerve.

Alternate Technique 2

a. Patient position
    i. Seated or supine with the wrist in a supinated position and the wrist in slight dorsiflexion over a small rolled towel
b. Transducer position (Figure 43-8A)
    i. Long axis to the median nerve at the distal wrist crease
c. Needle orientation relative to the transducer
    i. In plane
d. Needle approach (Figure 43-8B)
    i. Proximal to distal
e. Target (see Figure 43-8B)
    i. Superficial to the median nerve
f. Pearls and Pitfalls
    i. See "Pearls and Pitfalls" under "Author's Preferred Technique."

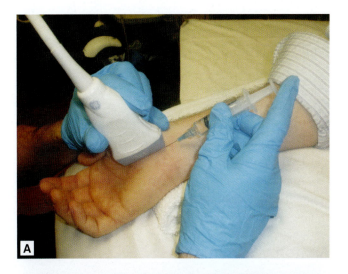

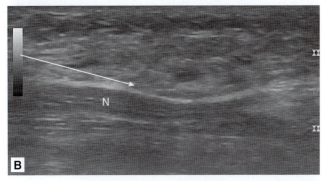

FIGURE 43-8 ■ (**A**) Surface and (**B**) ultrasound view of injection with *arrow* representing needle path for proximal to distal in plane approach. N, median nerve.

References

1. Dammers JW, Veering MM, Vermuelen M. Injection with methylprednisolone proximal to the carpal tunnel: randomized double blind trial. *Br Med J.* 1999;319:884–886.
2. Jamadar DA, Jacobson JA, Hayes CW. Sonographic evaluation of the median nerve at the wrist. *J Ultrasound Med.* 2001;20:1011–1014.
3. Propeck T, Quinn TJ, Jacobson JA, et al. Sonography and MR imaging of bifid median nerve with anatomic and histologic correlation. *AJR Am J Roentgenol.* 2000;175:1721–1725.
4. Racasan O, Dubert T. The safest location for steroid injection in the treatment of carpal tunnel syndrome. *J Hand Surg Br.* 2005;30:412–414.
5. Smith J, Wisniewski SJ, Finnoff JT, Payne JM. Sonographically guided carpal tunnel injection: the ulnar approach. *J Ultrasound Med.* Oct 2008;27(10):1485–1490.

Paul D. Tortland, DO, FAOASM

KEY POINTS

- Use a high-frequency, linear array transducer.
- Use a 25-gauge, 1- to 1.5-inch needle.
- Applying too much probe pressure will compress and obscure the view of the nerve.

- The nerve is easiest to track by starting more proximal and tracing its distal path.

Anatomy

The superficial branch of the radial nerve originates from the radial nerve just proximal and anterior to the radiocapitellar joint, between the brachialis and brachioradialis muscles (Figure 44-1). Roughly at the level of the radiocapitellar joint, the nerve bifurcates into a deep motor branch and a superficial sensory branch, the *cutaneous* or *superficial radial nerve* (Figure 44-2).

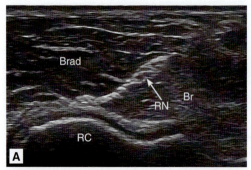

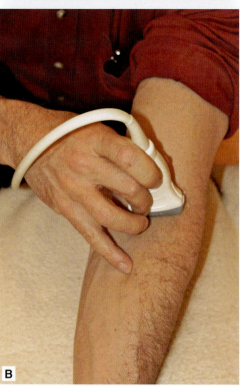

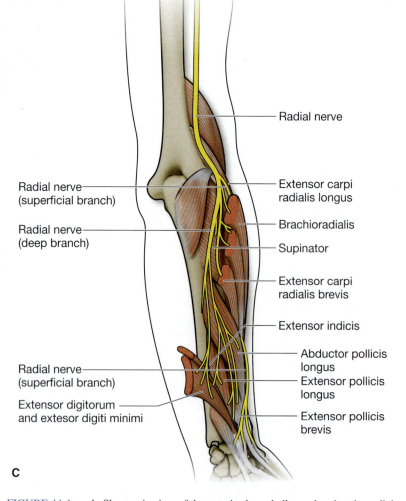

FIGURE 44-1 ■ **A.** Short-axis view of the anterior lateral elbow, showing the radial nerve (RN) lying between the brachialis (Br) and brachioradialis (Brad) muscles, anterior to the radiocapitellar joint (RC). **B.** Probe position for image seen in Figure 44-1A. **C.** Anatomy of the radial nerve and its main branches.

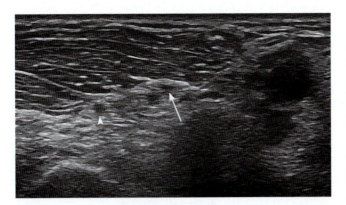

FIGURE 44-2 ▪ Short-axis view of the anterior elbow, just distal to Figure 44-1A, showing the beginning of the bifurcation of the radial nerve into the deep branch of the radial nerve (*arrow head*) and the superficial radial nerve (*arrow*). The left side of the screen is radial/lateral.

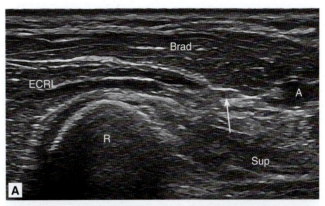

The superficial branch at first lies radial to the radial artery, beside which it travels, beneath the brachioradialis (Figure 44-3). Roughly 7 cm proximal to the wrist, the superficial branch diverges from the artery, passes beneath the tendon of the brachioradialis, and, piercing the deep fascia, ultimately emerges between that muscle and the extensor carpi radialis longus tendon at the junction of the proximal two-thirds to distal one-third of the forearm. The nerve then courses in a superficial subcutaneous plane before finally emerging even more superficially next to the tendons of the second dorsal wrist compartment just proximal to the intersection of the first and second dorsal wrist compartments (Figure 44-4).

The nerve provides sensation to the dorsal aspect of the hand from the thumb to the junction of the ring and long fingers. Sensation to the digits is provided up to the area of approximately the dorsal proximal interphalangeal joint.

Pathology

Symptoms of entrapment of the superficial radial nerve can include decreased sensation, paresthesia, and tingling in the distribution of the superficial radial nerve. A positive Tinel and compression sign may be present at the site of exit of the nerve. The symptoms are often provoked by extreme pronation of the wrist. The constellation of symptoms seen in superficial radial nerve entrapment is also known *Wartenberg syndrome.*

Repetitive movement, direct trauma, and compression all can affect the nerve. Compression occurs most commonly at one or more sites: by fascial bands in the subcutaneous tissue at the nerve's exit site; by the tendons of the brachioradialis; and by the extensor carpi radialis longus tendon.

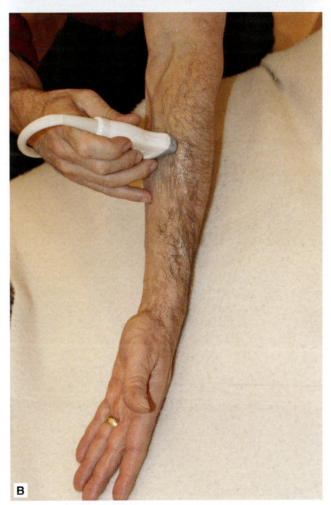

FIGURE 44-3 ▪ **A.** Short-axis view through the mid volar forearm, toward the radial side. The superficial branch of the radial nerve (*arrow*) can be seen lying in the fascia deep to the brachioradialis (Brad). A, radial artery; ECRL, extensor carpi radialis longus; R, radius; Sup, supinator. The left side of the image is radial/lateral. **B.** Probe position corresponding to the image seen in Figure 44-3A.

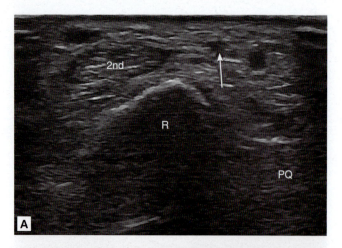

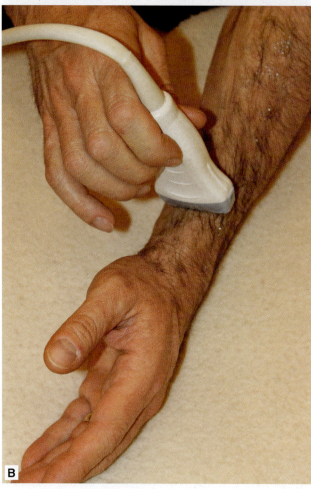

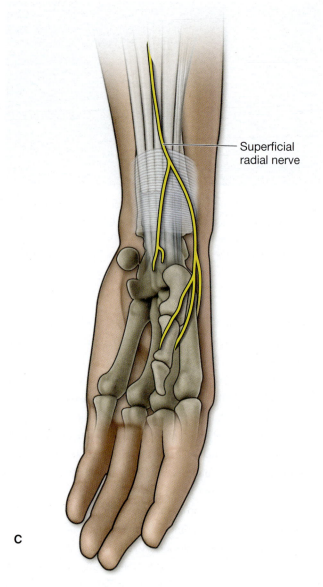

FIGURE 44-4 ■ **A.** Short-axis image through the distal volar radial forearm. The superficial branch of the radial nerve (*arrow*) is seen just prior to piercing the superficial fascia. 2nd, tendons of the second dorsal wrist compartment; PQ, pronator quadratus muscle; R, radius. **B.** Probe position corresponding to image seen in Figure 44-4A. **C.** Anatomy of the superficial radial nerve.

Ultrasound Image Findings

The superficial radial nerve normally is very small and can be difficult to find. As a result, a transverse or short-axis view is best; the nerve quickly gets lost in the surrounding connective tissue when attempting to view it in long axis. It is most easily located over the radial wrist lying between and just superficial to the first and second dorsal wrist compartments. Because the nerve lies so superficially, scanning is best done with a high-frequency linear array transducer at a depth typically of no more than 2 cm.

Start first by placing the transducer transverse to the wrist and locating Lister's tubercle. Use a light touch; moderate or heavy probe pressure will compress the subcutaneous tissue and fascial planes, obscuring landmarks and making the nerve indistinguishable from surrounding tissue.

Slowly perform a long-axis radial slide to bring both the first and second dorsal compartments into view. The nerve lies in a small superficial fascial pocket between the two compartments (more toward the first compartment), as seen in Figure 44-5A.

The nerve can be followed proximally by slowly performing a short-axis linear array slide with the transducer up the radial forearm. In so doing, the tendons of the first dorsal compartment will be seen sliding in the ulnar direction over the tendons of the second dorsal compartment (site of the *intersection syndrome*). Simultaneously, the overlying nerve moves in the *opposite* direction of the tendons of the first compartment (note the relative change in position of the nerve from (Figure 44-5A to 44-5B). Just proximal to the intersection the nerve starts to dive deeper.

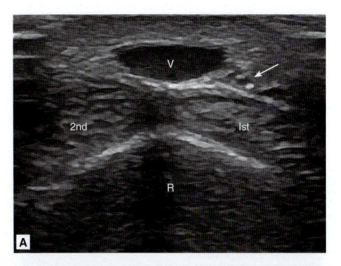

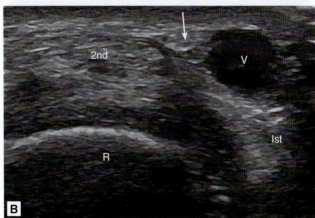

FIGURE 44-5 ■ **A** and **B.** Short-axis view of the dorsal wrist, just radial to Lister's tubercle. Note the different positions of the nerves in relation to the first and second dorsal compartment and overlying vessel. *Arrow,* superficial branch of the radial nerve; 1st, first dorsal wrist compartment; 2nd, second dorsal wrist compartment; R, radius; V, vein.

Equipment

- Needle: 25-gauge, 1.5-inch needle
- Injectate
  - Nerve block: 2 mL of local anesthetic ± injectable corticosteroids
  - Nerve hydrodissection and decompression: 5–10 mL of total solution (combination of normal saline, local anesthetic, ± dextrose solution)
- High-frequency linear array transducer

Author's Preferred Technique

a. Patient position
  i. Patient is seated across table from physician with affected arm resting on table, radius upward.
  ii. Alternate position: Patient lies prone on table, arm outstretched overhead, radial side up.
b. Transducer position (Figure 44-6)
  i. Short axis to superficial radial nerve at the target site
c. Needle orientation relative to the transducer (Figure 44-7)
  i. Out of plane
  ii. Use walk-down technique
d. Needle approach (see Figure 44-7)
  i. Distal to proximal
  ii. Once the needle is approximated to the center of the nerve in short axis, switch to long-axis view of nerve (in-plane view of needle)
e. Target
  i. Superficial radial nerve
f. Pearls and Pitfalls
  i. Most often the nerve is easier to find by initially identifying it more proximally in the forearm and then tracing it distally.
  ii. The nerve is extremely superficial. When using the walk-down technique, be sure to start at a very superficial trajectory.
  iii. Applying too much pressure with the transducer will distort the field of view, making it difficult to identify the nerve.

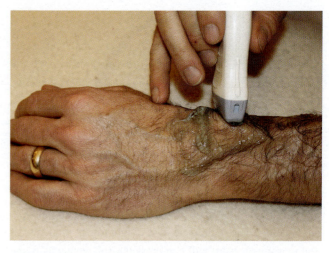

FIGURE 44-6 ▪ Probe position corresponding to image in Figure 44-5A with transducer short axis to nerve. Note that the probe has been moved in the radial direction from Figure 44-4B.

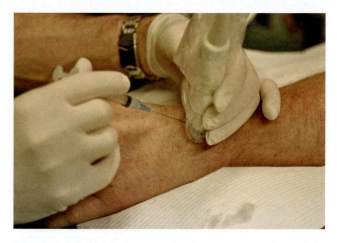

FIGURE 44-7 ▪ Out-of-plane approach to the superficial radial nerve.

Alternate Technique

a. Patient position
    i. Patient is seated across table from physician with affected arm resting on table, radius upward.
    ii. Alternate position: Patient lies prone on table, arm outstretched overhead, radial side up.
b. Transducer position (see Figure 44-6)
    i. Short axis to superficial radial nerve at the target site
c. Needle orientation relative to the transducer (Figure 44-8)
    i. In plane
d. Needle approach (see Figure 44-8)
    i. Posterior to anterior
e. Target
    i. Superficial radial nerve
f. Pearls and Pitfalls
    i. This technique allows visualization of the entire needle throughout the procedure.
    ii. It is easier to get to the undersurface of the nerve with this technique, but it does not allow as much room for hydrodissection as the first technique.
    iii. One must be more careful of neurovascular structures with this technique and plan the procedure accordingly.

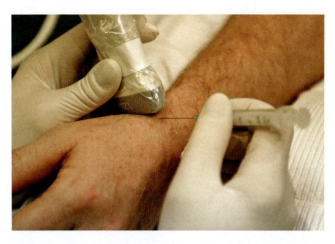

FIGURE 44-8 ▪ Alternate in-plane approach to the superficial radial nerve.

References

1. Bianchi S, Martinoli C. *Ultrasound of the Musculoskeletal System*. Berlin: Springer-Verlag; 2007.
2. Robson AJ, See MS, Ellis H. Applied anatomy of the superficial branch of the radial nerve. *Clin Anat.* 2008;21(1):38–45.

Pelvis

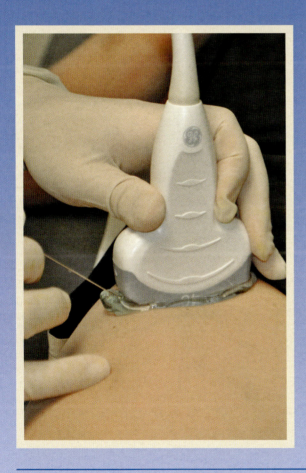

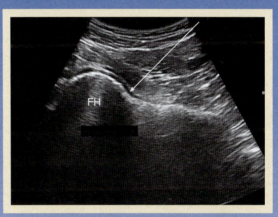

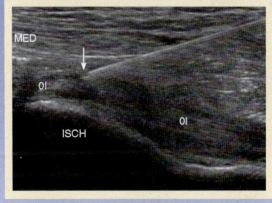

Mark-Friedrich Berthold Hurdle, MD

KEY POINTS

- Use a 25–23-gauge, 3.5-inch needle.
- A high-frequency curvilinear array transducer is required for most patients.
- The sacroiliac joint is usually most accessible at the caudal pole.
- The probe is placed in an axial plane over the joint.

Pertinent Anatomy

The sacroiliac joint is a diarthrodial joint consisting of the articulation of the lateral sacrum with posterior medial ilium (Figure 45-1A, B). The joint is stabilized by posterior sacroiliac ligament, sacrospinous ligament, sacrotuberous ligament (Figure 45-1C). The cephalad portion of the posterior joint contains the interosseous ligament and is not a true joint capsule.

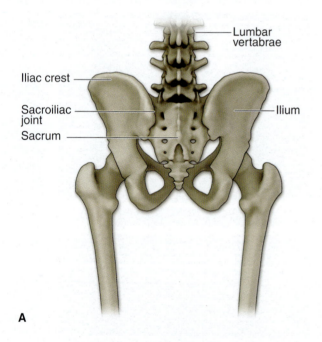

A

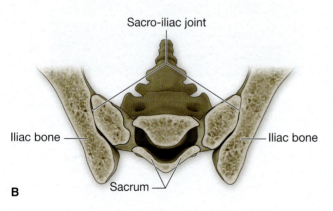

B

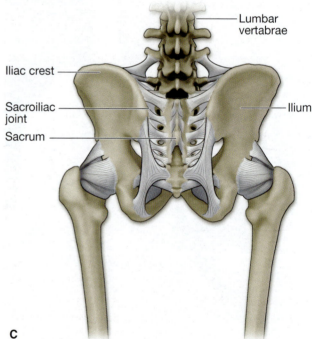

C

FIGURE 45-1 ■ **A** and **B.** Boney anatomy of the sacroiliac joint. **C.** Ligamentous structures about the sacroiliac joint.

Common Pathology

A host of conditions including degenerative changes, joint infections, structural abnormalities, inflammatory disorders, pregnancy, joint dysfunction, and metabolic conditions have been implicated in sacroiliac joint pain. Sacroiliac joint (SIJ) pain referral patterns may overlap other painful conditions involving the low back and lower extremities. Typically, sacroiliac pain involves the posterior superior iliac crest region of the affected side radiating distally. Although a host of provocative maneuvers are helpful in establishing the diagnosis, an intraarticular injection can help with confirmation.

Ultrasound Imaging Findings

The SIJ is best visualized using a curvilinear probe initially placed directly over the posterior superior iliac crest on the side of interest (Figure 45-2). The S1 foramen can be visualized medial to the cleft of the upper portion of the SIJ. The probe is then kept in the axial plane and slid distally until the lower pole is seen close to the posterior sacral foramen of S2.

Indications for Injections of the Sacroiliac Joint

Injection of the SIJ can be performed on patients with SIJ pain that does not respond to conservative interventions including physical therapy, relative rest, antiinflammatories, and modalities. Injection of the SIJ has been described based on palpation and fluoroscopic guidance. The success rate of unguided injections has been found to be 12% with fluoroscopy as the control.[1] Ultrasound-guided SIJ injections have been described by Klauser et al. and Pekkafahli et al. with an accuracy rate between 76% and 93%.[2,3] Clinical outcomes of ultrasound-guided versus fluoroscopically guided sacroiliac joints have not been described.

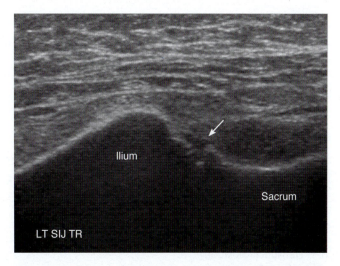

FIGURE 45-2 ▪ Ultrasound image of superior sacroiliac joint. *Arrow* points to joint opening.

Equipment

■ Needle: 25–23-gauge, 3.5-inch needle
■ Injectate
  • 1 mL local anesthetic
  • 1 mL of an injectable corticosteroid
■ High-frequency curvilinear array transducer

Author's Preferred Technique

a. Patient position
  i. Prone with pillow placed under pelvis for mild hip flexion
b. Transducer position
  i. Anatomic axial plane first over the posterior superior iliac spine (PSIS), then distally over the caudal one-third of the SIJ (Figure 45-3)
c. Needle orientation relative to the transducer
  i. In plane (see Figure 45-3)
d. Needle approach (Figure 45-4)
  i. Medial to lateral starting 2 cm medial to SIJ superficially
  ii. In-plane technique

Alternate Technique

a. Patient position
  i. Prone with pillow placed under the pelvis for mild hip flexion
b. Transducer position
  i. Anatomic axial plane first over the PSIS, then distally over the caudal one-third of the SIJ (see Figure 45-3)
c. Needle orientation relative to the transducer
  i. Out of plane
d. Needle approach
  i. Caudal to cephalad starting 1 cm caudal to SIJ
e. Pearls and Pitfalls
  i. Once the needle is in place, color Doppler can be used to visualize potential retrograde flow out of the hypoechoic clef between the ilium and sacrum.
  ii. Unfortunately, an intravascular injection would be difficult to detect once the needle tip is deep to the joint capsule.

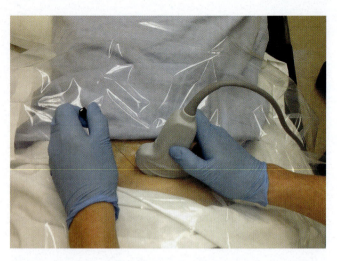

FIGURE 45-3 ■ Ultrasound probe position for sacroiliac joint injection.

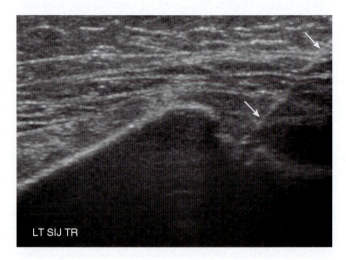

FIGURE 45-4 ■ Ultrasound image of needle positioned in the superior sacroiliac joint; in-plane, medial-to-lateral approach. *Arrows* point out needle as it enters SI joint.

References

1. Hanson HC. Is fluoroscopy necessary for sacroiliac joint injections? *Pain Physician* 2003;6(2):155–158.
2. Klauser A, De Zordo T, Feuchtner G, et al. Feasibility of ultrasound-guided sacroiliac joint injection considering sonoanatomic landmarks at two different levels in cadavers and patients. *Arthritis Rheum* 2008;59:1618–1624.
3. Pekkafahli MZ, Kiralp MZ, Basekim CC, et al. Sacroiliac joint injections performed with sonographic guidance. *J Ultrasound Med* 2003;22:553–559.

Jerod A. Cottrill, DO

KEY POINTS

- Use a low-frequency curvilinear array transducer.
- Use a long-axis, in-plane approach with a 22-gauge needle.
- Guided injection improves accuracy and has both diagnostic and therapeutic value.

- The anterior recess is the most accessible target for intraarticular hip injection on most patients, with optimal needle placement at or just proximal to the femoral head-neck junction.

Pertinent Anatomy

The hip joint is a ball and socket synovial joint with a thick surrounding extraarticular capsule, formed by the iliofemoral, ischiofemoral, and pubofemoral ligaments that extend over the femoral head and neck (Figure 46-1). The proximal femoral head articulates with the pelvic acetabulum, which is lined with a fibro-cartilaginous labrum.

Typically the labrum appears as a homogeneously hyperechoic triangular structure on ultrasound, with an appearance analogous to the knee meniscus. The iliofemoral ligament is appreciated superficial to the labrum anteriorly. The capsule originates from the acetabulum and acetabular labrum and inserts laterally at the intertrochanteric line. However, there is a deep layer that folds back from the intertrochanteric line and inserts at the femoral head-neck junction. Thus, the hip joint capsule is comprised of a single layer from the acetabular rim to the femoral head-neck junction, and two layers from the femoral head-neck junction to the intertrochanteric line.

The femoral neurovascular bundle descends through the femoral triangle formed by the sartorius laterally, adductor longus medially, and the inguinal ligament superiorly. It is separated from the hip joint by the iliopsoas muscle and tendon. The femoral artery feeds the deep femoral artery, which then divides into the medial and lateral circumflex arteries that supply the femoral head and neck. The posterior division of the obturator artery also contributes a branch that traverses the ligamentum teres to supply the femoral head. Innervation of the hip joint is provided by branches of the femoral, obturator and sciatic nerves.

Common Pathology

Hip pain is common, and the incidence of osteoarthrosis of weight-bearing joints is increasing in the United States, with an aging population and the rising prevalence of obesity. The hip joint is a common site of osteoarthrosis, both degenerative and

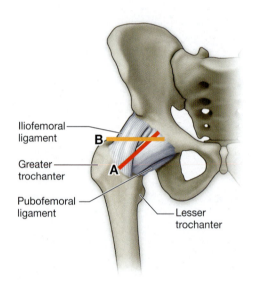

FIGURE 46-1 ■ Anterior view of the hip capsule. *Red line* (**A**), transducer position for first injection technique; *Yellow line* (**B**), transducer position for second injection technique.

traumatic, as well as a site that may be affected by inflammatory arthropathies. Hip osteoarthrosis is often symptomatic in weight-bearing activities, but as it advances, it can cause significant pain with transitional movements and at night. Management options include activity modification, physical therapy, weight loss, analgesics, intraarticular steroids, visco-supplementation, and total hip arthroplasty.[1] In the past, intraarticular hip injections have been performed with palpation guidance using anatomical landmarks, as well as under guidance using fluoroscopy, computed tomography (CT), and ultrasound.[2,3]

Indications for Intraarticular Hip Injection

Intraarticular injection of anesthetic can facilitate identification of the source of pain, and precision significantly increases the diagnostic value.[4] Intraarticular corticosteroid injections in the hip have clearly been shown to decrease pain and increase range of motion.[3] Based on the inherent deep location and variable body habitus, palpation-guided injections lack accuracy, as well as pose undue risk of damage or irritation to the neurovascular structures.[2] Fluoroscopy and CT guidance entail significant cost and result in radiation exposure. Fluoroscopy does not visualize the neurovascular bundle. Ultrasound is portable, inexpensive, and does not result in any radiation exposure to the practitioner or patient. It also provides delineation of the more superficial soft-tissue structures. Several studies have been published confirming the accuracy of ultrasound-guided intraarticular hip injections.[5-8]

Equipment

■ Needle: 22–25-gauge, 3.5-inch spinal needle
■ Injectate
  • 3–4 mL of anesthetic
  • 1–2 mL of injectable corticosteroids
■ Low-frequency curvilinear array transducer

Author's Preferred Technique

a. Patient position
   i. Supine with a pillow under knees for comfort and to relax the superficial structures around the joint
b. Transducer position (Figure 46-2A)
   i. Anteriorly in the oblique sagittal plane, parallel with the femoral neck
c. Needle orientation relative to the transducer
   i. In plane
d. Needle approach (see Figure 46-2B)
   i. Caudolateral to cephalomedial
e. Target (see Figure 46-2B)
   i. Anterior synovial recess, located at the junction of the femoral head and neck
f. Pearls and Pitfalls
   i. Use lower frequency probe for better visualization of deeper structures.
   ii. Always identify the presence of the lateral circumflex femoral artery (Figure 46-3) as it will often be in the projected trajectory of the needle.
   iii. Visualize the femoral neurovascular bundle medially.
   iv. Needle visualization may be difficult in deeper structures, especially if significant subcutaneous tissue is present, reducing the conspicuity of the target.

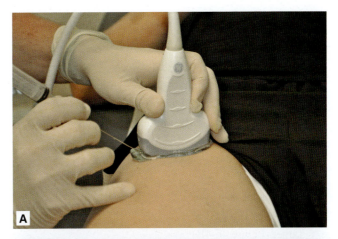

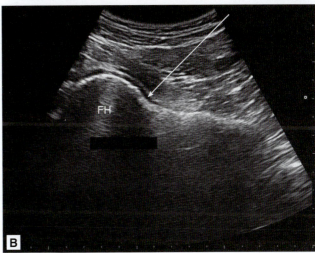

FIGURE 46-2 ■ Anterior sagittal oblique approach. **A.** Transducer position for in-plane approach to hip joint. **B.** Ultrasound image with target the anterior recess of the joint capsule at or just proximal to the femoral head-neck junction. *Arrow* indicates desired path of needle to target site. FH, femoral head.

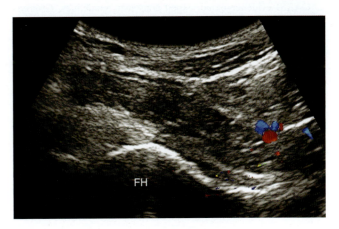

FIGURE 46-3 ■ Lateral femoral circumflex vasculature in anterior sagittal approach.

Alternate Technique

a. Patient Position

    i. Supine with a pillow under knees for comfort and to relax the superficial structures around the joint

b. Transducer position (Figure 46-4A)

    i. Anteriorly, slightly oblique with transducer short axis to the femoral head

c. Needle orientation relative to the transducer

    i. In plane

d. Needle approach

    i. Lateral to medial

e. Target (Figure 46-4B)

    i. Hip joint deep to the joint capsule

f. Pearls and Pitfalls

    i. This may be an easier technique with patients of larger body habitus as one can often better visualize the needle because of a more parallel trajectory with the transducer.

    ii. Be sure to maintain visualization of the tip of your needle at all times, especially to ensure you avoid the more medial neurovascular bundle.

    iii. See "Pearls and Pitfalls" under "Author's Preferred Technique."

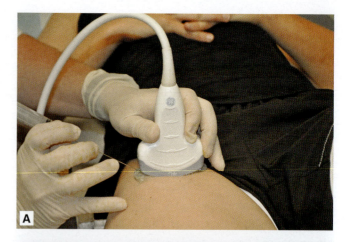

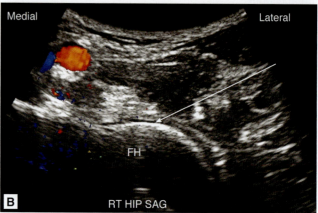

FIGURE 46-4 ■ Anterior transverse approach. **A.** Transducer position for alternate approach to hip joint. **B.** Ultrasound image with target the anterior recess of the joint capsule. *Arrow* indicates desired path of needle to target site. FH, femoral head.

References

1. Zhang W, Moskowitz RW, Nuki G, et al. OARSI recommendations for the management of hip and knee osteoarthritis, part II: OARSI evidence-based, expert consensus guidelines. *Osteoarthritis Cartilage* 2008;16(2):137–162.

2. Leopold SS, Battista V, Oliverio JA. Safety and efficacy of intraarticular hip injection using anatomic landmarks. *Clin Orthop Relat Res* 2001;391:192–197.

3. Kullenberg B, Runesson R, Tuvhag R, et al. Intraarticular corticosteroid injection: pain relief in osteoarthritis of the hip? *J Rheumatol* 2004;31(11)2265–2268.

4. Crawford RW, Lie GA, Ling RS, et al. Diagnostic value of intra-articular anaesthetic in primary osteoarthritis of the hip. *J Bone Joint Surg Br* 1998;80(2):279–281.

5. Robinson P, Keenan AM, Conaghan PG. Clinical effectiveness and dose response of image-guided intra-articular corticosteroid injection for hip osteoarthritis. *Rheumatology (Oxford)* 2007;46(2):285–291.

6. Sofka CM, Saboeiro G, Adler RS. Ultrasound-guided adult hip injections. *J Vasc Interv Radiol* 2005;16(8):1121–1123.

7. Smith J, Hurdle MF, Weingarten TN. Accuracy of sonographically guided intra-articular injections in the native adult hip. *J Ultrasound Med* 2009;28(3):329–335.

8. Pourbagher MA, Ozalay M, Pourbagher A. Accuracy and outcome of sonographically guided intra-articular sodium hyaluronate injections in patients with osteoarthritis of the hip. *J Ultrasound Med* 2005;24(10):1391–1395.

Marko Bodor, MD / Sean Colio, MD

KEY POINTS

- Use the highest possible frequency transducer that still permits adequate depth penetration to ensure accurate visualization of the paralabral cyst.
- A 18–22-gauge, 2.5–3.5-inch needle is recommended for the procedure.
- Visualize the cyst in at least two planes and with color Doppler to ensure accurate diagnosis and that it is not a vein, anisotropic psoas tendon, or solid tumor.

- Choose an inferior, inferior-lateral or lateral approach, whichever best visualizes the cyst and avoids neurovascular structures.
- If unable to aspirate the cyst, consider rupturing it with normal saline or perforating it several times to disperse its contents.

Pertinent Anatomy

The hip labrum is a continuous fibrocartilaginous structure, triangular in cross-section, attached to the bony rim of the acetabulum (Figure 47-1). The labrum is 2–3 mm thick and is composed of thick type I collagen fiber bundles arranged mostly parallel but also oblique to the acetabular rim.[1] The labrum increases the surface area of the acetabulum by 28%.[2] Synovium lines its edge, forming a sulcus and sealing the joint capsule. An intact labrum and joint capsule allows for maintenance of a fluid layer between the articular surfaces of the femoral head and acetabulum, reducing friction and shear on the cartilage, and for fluid pressurization, reducing focal loading.[1,2] The blood supply of the labrum enters its outermost capsular surface layer leaving its central articular margin less vascular, similar to a knee meniscus.

Common Pathology

Labral tears are classified as anterior, posterior, or superior-lateral, with the most common location being anterior. They can also be classified morphologically as radial flap, radial fibrillated, longitudinal peripheral, and unstable.[1,3] Labral tears may be caused by acute or repetitive trauma in conjunction with hip dysplasia, femoral-acetabular impingement, capsular laxity and osteoarthritis.[1,4] Labral tears can be asymptomatic or result in symptoms of groin, buttock, or lateral hip pain and clicking.

Paralabral cysts occur in the presence of labral tears and are caused by leakage of joint fluid through the tear (Figure 47-2). These cysts may contain synovial or mucinous fluid, depending on chronicity and whether there is active communication with the joint.[3] Paralabral cysts can be asymptomatic

(Figure 47-3) or impinge on adjacent structures, such as the iliopsoas tendon causing internal snapping hip,[5] or the femoral nerve, causing femoral neuropathy (Figure 47-4).

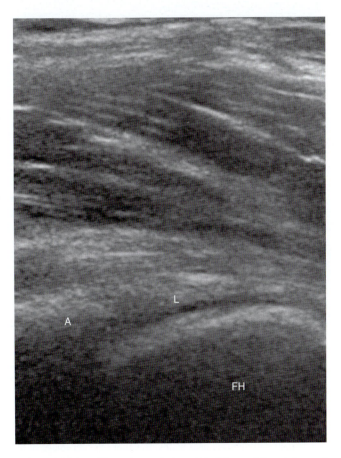

FIGURE 47-1 ■ Normal acetabulum (A), labrum (L) and femoral head (FH): Image with the transducer aligned with the long-axis of the thigh.

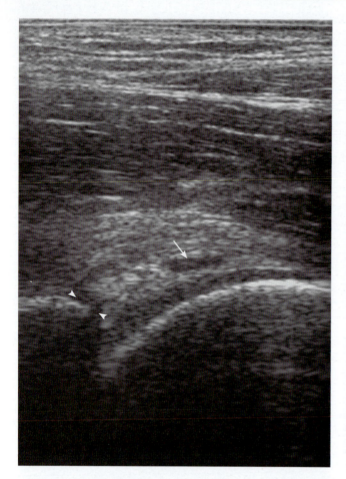

FIGURE 47-2 ■ Torn hip labrum (*arrowheads*) with paralabral cyst (*arrow*) in a symptomatic patient.

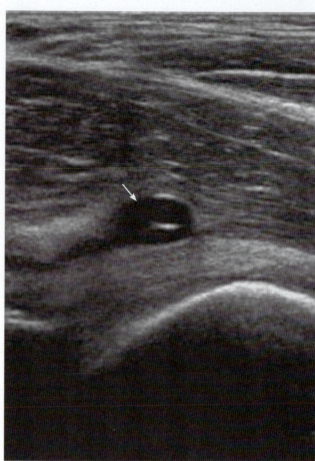

FIGURE 47-3 ■ Paralabral cyst (*arrow*) in an asymptomatic patient.

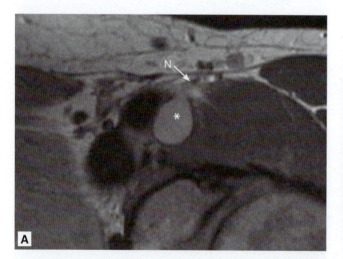

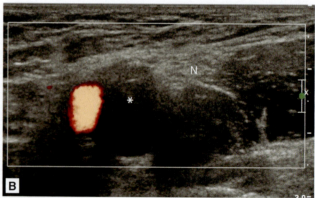

FIGURE 47-4 ■ **A.** Axial proton density magnetic resonance image shows a paralabral cyst (*asterisk*) contacting the femoral nerve (*N-arrow*) in a patient with femoral neuropathy. **B.** Color Doppler image of the cyst (*asterisk*) shows displacement of the femoral nerve (N) and artery (*bright signal*).

Ultrasound Imaging Findings

The presence of groin, buttock, or hip pain in the setting of normal hip radiographs and or magnetic resonance imaging raises the suspicion of a labral tear. Labral tears appear as thin hypoechoic or anechoic gaps between the acetabulum and the labrum (see Figure 47-2). Troelsen et al. reported a sensitivity of 94% and a positive predictive value of 94% in detecting anterior labral tears.[6] Using high-frequency linear array transducers, the authors have experienced a positive predictive value of 100% in diagnosing 27 consecutive arthroscopically confirmed anterior labral tears.

Paralabral cysts are typically round or fusiform fluid collections seen above the labrum. A thin stalk of fluid connecting the paralabral cyst with the labral tear and joint may be visualized (see Figure 47-2).

Indications for Aspiration of Paralabral Cyst of the Hip

The primary indication for aspiration of a hip paralabral cyst is suspicion that the patient's symptoms and findings, such as pain, a snapping iliopsoas tendon, or femoral neuropathy, are attributable to the cyst.

Equipment

- Needle
  - 25-gauge, 1.5–2-inch needle for local anesthetic
  - 18–22 gauge, 2.5–3.5-inch needle for aspiration and fenestration
- Injectate
  - 0.5 mL of local anesthesia
  - 0.5 mL of an injectable corticosteroid
  - For rupture of cyst, use 2–3 mL sterile saline
- Medium- to high-frequency linear array or curvilinear array transducer, depending on body habitus and depth of cyst

Author's Preferred Technique

a. Patient position
   i. Supine with pillow under the head and appropriate draping to expose the inguinal region (Figure 47-5)

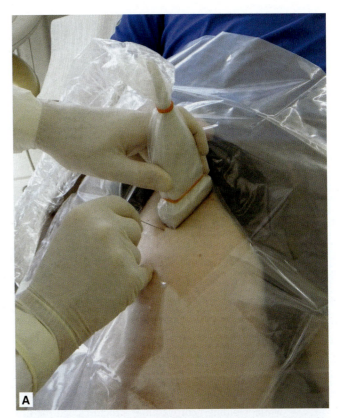

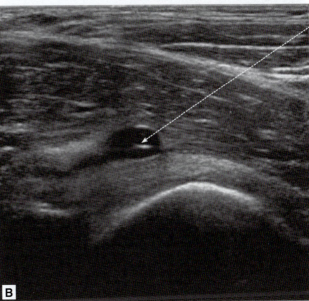

FIGURE 47-5 ■ **A.** Inferior-lateral approach for paralabral cyst aspiration. **B.** Image shows the paralabral cyst and needle trajectory (*segmented arrow*).

b. Transducer position
   i. Aligned with the long-axis of the thigh for an inferior, the femoral neck for an inferior-oblique (see Figure 47-5), or transverse to the thigh for a lateral approach (Figure 47-6), whichever best visualizes the cyst while avoiding neurovascular structures
c. Needle orientation relative to the transducer (Figure 47-5)
   i. In plane
d. Needle approach (Figure 47-5)
   i. Inferior, inferior-lateral, or lateral depending on cyst location
e. Target
   i. Middle of paralabral cyst
f. Pearls and Pitfalls
   i. Perform a preliminary scan to identify the paralabral cyst and the femoral nerve, artery and vein.
   ii. Confirm the cyst in at least two planes and use color Doppler to ensure it is not a vascular structure, anisotropic psoas tendon, or solid tumor.
   iii. Choose an approach, either inferior, inferior-lateral, or lateral, which provides the best view of the cyst while avoiding neurovascular structures and the hip labrum.
   iv. If unable to aspirate the cyst using a 22-gauge needle, attempt aspiration with an 18-gauge needle, or consider rupturing it with normal saline or fenestrating it to disperse its contents.

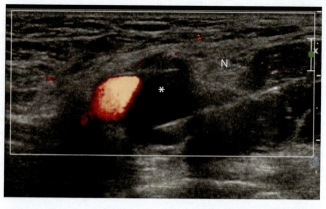

FIGURE 47-6 ■ Lateral approach for paralabral cyst aspiration (same patient as in Figure 47-4). Color Doppler image shows the tip of a 20-gauge needle within the cyst (*asterisk*) moments before successful aspiration. Notice proximity to neurovascular structures making precise guidance necessary for this procedure. N, nerve.

References

1. Groh MM, Herrera J. A comprehensive review of hip labral tears. *Curr Rev Musculoskelet Med* 2009;2(2):105–117.
2. Tan V, Seldes RM, Katz MA, et al. Contribution of acetabular labrum to articulating surface area and femoral head coverage in adult hip joints: an anatomic study in cadavera. *Am J Orthop* 2001;30(11):809–812.
3. Bharam S. Labral tears, extra-articular injuries, and hip arthroscopy in the athlete. *Clin Sports Med* 2006;25(2):279–292.
4. Robertson WJ, Kadrmas WR, Kelly BT. Arthroscopic management of labral tears in the hip: a systematic review. *Clin Orthop Relat Res* 2007;455:88–92.
5. Deslandes M, Guillin R, Cardinal E, et al. The snapping iliopsoas tendon: new mechanisms using dynamic sonography. *AJR Am J Roentgenol* 2008;190(3):576–581.
6. Troelsen A, Mechlenburg I, Gelineck J, et al. What is the role of clinical tests and ultrasound in acetabular labral tear diagnostics? *Acta Orthopaedica* 2009;80(3):314–318.

Ched Garten, MD

KEY POINTS

- Using 22–25-gauge needles with an out-of-plane approach is preferred.
- Use a high-frequency linear array transducer.
- The pubic symphysis is widest anteriorly.
- There will be some resistance while injecting the fibrocartilage disc in the joint.

Pertinent Anatomy

The pubic symphysis is a nonsynovial amphiarthrodial joint connecting the left and right superior rami of the pelvis. The anterior portion of the joint is 3–5 mm wider than the posterior portion. The joint is connected by fibrocartilage and surrounded by ligaments. The superior and inferior ligaments provide most of the joint's stability. In normal adults, the joint has approximately 2 mm of translation and 1 degree of rotation (Figure 48-1).

Common Pathology

The pubic symphysis may be subject to a painful, noninfectious, inflammatory condition called *osteitis pubis*. Osteitis pubis is usually a pelvic stress injury. In general, there is no direct trauma that initiates the onset of pain. Biomechanical factors may place undo strain across the joint leading to chronic inflammation and persistent symptoms. This condition is most commonly seen in athletes that participate in sports that involve quick changes of direction (eg, football, soccer, ice hockey, etc.). On occasion, a sudden, forceful distraction of the legs may cause a traumatic injury to the joint.

In osteitis pubis, radiographs of the pelvis may reveal widening of the joint and cortical irregularity. Magnetic resonance imaging may reveal subchondral bone marrow edema, fluid in the joint, and periarticular edema in acute osteitis pubis, while subchondral sclerosis may also be seen in more chronic cases.[1] The pubic symphysis is also subject to infection in postoperative or postpartum patients. In patients with ankylosing spondylitis, bony fusion of the pubic symphysis may occur.

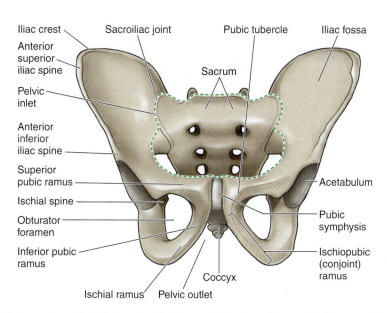

FIGURE 48-1 ■ Anatomy of the anterior pelvis. (Reproduced with permission from Morton DA, Foreman KB, Albertine KH, eds. *The Big Picture: Gross Anatomy*. New York: McGraw-Hill; 2011: figure 6-1B.)

Ultrasound Imaging Findings

The pubic symphysis is best visualized in long axis using a high-frequency linear array transducer and a depth of less than 3 cm in patients of normal body habitus (Figure 48-2). Common findings include thickening of the superior joint capsule, cortical irregularities, widening of the joint, and enthesopathies of the superior ligament.

Indications for Injections of the Symphysis Pubis

An injection of the pubic symphysis may be performed for patients with ongoing pain from osteitis pubis that has not responded to activity modification, icing, antiinflammatories, and physical therapy.

Injection of the pubic symphysis with fluoroscopic guidance has been described for the diagnosis and treatment of osteitis pubis in athletes.[2] A technique for palpation-guided injection of the pubic symphysis in athletes with osteitis pubis has also been described.[3] Both fluoroscopically guided and palpation-guided injections for osteitis pubis in the athlete have been found to promote a more rapid return to play. One study reported 87.5% of athletes having immediate relief and the ability to return to play 48 hours post procedure.[2] Desmond and Harmon have described ultrasound-guided pubic symphysis injection in pregnancy.[4] Clinical outcomes of palpation-guided versus image-guided injections of the symphysis pubis have not been described.

Equipment

- Needle: 22-gauge, 1.5-inch needle
- Injectate: 1 mL local anesthetic and 0.5–1 mL of injectable corticosteroid
- High-frequency linear array transducer

Author's Preferred Technique

a. Patient position
   i. Supine
b. Transducer position (Figure 48-3)
   i. Anatomic transverse plane over the anterior aspect of the pubic symphysis
c. Needle orientation relative to the transducer
   i. Out of plane
d. Needle approach (see Figure 48-3)
   i. Anterosuperior to posteroinferior
   ii. Use walk-down technique

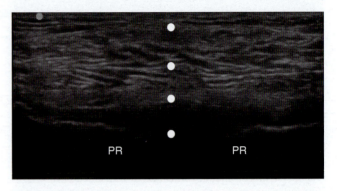

FIGURE 48-2 ▪ Long-axis view of pubic symphysis joint. *Dots represent walk-down technique into the joint space for out-of-plane injection. PR, pubic ramus.*

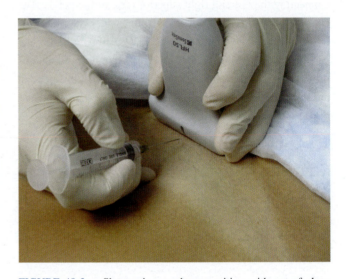

FIGURE 48-3 ▪ Short-axis transducer position with out-of-plane needle approach.

e. Target (Figure 48-2)

   i. Anterior pubic symphysis joint

f. Pearls and Pitfalls

   i. Because this joint is a nonsynovial joint, it is important to inject the fibrocartilage disc within the joint. Entering the fibrocartilage disc will give the clinician performing the injection the sensation of puncturing a block of cheese. If preferred, a 25-gauge needle may be used to anesthetize the soft tissue down to the joint; however, a 22-gauge needle is often needed to enter the joint.

   ii. Shaving the injection site will greatly improve the ease of preparation and injection.

   iii. An anterosuperior to posteroinferior approach is recommended to avoid vascular structures of the genitalia that are inferior to the joint.

   iv. Be sure not to puncture posterior to the joint as this may cause injury to the bladder.

Alternate Technique

a. Patient position

   i. Supine

b. Transducer position (Figure 48-4)

   i. Anatomic sagittal plane over the anterior aspect of the pubic symphysis

c. Needle orientation relative to the transducer

   i. In plane

d. Needle approach (see Figure 48-4)

   i. Anterosuperior to posteroinferior

   ii. Use a large amount of sterile gel for the oblique standoff approach. This will allow for easier entry of the needle using the in-plane approach.

e. Target (Figure 48-5)

   i. Anterior pubic symphysis joint

f. Pearls and Pitfalls

   i. A longer needle may be needed to reach the joint space when taking this approach.

   ii. To locate the fibrocartilage disc, find the pubic ramus in short axis and slide medially over the joint space. A hypoechoic region will appear, which represents the fibrocartilage disc. Entering the disc will give the clinician performing the injection the sensation of puncturing a block of cheese.

   iii. See "Pearls and Pitfalls" under "Author's Preferred Technique."

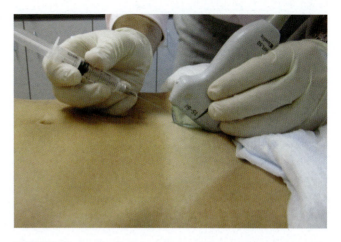

FIGURE 48-4 ▪ Sagittal transducer position with in-plane needle approach.

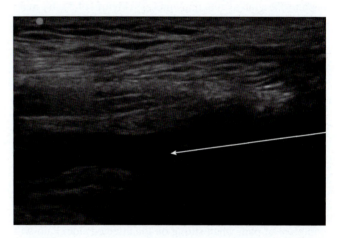

FIGURE 48-5 ▪ Short-axis view of pubic symphysis joint. *Arrow* indicates needle entry into the joint space Note the absence of cortical bone in the picture as this indicates the best view of the pubic symphysis joint for this technique.

References

1. Kunduracioglu B, et al. Magnetic resonance findings of osteitis pubis. *J Magn Reson Imaging* 2007;25:535–539.
2. O'Connell MJ, Powell T, McCaffrey NM, O'Connell D, Eustace SJ. Symphyseal cleft injection in the diagnosis and treatment of osteitis pubis in athletes. *AJR Am J Roentgenol* 2002;179(4):955–959.
3. Holt MA, Keene JS, Graf BK, Helwig DC. Treatment of osteitis pubis in athletes. Results of corticosteroid injections. *Am J Sports Med* 1995;23(5):601–606.
4. Desmond FA, Harmon D. Ultrasound-guided symphysis pubis injection in pregnancy. *Anesth Analg* 2010;111(5):1329–1330.

Steve J. Wisniewski, MD / Jay Smith, MD

KEY POINTS

- A medium-frequency linear array transducer or a low-frequency curvilinear array transducer will allow adequate visualization of the piriformis muscle with an axial oblique image from cephalomedial to caudolateral.
- Use a 22-gauge, 3.5-inch needle.

- The sciatic nerve must be identified during preprocedure scanning. It will most commonly be found deep to the piriformis muscle.
- The piriformis muscle can be injected with an in-plane, medial-to-lateral or lateral-to-medial approach.

Pertinent Anatomy

The piriformis muscle is a relatively small muscle that lies deep to the gluteus maximus muscle (Figure 49-1). Its main function is to externally rotate the hip. It originates on the anterior lateral sacrum, passes through the greater sciatic foramen, and inserts onto the superior greater trochanter. The sciatic nerve normally is found deep to the piriformis muscle, but occasionally the sciatic nerve or its peroneal division may pierce the piriformis muscle or be found superficial to it.

Common Pathology

The piriformis muscle is a potential cause of myofascial pain in patients presenting with gluteal pain. Patients will often complain of pain when sitting on the affected side. Pain will often be reproduced with stretching of the muscle and with focal palpation of the muscle in the sciatic notch. In addition, piriformis syndrome is a clinical condition characterized by gluteal pain and radicular leg pain, presumably due to involvement of the adjacent sciatic nerve.[1] This is often a diagnosis of exclusion, and may be confirmed with a diagnostic injection.

Ultrasound Imaging Findings

The piriformis muscle is best imaged in its long axis.[2,3] A low-frequency curvilinear array transducer will often be required to adequately visualize the muscle because of its deep location beneath the gluteus maximus muscle. Alternatively, a medium-frequency linear array transducer may suffice for some patients. The ultrasound transducer is initially placed horizontally across the posterior superior iliac spine. The transducer is then slowly moved caudally until the posterior

inferior iliac spine is visualized. As the transducer is moved just inferior to this, the ilium will disappear from view and the transducer will be over the greater sciatic notch. The medial end of the transducer remains on the sacrum while

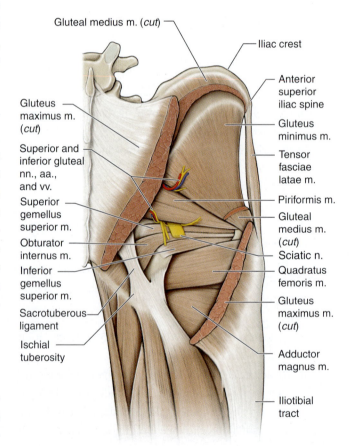

FIGURE 49-1 ■ Image of the gluteal region illustrating the deep gluteal muscles, including the piriformis muscle. (Reproduced with permission from Morton DA, Foreman KB, Albertine KH, eds. *The Big Picture: Gross Anatomy.* New York: McGraw-Hill; 2011: figure 35-1C.)

the lateral end of the transducer is then rotated caudally to visualize the piriformis muscle. The piriformis muscle will be found originating off the sacrum extending caudolaterally to insert onto the greater trochanter. Passive hip internal and external rotation is helpful to identify the piriformis muscle as it moves relative to the overlying gluteus maximus. The final ultrasound transducer position will be over the greater sciatic foramen, with an axial oblique image from cephalomedial to caudolateral (Figure 49-2).

Indications for Injections of the Piriformis Muscle

The diagnosis of piriformis syndrome is often a diagnosis of exclusion. In patients with persistent gluteal pain and/or radicular leg pain that has failed other conservative treatment options (medications, physical therapy, etc.), the piriformis muscle may be accurately injected under ultrasound guidance for diagnostic and therapeutic purposes. Injection of the piriformis muscle has previously been described with electrophysiologic guidance, computed tomography, magnetic resonance imaging, and fluoroscopy to ensure proper needle placement. However, a previous cadaveric study showed that ultrasound may be significantly more accurate than fluoroscopy.[3]

Equipment

- Needle: 22-gauge, 3.5-inch needle
- Injectate: local anesthetic with or without corticosteroid (total volume 3–4 mL)
- Medium-frequency linear array transducer or low-frequency curvilinear array transducer depending on body habitus and desired field of view

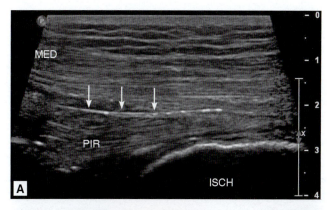

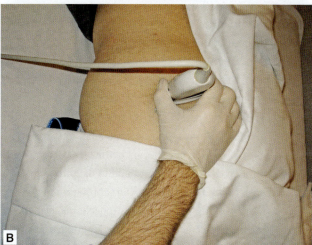

FIGURE 49-2 ▪ **A.** Long-axis ultrasound image of the piriformis muscle. *Arrows* indicate the piriformis muscle just deep to the gluteus maximus muscle. ISCH, ischium; MED, medial; PIR, piriformis muscle. **B.** Example of ultrasound probe position to visualize the piriformis muscle. The transducer is positioned from cephalomedial to caudolateral. Top of the picture is cephalad, left side of the picture is lateral.

Author's Preferred Technique

a. Patient position
   i. Prone
b. Transducer position (Figure 49-2)
   i. Axial oblique from cephalomedial to caudolateral over the piriformis muscle
c. Needle orientation relative to the transducer
   i. In plane
d. Needle approach
   i. Lateral to medial (or medial to lateral) (Figure 49-3)
e. Target (Figure 49-3)
   i. Piriformis muscle sheath and/or piriformis muscle
f. Pearls and Pitfalls
   i. The sciatic nerve position relative to the piriformis muscle should be identified with preprocedure scanning.
   ii. The sciatic nerve will most often be found deep to the piriformis muscle, but anatomic variations exist where the nerve or its peroneal division passes through or is found superficial to the piriformis.
   iii. Passive hip internal and external rotation may assist in identifying the piriformis muscle because of the relative movement of the muscle compared to the overlying gluteus maximus muscle.

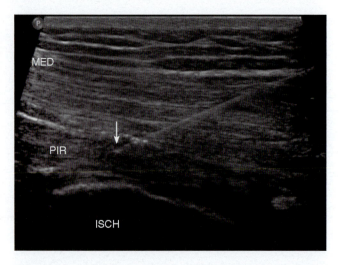

FIGURE 49-3 ■ Ultrasound image of intrapiriformis muscle needle placement. *Arrow* indicates needle tip. ISCH, ischium; MED, medial; PIR, piriformis muscle.

References

1. Windisch G, Braun EM, Anderhuber F. Piriformis muscle: clinical anatomy and consideration of the piriformis syndrome. *Surg Radiol Anat* 2007;29:37–45.
2. Smith J, Hurdle MF, Locketz AJ, et al. Ultrasound-guided piriformis injection: technique description and verification. *Arch Phys Med Rehabil* 2006;87:1664–1667.
3. Finnoff JT, Hurdle MFB, Smith J. Accuracy of ultrasound-guided versus fluoroscopically guided contrast–controlled piriformis injections: a cadaveric study. *J Ultrasound Med* 2008; 27:1157–1163.

Steve J. Wisniewski, MD / Jay Smith, MD

KEY POINTS

- Use a 22-gauge, 3.5-inch needle.
- A low-frequency curvilinear array transducer is preferred, although a medium-frequency linear array transducer may be used depending on body habitus and desired field of view.
- The obturator internus muscle and tendon can be visualized with ultrasound with the probe in an anatomic transverse plane over the posterior gluteal region.

- The sciatic nerve must be identified during preprocedure scanning. It will most commonly be found superficial to the lateral part of the obturator internus tendon.
- The obturator internus can be injected with an in-plane, medial-to-lateral or lateral-to-medial approach into the muscle or tendon sheath. The needle may also be guided to the region of the bursa, which lies between the tendon and ischium.

Pertinent Anatomy

The obturator internus muscle is a relatively small muscle that lies deep to the gluteus maximus muscle (Figure 50-1). It originates from the inner margin of the obturator foramen, obturator membrane, iliac bone, and base of the ischial spine, passes through the lesser sciatic foramen, and courses laterally to an insertion point on the medial greater trochanter.[1] The obturator internus bursa is located between the ischium and the overlying tendon. Along with the gluteus maximus and other short external rotators (eg, piriformis, quadratus femoris), the obturator internus functions as an external rotator of the thigh. The sciatic nerve normally is found superficial to the tendon.

Common Pathology

Obturator internus myofascial pain, tendinitis, tendinosis, and bursitis have been reported to be associated with gluteal and posterior hip pain.[1,2] Symptoms may be vague and poorly localized. The small size and deep location of the muscle or tendon may make accurate palpation and diagnosis difficult. Thus, a diagnostic injection of the muscle, tendon sheath, or bursa may be helpful to confirm the pain generator when clinically indicated.

Ultrasound Imaging Findings

Because of the small size and deep location of the obturator internus, the ability to visualize this muscle-tendon unit is dependent on patient body habitus and the specific ultrasound equipment used. The obturator internus muscle-tendon is best imaged in its long axis. A low-frequency, curvilinear array transducer will often be required to adequately visualize the muscle-tendon because of its deep location beneath the

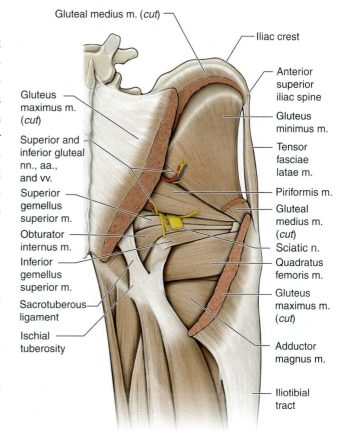

FIGURE 50-1 ■ Image of the gluteal region illustrating the deep gluteal muscles, including the obturator internus muscle. (Reproduced with permission from Morton DA, Foreman KB, Albertine KH, eds. *The Big Picture: Gross Anatomy*. New York: McGraw-Hill; 2011: figure 35-1C.)

gluteus maximus muscle, but thinner patients may be imaged with medium-frequency linear array transducers. The obturator internus may be best localized by first locating the piriformis muscle (see Chapter 49), then scanning caudad into the lesser sciatic foramen. As one scans caudad below the inferior border of the piriformis, the obturator internus will be seen emerging from the pelvis, passing over the ischium. Passively rotating the hip will produce motion in the obturator internus and assist in its identification. The sciatic nerve will usually be located just superficial to the lateral part of the tendon.

Indications for Injections of the Obturator Internus

The obturator internus muscle, tendon sheath, or bursa may be injected under ultrasound guidance to assist in the diagnostic evaluation and management of patients presenting with gluteal and posterior hip pain syndromes. Recently, Smith et al. validated sonographically guided techniques for injecting the obturator internus (OI) muscle or bursa using a cadaveric model.[3] They evaluated three different techniques of injecting the OI. They found that all 10 OI region injections accurately placed latex into the primary target site. Two of the four OI tendon sheath injections produced overflow into the underlying OI bursa. Both OI intramuscular injections delivered 100% of the latex within the OI. All four OI bursa injections (two trans tendinous and two short axis) delivered 100% of the latex into the OI bursa, with the exception that one OI bursa trans-tendinous injection produced minimal overflow into the OI itself. No injection resulted in injury to the sciatic nerve or gluteal arteries, and no injectate overflow occurred outside the confines of the OI or its bursa.

Equipment

- Needle: 22-gauge, 3.5-inch needle
- Injectate: local anesthetic with or without corticosteroid (total volume 3–4 mL)
- Low-frequency curvilinear array transducer; a medium-frequency linear array transducer depending on body habitus and desired field of view

Author's Preferred Technique

a. Patient position
   i. Prone
b. Transducer position (Figure 50-2)
   i. Long axis to the obturator internus muscle-tendon, in an anatomic transverse or axial plane

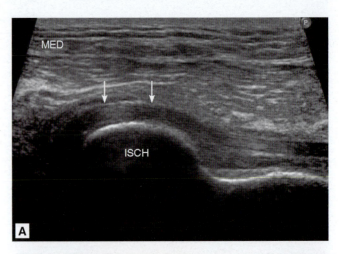

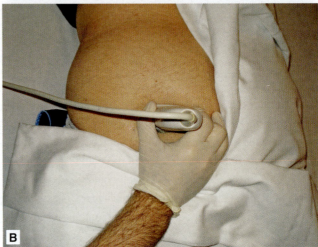

FIGURE 50-2 ■ **A.** Long-axis ultrasound image of the obturator internus. *Arrows* indicate obturator internus tendon. ISCH, ischium; MED, medial. **B.** Example of ultrasound probe position to visualize the obturator internus. The transducer is positioned long axis to the obturator internus muscle-tendon, in an anatomic transverse or axial plane. Top of the picture is cephalad, left side of the picture is lateral.

c. Needle orientation relative to the transducer
   i. In plane
d. Needle approach
   i. Medial to lateral or lateral to medial
e. Target (Figures 50-3 and 50-4)
   i. Obturator internus muscle, tendon sheath, or bursa. To access the bursa, the needle is passed through the muscle-tendon to the space between the obturator internus and the underlying ischium.
f. Pearls and Pitfalls
   i. The sciatic nerve must be identified in preprocedure scanning and avoided during the injection.
   ii. The nerve will most commonly be found just superficial to the lateral obturator internus tendon.

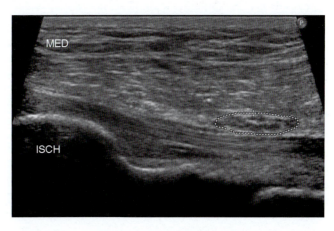

FIGURE 50-3 ■ Long-axis ultrasound image of the obturator internus. The sciatic nerve (*circled*) is seen just superficial to the lateral obturator internus tendon. ISCH, ischium; MED, medial.

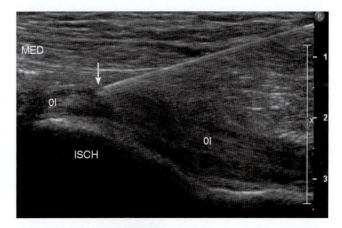

FIGURE 50-4 ■ Ultrasound image of obturator internus tendon sheath injection. *Arrow* indicates needle tip. ISCH, ischium; MED, medial; OI, obturator internus tendon.

References

1. Hwang JY, Lee SW, Kim JO. MR imaging features of obturator internus bursa of the hip. *Korean J Radiol* 2008;9:375–378.
2. Rohde RS, Ziran BH. Obturator internus tendinitis as a source of chronic hip pain. *Orthopedics* 2003;26(4):425–426.
3. Smith J, Wisniewski SJ, Wempe MK, Landry BW, Sellon JL. Sonographically guided obturator internus injections techniques and validation. *J Ultrasound Med* 2012;31:1597–1608.

Kimberly G. Harmon, MD

KEY POINTS

- Use a 27-gauge, 1.5-inch needle.
- Use a high-frequency linear array or curvilinear array transducer.

- The ischial bursae is not always visible on ultrasound or magnetic resonance imaging (MRI).
- The approach to the hamstring is difficult; patient positioning is key.

Pertinent Anatomy

There are three hamstring muscles that work to extend the hip and flex the knee. They are all diarthrodial (cross two joints) and all originate from the ischial tuberosity; the semimembranosus, the semitendinosus, and the long head of the biceps femoris. The short head of the biceps femoris originates from the linea aspera of the femur and joins the long head in the distal portion of the leg. Counterintuitively, the semimembranosus, whose muscle belly runs medially, originates on the superolateral aspect of the ischial tuberosity beneath the proximal half of the semitendinosus. The top half of the muscle is primarily aponeurosis turning into muscle more distal in the leg. The semimembranosus attaches in several places on the medial tibia via five fibrous attachments. The conjoint tendon attaches to the inferomedial facet of the ischial tuberosity and is composed of fibers of the semitendinosus and the biceps femoris. The semitendinosus is a bulbous muscle proximally ending in a long, thin tendon overlying the semimembranosus and inserting with the gracilis and sartorius as part of the pes anserine. The biceps femoris runs more laterally and inserts on the fibular head.[1-4] The ischial bursae lies just inferior to the ischium (Figure 51-1). It is generally only visible on ultrasound and MRI if it is inflamed.

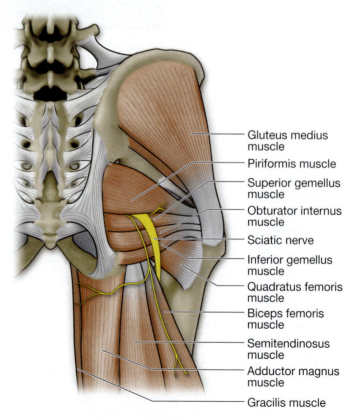

Gluteus medius muscle
Piriformis muscle
Superior gemellus muscle
Obturator internus muscle
Sciatic nerve
Inferior gemellus muscle
Quadratus femoris muscle
Biceps femoris muscle
Semitendinosus muscle
Adductor magnus muscle
Gracilis muscle

FIGURE 51-1 ■ Anatomy of the hamstring tendon origin and ischial bursa.

Common Pathology

The proximal hamstring is a common location for pathology. Tendinitis can occur at the proximal hamstrings after acute overuse. Tendinopathy, or chronic degenerative changes, typically begin gradually. Ultrasound imaging findings of tendinopathy show thickened tendons with hypoechoic areas with loss of the normal fibrillar architecture sometimes with a peritendinous fluid collection and are often accompanied by cortical irregularity of the ischial tuberosity. The proximal hamstring is best visualized in long axis using a high-frequency linear array transducer at a frequency of 8–12 Hz and depth of between 3 and 6 cm (Figure 51-2). In heavier patients it may be necessary to use a curvilinear array transducer. Pressing on the transducer to compress and decrease the depth of the overlying soft tissue can also compress the tendon and mask thickening or peritendinitis. Because of the challenges, in this area, MRI can be helpful to further define pathology.

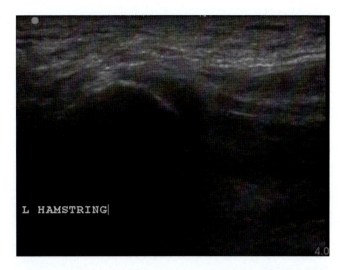

FIGURE 51-2 ■ Ultrasound of tendinopathic proximal hamstring long-axis view.

Indications for Injection of the Ischial Bursae or Peritendinous Injection

Peritendinous injection of the proximal hamstring complex can be performed for patients with recalcitrant tendinopathy that is unresponsive to rest, icing, antiinflammatories, and physical therapy including eccentric exercises. Injection of corticosteroids into tendons should be avoided,[5] however, peritendinous injection is hypothesized to limiting chronic inflammation, which leads to tendon scarring and adhesion.[4] It has been suggested that ultrasound guidance not only ensures accurate localization of the needle to the hamstring tendon complex, but can decrease the chance of potentially deleterious intratendinous injection. Injection into the ischial bursae is indicated for bursitis.

Injection of the proximal hamstring complex has been described based on palpation, but the accuracy of unguided injection is unknown. Ultrasound allows direct visualization of the hamstring complex and the injectate without exposure to ionizing radiation. The needle can be seen just adjacent to the hamstring tendons and the injectate can be seen flowing up and down the peritendinous area. Clinical outcomes at 1 and 6 months of ultrasound-guided peritendinous corticosteroid are favorable.[4]

Equipment

- For skin and superficial soft tissue
  - Needle: 27-gauge, 1.5-inch needle
  - Injectate: 1% lidocaine without epinephrine
- For injectate
  - Needle: 22-gauge, 3-inch needle
  - Injectate: 1 mL of an injectable corticosteroid and 2-5 mL of a local anesthetic
- High-frequency linear array or curvilinear array transducer

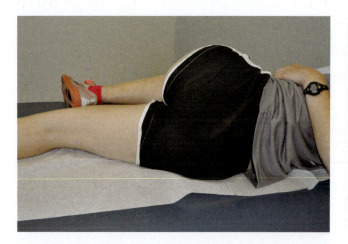

FIGURE 51-3 ■ Patient in side-lying position for proximal hamstring injection.

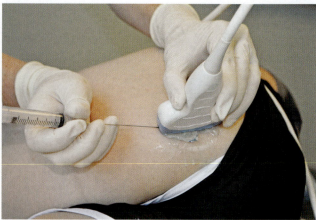

FIGURE 51-4 ■ Injection technique for long-axis approach to hamstring tendon origin and ischial bursa from distal to proximal.

Author's Preferred Technique

a. Patient position
    i. Prone (Figure 51-6): The examination table can be inverted or the patient's mid-section propped up with pillows to reduce the angle between the buttock on the upper leg making injection easier.
    ii. Alternate position (Figure 51-3): side-lying with affected side superior and hip and knee flexed (Figure 51-4).

b. Transducer position
    i. Sagittal, long axis to the hamstring tendon complex

c. Needle orientation relative to the transducer
    i. In plane

d. Needle approach (Figures 51-4 and 51-5)
    i. Distal to proximal

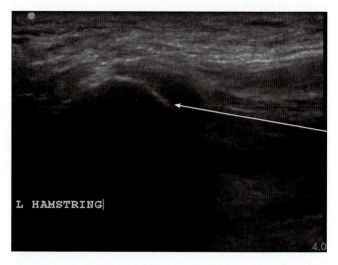

FIGURE 51-5 ■ Ultrasound image of long-axis, in plane approach to hamstring tendon origin and ischial bursa from distal to proximal. *Arrow* represents needle approach to tendon.

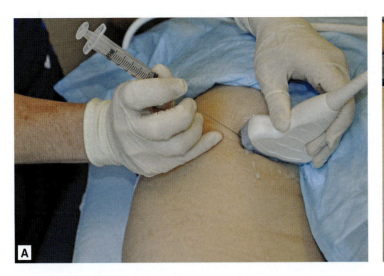
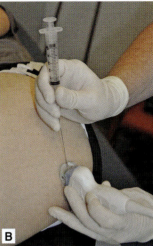

FIGURE 51-6 ■ Injection technique for short-axis approach to hamstring tendon origin and ischial bursa from lateral to medial: (**A**) is in prone position and (**B**) is in side-lying position.

e. Target
  i. Peritendon
  ii. Ischial bursae
f. Pearls and Pitfalls
  i. The sciatic nerve is just lateral to the hamstring tendons. The nerve should be identified in the axial view prior to injection and avoided.
  ii. As the corticosteroid is injected, you should see it flow up and down the tendon when performing a peritendinous injection. If this is not visible, reposition the needle tip, usually by slightly withdrawing and inject until the flow is seen.
  iii. The bursae will enlarge when injecting.

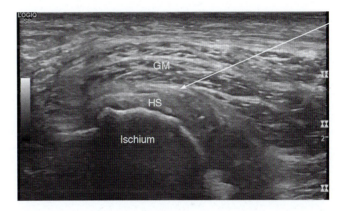

FIGURE 51-7 ■ Ultrasound image of short-axis approach to hamstring tendon origin and ischial bursa from lateral to medial. GM, gluteus maximus; HS, hamstring tendon, also in caption write arrow represents needle approach to peritendon region.

Alternate Technique

a. Patient position
  i. Prone
b. Transducer position
  i. Short axis to the hamstring tendon complex and bursa
c. Needle orientation relative to the transducer
  i. In plane
d. Needle approach (Figure 51-6)
  i. Lateral to medial
e. Target
  i. Peritendon (Figure 51-7)
  ii. Ischial bursae
f. Pearls and Pitfalls
  i. See "Pearls and Pitfalls" under "Author's Preferred Technique."

References

1. De Smet AA, Blakenbaker DG, Alsheik NH, Lindstrom MJ. MRI appearance of the proximal hamstring tendons in patients with and without symptomatic proximal hamstring tendinopathy. *AJR Am J Roentgenol* 2012;198:418–422.

2. Koulouris G, Connell D. Hamstring muscle complex: an imaging review. *Radiographics* 2005;25:571–586.

3. Lempainen L, Sarimo J, Mattila K, Vaittinen S, Orava S. Proximal hamstring tendinopathy: results of surgical management and histopathologic findings. *Am J Sports Med* 2009;37:727–734.

4. Zissen MH, Wallace G, Stevens KJ, Fredericson M, Beaulieu CF. High hamstring tendinopathy: MRI and ultrasound imaging and therapeutic efficacy of percutaneous corticosteroid injection. *AJR Am J Roentgenol* 2010;195:993–998.

5. Fredberg U. Local corticosteroid injection in sport: Review of literature and guidelines for treatment. *Scand J Med Sci Sports* 1997;7:131–139.

Kimberly G. Harmon, MD

KEY POINTS

- Use a 22-gauge, 3-inch needle.
- Use a high-frequency linear array or curvilinear array transducer.

- The hamstring tendons are deep and curved and may be challenging to image and treat.
- The approach to the hamstring is difficult; patient positioning is key.

Pertinent Anatomy

There are three hamstring muscles that work to extend the hip and flex the knee. They are all diarthrodial (cross two joints) and all originate from the ischial tuberosity; the semimembranosus, the semitendinosus, and the long head of the biceps femoris (Figure 52-1A). The short head of the biceps

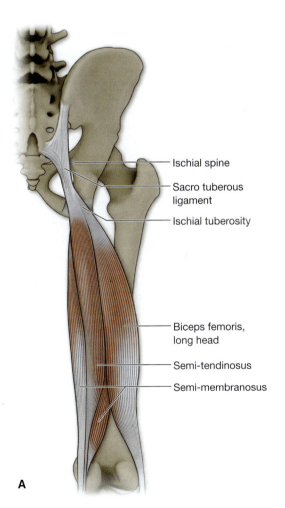

Ischial spine

Sacro tuberous ligament

Ischial tuberosity

Biceps femoris, long head

Semi-tendinosus

Semi-membranosus

A

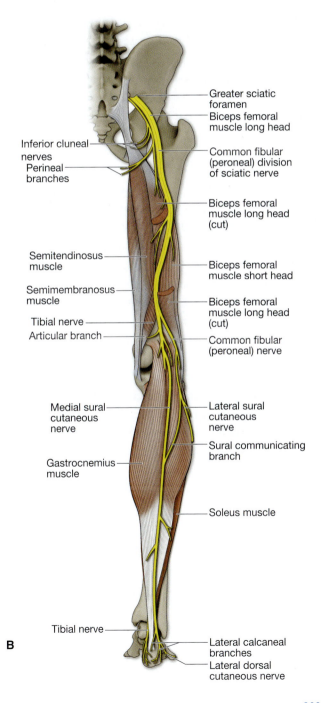

Greater sciatic foramen

Biceps femoral muscle long head

Inferior cluneal nerves

Perineal branches

Common fibular (peroneal) division of sciatic nerve

Biceps femoral muscle long head (cut)

Semitendinosus muscle

Biceps femoral muscle short head

Semimembranosus muscle

Tibial nerve

Biceps femoral muscle long head (cut)

Articular branch

Common fibular (peroneal) nerve

Medial sural cutaneous nerve

Lateral sural cutaneous nerve

Sural communicating branch

Gastrocnemius muscle

Soleus muscle

Tibial nerve

Lateral calcaneal branches

Lateral dorsal cutaneous nerve

B

FIGURE 52-1 ■ Anatomy of hamstrings.

femoris originates from the linea aspera of the femur and joins the long head in the distal portion of the leg. Counter-intuitively, the semimembranosus, whose muscle belly runs medially, originates on the superolateral aspect of the ischial tuberosity beneath the proximal half of the semitendinosus. The top half of the muscle is primarily aponeurosis turning into muscle more distal in the leg. The semimembranosus attaches in several places on the medial tibia via five fibrous attachments. The conjoint tendon attaches to the inferomedial facet of the ischial tuberosity and is composed of fibers of the semitendinosus and the biceps femoris. The semitendinosus is a bulbous muscle proximally ending in a long, thin tendon overlying the semimembranosus and inserting with the gracilis and sartorius as part of the pes anserine. The biceps femoris runs more laterally and inserts on the fibular head.[1-4] The sciatic nerve lies just lateral to the hamstring tendons and is important to identify when performing ultrasound evaluation of the proximal hamstring tendons (Figure 52-1B).

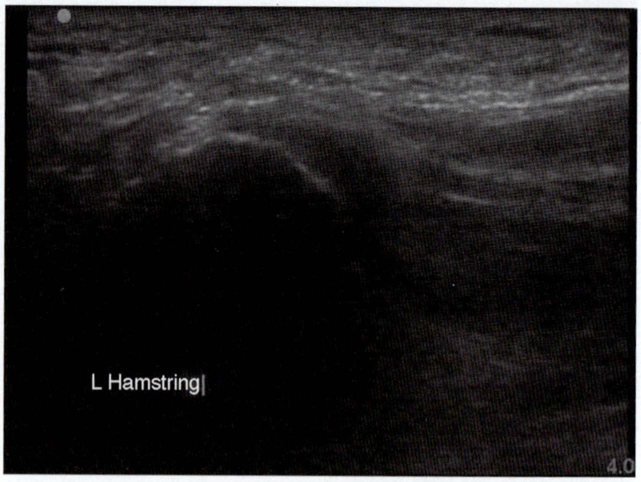

FIGURE 52-2 ■ Ultrasound of tendinopathic proximal hamstring in long-axis view.

Common Pathology

The proximal hamstring is a common location for tendinopathy. Tendinopathy is most common in distance runners and typically begins gradually. Injury can also occur more acutely, particularly when someone slips or uses the leg in a ballistic motion like kicking. Ultrasound imaging findings of tendinopathy show thickened tendons with hypoechoic areas with loss of the normal fibrillar architecture. It is not unusual for hyperechoic foci of calcific tendinosis to be present. Partial tears, either acute or more chronic and related to degenerative tendinopathy, can be seen as gaps in the tendon. Tendinopathy is often accompanied by cortical irregularity of the ischial tuberosity. The proximal hamstring is best visualized in long axis using a high-frequency linear array transducer at a depth of between 3 and 6 cm (Figure 52-2). In heavier patients, it may be necessary to use a curvilinear array transducer. Pressing on the transducer to compress and decrease the depth of the overlying soft tissue can also compress the tendon and mask changes. Because of the challenges, in this area, magnetic resonance imaging can be helpful to further define pathology.

Indications for Injection and Fenestration of the Proximal Hamstring Complex

Injection and fenestration of the proximal hamstring can be performed for patients with recalcitrant tendinopathy that is unresponsive to rest, icing, antiinflammatories, and physical therapy including eccentric exercises. Fenestration of the tendon, or repetitive needling, is done in an attempt to stimulate healing.[5] Injection of corticosteroids into tendons should be avoided;[6] however, injection of autologous blood, platelet-rich plasma, and dextrose have been proposed as possible intratendinous treatment to stimulate healing in tendinopathy.[7]

Injection of the proximal hamstring complex has been described based on palpation, but the accuracy of unguided injection is unknown. Because of the depth of the tissue and concern for accuracy, hamstring injections are often done with ultrasound or fluoroscopic guidance. Ultrasound allows direct visualization of the hamstring complex and the injectate without exposure to ionizing radiation. Clinical outcomes of guided versus unguided injection have not been described.

Equipment

■ Needle: 22-gauge, 3-inch needle
■ Injectate
  • Local anesthetic without epinephrine
  • Can use autologous blood, platelet-rich plasma, or dextrose as described above, but not required
■ High-frequency linear array or curvilinear array transducer

Author's Preferred Technique

a. Patient position
   i. Prone: The examination table can be inverted or the patient's midsection propped up with pillows to reduce the angle between the buttock on the upper leg, making injection easier.
   ii. Alternate position: side-lying with affected side superior and hip and knee flexed (Figure 52-3).
b. Transducer position
   i. Sagittal, long axis to the hamstring tendon complex (Figure 52-4)
c. Needle orientation relative to the transducer
   i. In plane
d. Needle approach
   i. Distal to proximal (Figure 52-5)
   ii. Alternate approach proximal to distal
e. Target
   i. Hamstring tendon origin complex
f. Pearls and Pitfalls
   i. The sciatic nerve is just lateral to the hamstring tendons. The nerve should be identified in the axial view prior to injection and avoided.
   ii. Use just enough local anesthetic to reduce pain during the procedure and avoid excess local injectate directly into the tendons.
   iii. While injecting, the ultrasound probe can be changed to a short-axis view and the needle tip shown in an out-of-plane view to visualize the needle position in a medial to lateral plane.

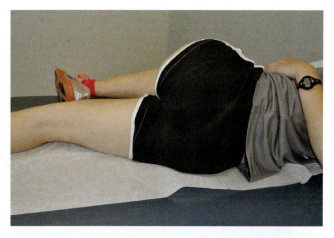

FIGURE 52-3 ■ Side-lying position for performing proximal hamstring injection.

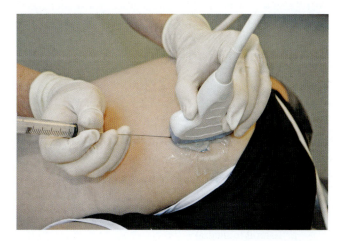

FIGURE 52-4 ■ Long-axis, in-plane approach for injecting the proximal hamstring tendon.

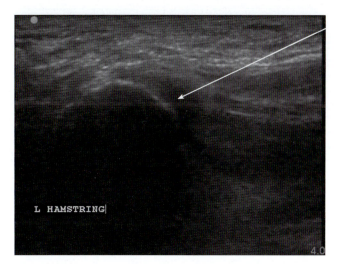

FIGURE 52-5 ■ Ultrasound image of needle position (*arrow*) for performing a long-axis, in-plane, distal to proximal needle approach to the proximal hamstring tendon.

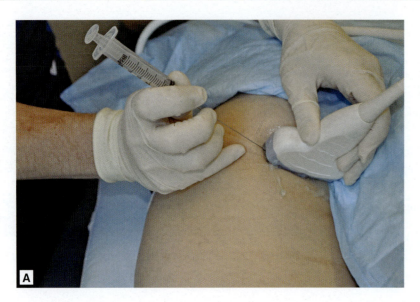
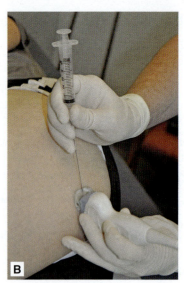

FIGURE 52-6 ■ **A** and **B.** Short-axis, in-plane approach for injecting the proximal hamstring tendon.

Alternate Technique

a. Patient position
    i. Prone
b. Transducer position
    i. Short axis to the hamstring tendon complex
        (Figure 52-6A, B)
c. Needle orientation relative to transducer
    i. In plane
d. Needle approach
    i. Lateral to medial
e. Target
    i. Proximal hamstring tendons
f. Pearls and Pitfalls
    i. Keep the sciatic nerve visualized and avoid injection
        of it.

References

1. De Smet AA, Blakenbaker DG, Alsheik NH, Lindstrom MJ. MRI appearance of the proximal hamstring tendons in patients with and without symptomatic proximal hamstring tendinopathy. *AJR Am J Roentgenol* 2012;198:418–422.
2. Koulouris G, Connell D. Hamstring muscle complex: an imaging review. *Radiographics* 2005 May-Jun;25(3):571–586.
3. Lempainen L, Sarimo J, Mattila K, Vaittinen S, Orava S. Proximal hamstring tendinopathy: results of surgical management and histopathologic findings. *Am J Sports Med* 2009 Apr;37(4):727–734.
4. Zissen MH, Wallace G, Stevens KJ, Fredericson M, Beaulieu CF. High hamstring tendinopathy: MRI and ultrasound imaging

and therapeutic efficacy of percutaneous corticosteroid injection. *AJR Am J Roentgenol* 2010 Oct;195(4):993–998.
5. Housner JA, Jacobson JA, Misko R. Sonographically guided percutaneous needle tenotomy for the treatment of chronic tendinosis. *J Ultrasound Med* 2009 Sep;28(9):1187–1192.
6. Fredberg U. Local corticosteroid injection in sport: review of literature and guidelines for treatment. *Scand J Med Sci Sports* 1997 Jun;7(3):131–139.
7. Linklater JM, Hamilton B, Carmichael J, Orchard J, Wood DG. Hamstring injuries: anatomy, imaging, and intervention. *Semin Musculoskelet Radiol* 2010 Jun;14(2):131–161.

Marko Bodor, MD / John M. Lesher, MD, MPH

KEY POINTS

- Use a 22-gauge, 3.5-inch spinal needle inserted in plane.
- Subgluteus maximus bursitis (trochanteric bursitis) is less common than gluteal tendon tears and tendinosis.
- A medium- or high-frequency linear array transducer, rotated approximately 37 degrees posterior to the long axis of the femur best visualizes the lateral facet.
- Rotation of the hip while scanning identifies the plane between the gluteus medius and the gluteus maximus.

Pertinent Anatomy

The word "trochanter" means "runner" in Greek, leading us to believe that the ancient Greeks were familiar with greater trochanteric pain syndrome (GTPS) and running as one of its causes. GTPS is a common regional pain syndrome characterized by chronic, intermittent pain over the greater trochanter, buttock, and lateral aspect of the thigh.[1]

The greater trochanter has anterior, lateral, and superoposterior facets, to which are attached the gluteus minimus, anterior gluteus medius, and posterior gluteus medius tendons, respectively (Figure 53-1). The lateral facet has the largest attachment area, on average 34 mm long by 10 mm wide, angled approximately 37 degrees posterior relative to the long axis of the femur.[2]

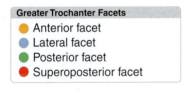

Greater Trochanter Facets
- ● Anterior facet
- ● Lateral facet
- ● Posterior facet
- ● Superoposterior facet

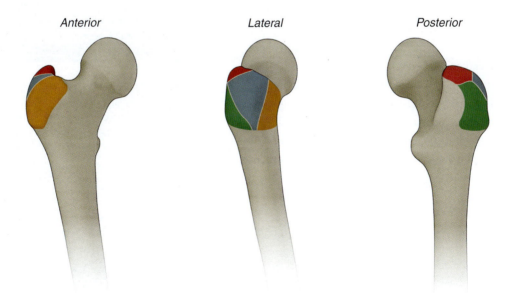

Anterior   Lateral   Posterior

FIGURE 53-1 ■ Schematic drawing of the four facets of the greater trochanter: the anterior facet, lateral facet, posterior facet, and superoposterior facet, which represent the osseous attachment sites of the gluteus medius and gluteus minimus tendons.

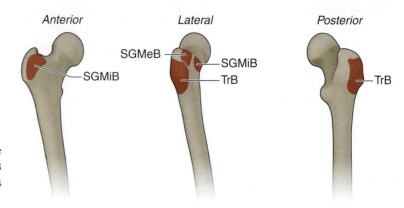

FIGURE 53-2 ■ Locations of the bursae around the greater trochanter: TrB (trochanteric bursa), SGMeB (subgluteus medius bursa), and SGMiB (subgluteus minimus bursa).

The gluteus minimus and anterior and posterior gluteus medius tendons make up the "rotator cuff" of the hip,[3] and the gluteus maximus and fascia lata are comparable to the deltoid muscle of the shoulder.[4] The subgluteus maximus bursa (trochanteric bursa) lies between the gluteus maximus and the posterior part of gluteus medius. The subgluteus medius and minimus bursae are located under their respective tendons. Figure 53-2 demonstrates the relationships of the bursa to the bony landmarks.

Common Pathology

Excessive friction between the tendon layers can cause inflammation, thickening, and fluid accumulation in the subgluteus maximus bursa, which can be diagnosed via ultrasound (Figure 53-3A, B). Trochanteric bursitis is no longer the preferred medical description given that true inflammation of the subgluteus maximus bursa, with redness, heat, swelling, and tenderness is rare.[5]

Common imaging and surgical findings include interstitial, partial-thickness, or full-thickness tears of the gluteus medius and minimus tendons. The most common location of pathology is seen in the anterior gluteus medius tendon.[3,6] In these cases, the primary source of pain is felt to be the tendon tear and its associated repair response rather than friction-induced bursitis.

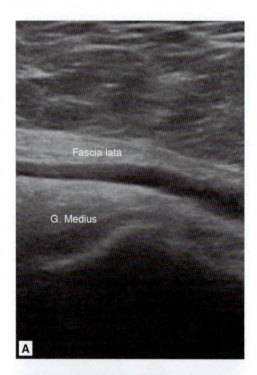

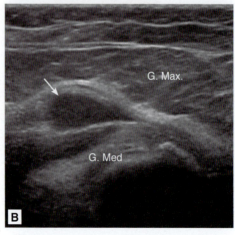

FIGURE 53-3 ■ Subgluteus maximus bursitis (arrow). **A** and **B.** Long-axis views of bursal fluid collections.

Ultrasound Imaging Findings

Initial scanning begins over the greater trochanter with the transducer superficial and parallel to the lateral facet. Next, slide the transducer anteriorly to visualize the "rooftop" appearance of the anterior and lateral facets and the round profile of the gluteus minimus tendon. Then slide posteriorly and carefully scan the broad flat anterior gluteus medius tendon and the ovoid-appearing posterior gluteus medius (Figure 53-4A–E). Gentle hip rotation while scanning facilitates visualization of the gluteus medius and minimus rotating under the gluteus maximus and fascia lata. Fluid accumulation or thickening of the bursa between the gluteus maximus and gluteus medius tendons suggests bursal inflammation (see Figure 53-3A, B). Hypoechoic or anechoic areas within the tendon, cortical irregularities, or absence of a visible tendon indicates partial- or full-thickness tendon tears, whereas reduced echogenicity with diffuse tendon enlargement is a hallmark of tendinosis.[4,6] This is discussed further in Chapter 54.

Indications for Injections of the Greater Trochanteric Bursae

It is important to establish an accurate diagnosis prior to any injection, particularly one involving corticosteroids, which could improve symptoms temporarily while exacerbating long-term tendon pathology.

A primary indication for an anesthetic lateral hip injection (lidocaine or bupivacaine only) is to confirm the diagnosis of GTPS. Corticosteroid injections are used to treat recalcitrant GTPS unresponsive to conservative care and can help reduce symptoms of bursitis. Increasingly, platelet-rich plasma and other biologic injections are being performed for gluteal tendon tears and tendinosis so special attention is needed not to miss this diagnosis.

Equipment

- Needle: 22–25-gauge, 2–3.5-inch needle
- Injectate
  - 1–2 mL of local anesthetic
  - 0.5–1 mL of injectable corticosteroid
- Medium- to high-frequency linear array transducer; or if necessary low-frequency curvilinear array transducer

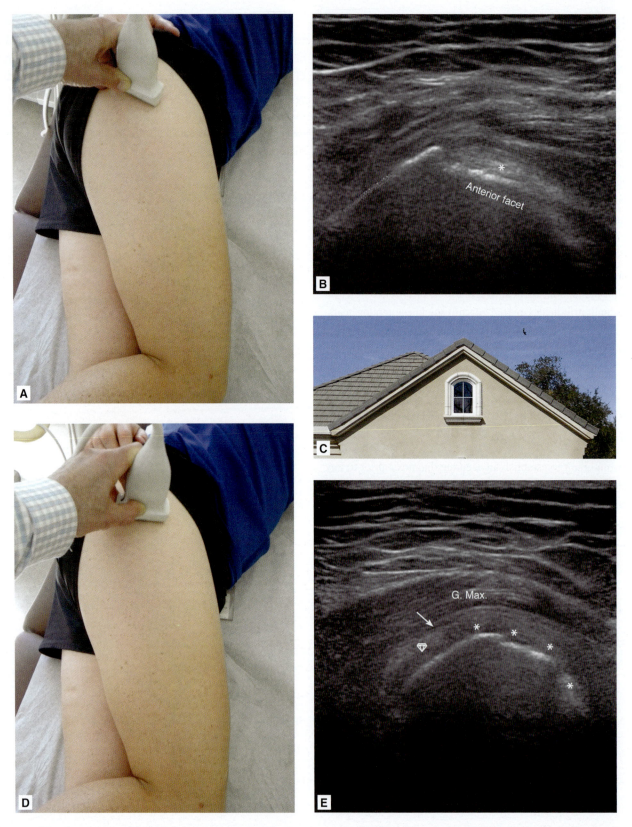

FIGURE 53-4 ■ Normal sonographic appearance of the gluteal tendons: (**A**) transducer position and (**B**) short-axis image of the round profile of the gluteus minimus tendon (*asterisk*) sitting on top of the anterior facet. Notice the "rooftop" appearance (**C**) of the anterior and lateral facets at this location; (**D**) transducer position, and (**E**) short-axis image of the posterior and lateral facets with the posterior (*diamond*) and anterior (*asterisks*) gluteus medius and minimus (*asterisk*) tendons. The *white arrow* points to the location of the subgluteus maximus bursa in a normal, noninflamed state.

Author's Preferred Technique

a. Patient position
    i. Side-lying with pillows under the head and between the legs.

b. Transducer position for the subgluteus maximus bursa (Figure 53-5A)
    i. Superficial and slightly posterior to the lateral facet, approximately 37 degrees posterior rotation relative to the long axis of femur.
    ii. If the bursa is not visible, its location in the potential space between the gluteus maximus and medius muscle-tendon layers can be identified by gentle internal and external hip rotation.

c. Transducer position for the subgluteus medius and minimus bursa
    i. Superficial to the junction of the anterior and lateral facets aligned with the long axis of the femur for subgluteus medius bursa injection.
    ii. Superficial to the anterior facet aligned with the subgluteus medius tendon for subgluteus minimus bursa injection.

d. Needle orientation relative to the transducer (see Figure 53-5A)
    i. In plane

e. Needle approach (Figure 53-5B)
    i. Anterior or posterior for subgluteus maximus bursa injection
    ii. Inferior or superior for subgluteus medius or minimus bursa injection

f. Target
    i. Subgluteus maximus bursa, or its location between the gluteus maximus-fascia lata and gluteus medius muscle-tendon layers.
    ii. Subgluteus medius or minimus bursa, or its location between tendon and bone.

g. Pearls and Pitfalls
    i. If the subgluteus maximus bursa is not visible, its location in the potential space between the gluteus maximus and medius muscle-tendon layers can be identified by gentle hip rotation.
    ii. Avoid injection of corticosteroid into the gluteal tendons or in the presence of tendon tears or tendinosis.
    iii. If bursitis is present, be extra careful scanning for presence of gluteal tendon tear. If tear is seen, you will likely need to address it with additional treatment, possibly biological, for attempted healing.

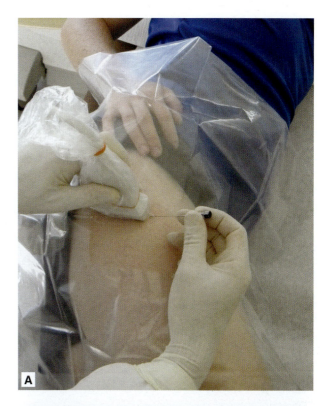

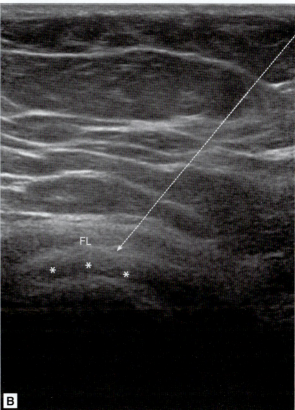

FIGURE 53-5 ▪ Subgluteus maximus bursa injection: (**A**) in-plane approach, short axis and slightly oblique to the tendon with same transducer orientation as in Figure 53-4; (**B**) image with enhanced needle trajectory (*dotted arrow*), fascia lata (FL), and gluteus medius tendon (*asterisks*).

References

1. Shbeeb MI, Matteson EL. Trochanteric bursitis (greater trochanter pain syndrome). *Mayo Clin Proc* 1996;71:565–569.

2. Robertson WJ, Gardner MJ, Barker JU, et al. Anatomy and dimensions of the gluteus medius tendon insertion. *Arthroscopy* 2008 Feb;24(2):130–136.

3. Bunker TD, Esler CAN, Leach WJ. Rotator cuff tear of the hip. *J Bone Joint Surg Br* 1997;79:618–620.

4. Martinoli C, Bianchi S. Hip. In: Bianchi S, Martinoli C. *Ultrasound of the Musculoskeletal System.* 1st ed. Heidelberg DE: Springer; 2007:551–610.

5. Silva F, Adams T, Feinstein J, et al. Trochanteric bursitis: refuting the myth of inflammation. *J Clin Rheumatol* 2008;14(2): 82–86.

6. Kong A, Van derVliet A, Zadow S. MRI and US of gluteal tendinopathy in greater trochanter pain syndrome. *Eur Radiol* 2007 Jul;17(7):1772–1783.

Jon A. Jacobson, MD

KEY POINTS

- For gluteus medius and minimus tendon procedures, use a 20-gauge spinal needle, in-plane, inferior-to-superior technique.
- The procedure may require anything from a high-frequency linear array transducer to a low-frequency curvilinear array transducer depending on body habitus.
- Greater trochanter osseous landmarks are key for orientation.
- Several bursae can be found about the greater trochanter.
- Greater trochanteric pain syndrome is more likely from gluteus tendon abnormality rather than from bursitis.

Pertinent Anatomy

The gluteus medius originates from the ilium and inserts onto the posterosuperior and lateral facets of the greater trochanter of the proximal femur.[1] The gluteus minimus also originates from the ilium but is located deep to the gluteus medius and inserts onto the anterior facet of the greater trochanter of the proximal femur. Figure 54-1A and B demonstrates these muscles, as well as the landmarks, on the greater trochanter where these tendons insert. The larger gluteus maximus is located more posterior and does not insert, but rather passes over the posterior facet of the greater trochanter to insert onto the gluteal tuberosity of the posterior femur.

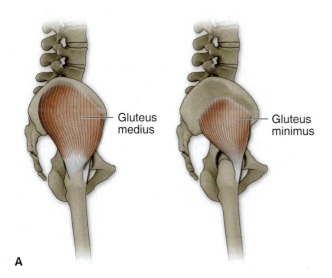

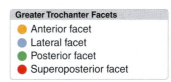

Greater Trochanter Facets
- Anterior facet
- Lateral facet
- Posterior facet
- Superoposterior facet

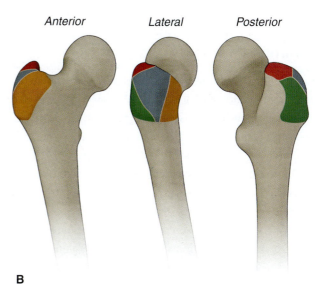

Anterior   Lateral   Posterior

FIGURE 54-1 ■ **A.** Anatomy of the gluteus medius and minimus muscles. **B.** Schematic drawing of the four facets of the greater trochanter: the anterior facet, lateral facet, posterior facet, and superoposterior facet, which represent the osseous attachment sites of the gluteus medius and gluteus minimus (AF) tendons; and locations of the bursae.

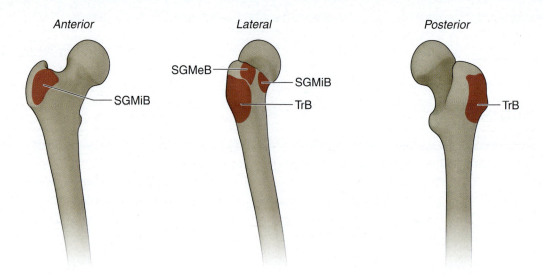

FIGURE 54-2 ■ Locations of the bursae around the greater trochanter: SGMeB, subgluteus medius bursae; SGMiB, subgluteus minimus bursa; TrB, trochanteric bursa.

There are several bursae that are found about the greater trochanter and gluteal tendons.[1] The largest trochanteric (or subgluteus maximus) bursa is located between the posterior facet of the greater trochanter and extends anterior over the lateral aspect of the gluteus medius. The subgluteus medius bursa is located between the lateral facet of the greater trochanter and the gluteus medius tendon. The subgluteus minimus bursa is located between the anterior facet of the greater trochanter and the gluteus minimus tendon. Figure 54-2 demonstrates the relationships of the bursae to the bony landmarks.

Common Pathology

Both the gluteus medius and minimus may demonstrate tendinosis and tendon tear at the insertion sites on the greater trochanter.[2] In the clinical setting of greater trochanteric pain syndrome, gluteus medius and minimus tendon tears are common findings.[3,4] In contrast, an isolated bursitis as a cause of greater trochanteric pain syndrome is rare and when a bursa is present, inflammation is usually lacking.[5] Gluteus medius and minimus abnormalities may also occur after hip replacement surgery.[6] Calcium deposition in the form of calcium hydroxyapatite may cause calcific tendinosis. Gluteus minimus and medius tendon abnormalities may be associated with adjacent bursal distention.

Ultrasound Imaging Findings

Evaluation for gluteus minimus and medius tendon abnormalities can be completed with a high-frequency linear array transducer, although a lower frequency transducer may be needed in patients with a large body habitus. A curvilinear array transducer is often helpful as this increases the field of view. For orientation, it is often helpful to begin ultrasound scanning short axis to the femur over the lateral hip with patients lying on their contralateral side. In this position, the characteristic contours of the greater trochanter can be seen with the flat anterior and lateral facets separated by a cortical apex. The gluteus minimus will be seen over the anterior facet and the gluteus medius over the lateral facet. The curved posterior facet is seen more posterior with the overlying gluteus maximus muscle. Once the gluteus minimus and medius tendons are evaluated in short axis, the transducer is turned 90 degrees over each facet to image each respective gluteal tendon in long axis. When imaging the gluteus medius tendon in long axis over the lateral facet, the transducer should also be moved superior and posterior to visualize the gluteus medius tendon attachment onto the superoposterior facet of the greater trochanter. The soft tissues between the various greater trochanter facets and the overlying gluteal tendons are also evaluated for abnormal bursal distention.

Tendinosis will appear as abnormal hypoechogenicity and tendon swelling (Figure 54-3).[2] One must be careful not to mistake anisotropy as tendinosis when the tendon is not imaged perpendicular to the sound beam. To avoid this artifact, the cortical bone underlying the tendon being imaged should be parallel to the transducer face and echogenic. Tendon tears will appear as hypoechoic or anechoic tendon fiber disruption. Cortical irregularity of the greater trochanter may be an associated finding.[7] Calcium deposition in tendon will appear as hyperechoic foci with variable shadowing. Adjacent bursal distention may range from anechoic (if simple fluid) to isoechoic or hyperechoic (if complex fluid or synovial hypertrophy).

Indications for Gluteus Medius and Minimus Percutaneous Tenotomy

Gluteus medius and/or minimus tendon pathology can be treated with a number of percutaneous options. Ultrasound-guided injection of corticosteroids over the surface of gluteus medius tendinopathy has shown short-term effectiveness with 72% clinical improvement in pain at 1 month after injection.[8] Ultrasound-guided fenestration (also termed *tenotomy* or *dry-needling*) has been used effectively at many sites about the body, but only preliminary results have been reported for gluteal tendons.[9] Other forms of tendon injections for the treatment of tendinosis and tendon tear include injection of whole blood and platelet-rich plasma, but there are few studies evaluating their use for gluteal tendon abnormalities. When calcific tendinosis is identified, ultrasound-guided lavage and aspiration may be completed, similar to what is described in the rotator cuff.[10]

Equipment

- ▪ Needle: 20-gauge, 3.5-inch needle
- ▪ Injectate: Limited amount of local anesthesia to allow for adequate pain control during needle fenestration of the tendon
- ▪ High-to-low range transducer utilized depending on body habitus

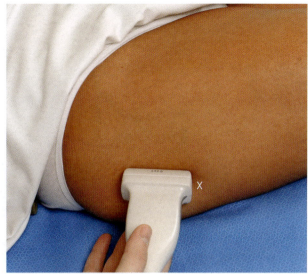

FIGURE 54-3 ▪ Close up approach of linear array transducer with needle entry (*X*) for in-plane, distal to proximal approach.

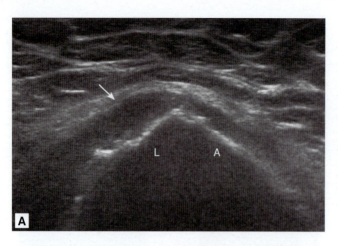
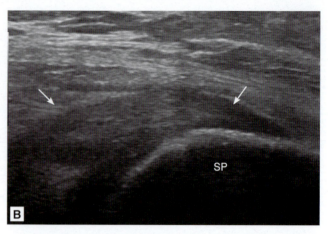

FIGURE 54-4 ■ Gluteus medius tendinosis. Ultrasound images (**A**) short axis and (**B**) long axis to gluteus medius tendon (*arrows*) show hypoechoic thickening (*arrows*) over lateral (L) and superoposterior (SP) facets of the greater trochanter. Note relative thickness of the gluteus minimus tendon over the anterior facet (A). The left side of image A is posterior, and the left side of B is superior.

Author's Preferred Injection Technique

a. Patient position (Figure 54-4)
   i. Patient lies on contralateral hip.
   ii. Hip in neutral or slight flexion position.
b. Transducer position (see Figure 54-4)
   i. Long axis to gluteus tendon
c. Needle orientation relative to the transducer (Figure 54-5)
   i. In plane
d. Needle technique (Figure 54-6)
   i. Inferior to superior
e. Target
   i. Abnormal segment of gluteus minimus/medius tendon
f. Pearls and Pitfalls
   i. With stylet removed, the needle is repeatedly passed through the abnormal tendon. The needle is retracted just out of the tendon with each pass to redirect the needle in a slightly different angle. The goal is to cover all areas where the tendon appears abnormal by ultrasound.
   ii. The transducer should be turned 90 degrees to ensure the entire area of abnormal tendon is treated.
   iii. The number of passes varies depending on the size of the abnormal tendon area and is usually between 15 and 30 needle passes. The transducer sound beam should be perpendicular to the underlying greater trochanter facet being imaged to eliminate potential anisotropy of the overlying gluteus tendons that may be mistaken as tendinosis.

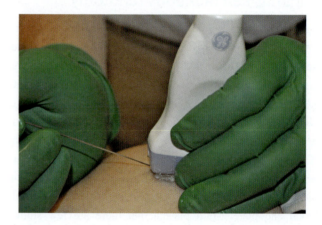

FIGURE 54-5 ■ Patient and needle positioning. For gluteus tendon injection, the patient lies on the contralateral side with hip in neutral position, the transducer is long axis to the targeted gluteal tendon, and needle is directed in plane with the transducer from inferior to superior.

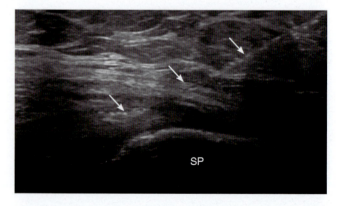

FIGURE 54-6 ■ Gluteus medius fenestration. Ultrasound image long axis to the gluteus medius over the superoposterior (SP) facet of the greater trochanter shows 20-gauge needle and needle tip (*arrows*) within hypoechoic and thickened tendon segment (left side of image is superior).

iv. The superoposterior facet of the greater trochanter must be evaluated for a complete assessment of the gluteus medius tendon.

v. The gluteus medius tendon normally is somewhat thicker over the superoposterior facet compared to the tendon attachment at the lateral facet.

vi. If a calcific deposit is identified, an 18–20-gauge needle is inserted once into the center of the calcification in plane with the transducer either short axis or long axis to the tendon. This is followed by lavage and aspiration with minimal local anesthetic, similar to the technique that is most commonly used in the rotator cuff.[10]

References

1. Pfirrmann CW, Chung CB, Theumann NH, Trudell DJ, Resnick D. Greater trochanter of the hip: attachment of the abductor mechanism and a complex of three bursae—MR imaging and MR bursography in cadavers and MR imaging in asymptomatic volunteers. *Radiology* 2001;221:469–477.

2. Connell DA, Bass C, Sykes CA, Young D, Edwards E. Sonographic evaluation of gluteus medius and minimus tendinopathy. *Eur Radiol* 2003;13:1339–1347.

3. Fearon AM, Scarvell JM, Cook JL, Smith PN. Does ultrasound correlate with surgical or histologic findings in greater trochanteric pain syndrome? A pilot study. *Clin Orthop Relat Res* 2010;468:1838–1844.

4. Kong A, Van der Vliet A, Zadow S. MRI and US of gluteal tendinopathy in greater trochanteric pain syndrome. *Eur Radiol* 2007;17:1772–1783.

5. Silva F, Adams T, Feinstein J, Arroyo RA. Trochanteric bursitis: refuting the myth of inflammation. *J Clin Rheumatol* 2008;14:82–86.

6. Garcia FL, Picado CH, Nogueira-Barbosa MH. Sonographic evaluation of the abductor mechanism after total hip arthroplasty. *J Ultrasound Med* 2010;29:465–471.

7. Steinert L, Zanetti M, Hodler J, et al. Are radiographic trochanteric surface irregularities associated with abductor tendon abnormalities? *Radiology* 2010;257:754–763.

8. Labrosse JM, Cardinal E, Leduc BE, et al. Effectiveness of ultrasound-guided corticosteroid injection for the treatment of gluteus medius tendinopathy. *AJR Am J Roentgenol* 2010;194:202–206.

9. Housner JA, Jacobson JA, Misko R. Sonographically guided percutaneous needle tenotomy for the treatment of chronic tendinosis. *J Ultrasound Med* 2009;28:1187–1192.

10. Lee KS, Rosas HG. Musculoskeletal ultrasound: how to treat calcific tendinitis of the rotator cuff by ultrasound-guided single-needle lavage technique. *AJR Am J Roentgenol* 2010; 195:638.

Jon A. Jacobson, MD

KEY POINTS

- A 20–25-gauge spinal needle, in-plane, lateral-to-medial approach is used for iliopsoas bursa and peritendon procedures.
- Use a medium- to low-frequency transducer, depending on patient body habitus.
- Iliopsoas bursa distention is uncommon.

- The iliopsoas bursa communicates with the hip joint in 15% of normal subjects.
- Iliopsoas bursal abnormalities are frequently related to the hip joint.
- Dynamic evaluation for iliopsoas snapping should be considered.

Pertinent Anatomy

The iliopsoas musculotendinous unit is comprised of the psoas major, iliacus, and psoas minor (Figure 55-1).[1] The psoas major originates from the twelfth thoracic through fifth lumbar vertebrae transverse processes, lateral vertebral margins, and intervening disks. The iliacus originates from the iliac wing and merges with the psoas major near the inguinal ligament to form the iliopsoas muscle. The psoas minor originates from the twelfth thoracic through first lumbar vertebral bodies, is located anterior to the psoas major, and is absent in up to 40% of the population.[1]

The distal iliopsoas anatomy is complex with five distal components described.[2] Of these components, the medial fibers of the iliacus muscle form an accessory tendon, which merges with the psoas major tendon to attach to the lesser trochanter. Lateral muscle fibers of the iliacus may insert directly onto the proximal femur.[3] The iliopsoas tendon may also be bifid.

The iliopsoas bursa is a synovial-lined space located anterior to the hip joint. This bursa communicates with the hip joint in 15% of the normal population.[4] Abnormal distention of the iliopsoas bursa is usually related to adjacent hip joint pathology. A distended iliopsoas bursa is located directly anterior to the hip joint, posterior or posteromedial to the iliopsoas tendon, and may extend anterior and lateral to the iliopsoas tendon. A markedly distended iliopsoas bursa may extend into the pelvis.[5]

Common Pathology

The iliopsoas may demonstrate tendinosis or less commonly tendon tear with repetitive injury or acute trauma. While iliopsoas bursal distention may accompany iliopsoas tendon pathology or may be uncommonly an isolated finding, bursal

distention is more frequently related to pathologic process that involves the hip joint, where joint fluid and/or synovial processes extend into the bursa from the hip joint. Examples of such hip joint pathology include osteoarthritis, rheumatoid arthritis, and septic arthritis. Communication between an iliopsoas bursal and the hip joint may also occur after hip

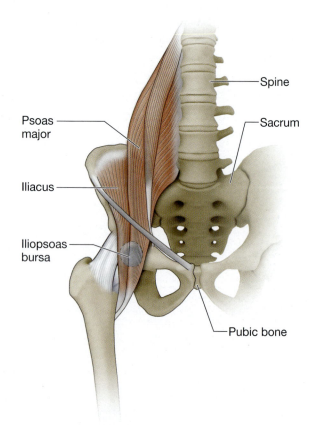

FIGURE 55-1 ■ Anterior hip anatomy. Illustration shows iliacus and psoas major muscles joining together to form iliopsoas tendon with the right side illustration showing approximate location of the iliopsoas bursa.

replacement if the joint capsule is resected. In the setting of a hip replacement, the anterior aspect of the acetabular cup or femoral collar may cause iliopsoas tendon impingement. Lesser trochanter avulsion at the iliopsoas tendon attachment may occur after trauma in children; however, lesser trochanter avulsion in the adult should raise concern for pathologic fracture, such as with a lung cancer metastasis. Abnormal snapping of the iliopsoas may also be seen dynamically.[2]

Ultrasound Imaging Findings

Evaluation of the iliopsoas can be completed with a high-frequency linear array transducer; although a lower frequency transducer may be needed in patients with a large body habitus. A curvilinear transducer is often helpful as this increases the field of view. The iliopsoas tendinosis will appear as abnormal hypoechogenicity and tendon tear will appear as anechoic or hypoechoic tendon disruption. Abnormal iliopsoas bursal distention can range from anechoic (if simple fluid) to isoechoic or hyperechoic (if complex fluid and synovial hypertrophy) (Figure 55-2). Evaluation for snapping iliopsoas is completed with the transducer short axis to the iliopsoas tendon parallel to the inguinal ligament. Abnormal snapping or abrupt motion of the iliopsoas tendon can be seen dynamically when moving the hip from flexion-external rotation or frog leg position to a straightened position.

Indications for Iliopsoas Peritendon and Bursa Procedures

Patients with groin pain and clinically suspected snapping iliopsoas can benefit from injection of corticosteroids and anesthetic agents into the iliopsoas bursa, where pain relief can also predict good outcome after surgical iliopsoas tendon release.[6] Ultrasound-guided iliopsoas peritendon injection has also been described in patients with pain after hip replacement when iliopsoas tendon impingement is suspected.[7,8] Ultrasound-guided aspiration and injection of a distended iliopsoas bursa may also be completed, although the cause of the bursal distention, such as hip joint pathology, must be addressed.

Equipment

- Needle: 20–22 gauge, 3.5-inch needle
- Injectate: 3 mL local anesthetic and 1 mL of an injectable corticosteroid
- Medium- to low-frequency linear array transducer, depending on patient body habitus

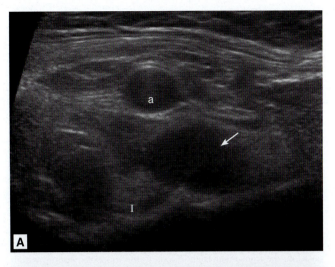

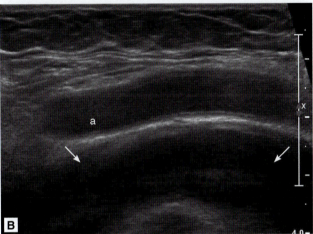

FIGURE 55-2 ■ Iliopsoas bursal distention. Ultrasound images (**A**) short axis and (**B**) long axis to iliopsoas tendon (I) show hypoechoic iliopsoas bursal distention (*arrows*). The left side of image A is lateral. a, femoral artery.

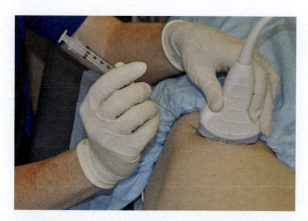

FIGURE 55-3 ▪ Patient and needle positioning. For iliopsoas bursa and peritendon injection, the patient lies supine with hip in neutral position, the transducer is short axis to the iliopsoas tendon, which is approximately parallel to the inguinal ligament, and the needle is directed in plane with the transducer from lateral to medial.

Author's Preferred Technique

a. Patient position (Figure 55-3)
   i. Supine
   ii. Hip in neutral position
b. Transducer position
   i. Oblique axial plane parallel to inguinal ligament and superior to femoral head
c. Needle orientation relative to the transducer
   i. In plane
d. Needle approach (Figure 55-4)
   i. Lateral to medial
e. Target
   i. Iliopsoas bursa (if distended) or between iliopsoas tendon and ilium (if bursa not identified)
f. Pearls and Pitfalls
   i. While imaging the iliopsoas tendon in short axis, toggle the transducer to angle the ultrasound beam superior and inferior to eliminate anisotropy and improve visualization of the tendon.
   ii. When injecting deep to the iliopsoas tendon, the femoral head should not be in view. This will ensure that the injectate is located adjacent to the iliopsoas tendon or in the iliopsoas bursa and not accidentally injected into the hip joint.
   iii. Beam-steering (if available) to remove needle anisotropy can make the needle more echogenic and assist in needle visualization (Figure 55-4B).
   iv. Limited ultrasound evaluation of the hip prior to the procedure is essential to screen for snapping hip syndrome and other causes for anterior hip pain, such as paralabral cyst.

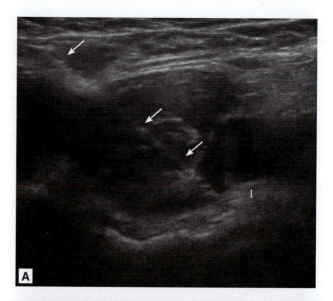

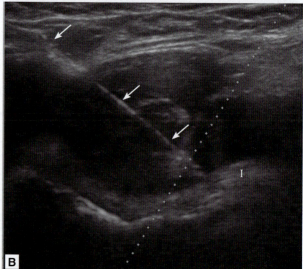

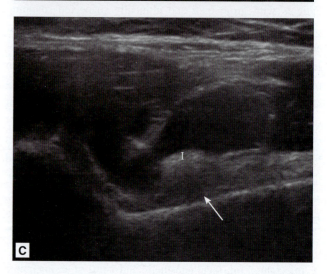

FIGURE 55-4 ▪ Iliopsoas peritendon injection. Ultrasound images in the oblique axial plane parallel to the inguinal ligament show echogenic needle (*arrows*) (**A**) without and (**B**) with beam steering. Ultrasound image postinjection shows (**C**) hypoechoic injectate (*long arrow*).

References

1. Blankenbaker DG, Tuite MJ. Iliopsoas musculotendinous unit. *Semin Musculoskelet Radiol* 2008;12:13–27.

2. Guillin R, Cardinal E, Bureau NJ. Sonographic anatomy and dynamic study of the normal iliopsoas musculotendinous junction. *Eur Radiol* 2009;19:995–1001.

3. Polster JM, Elgabaly M, Lee H, et al. MRI and gross anatomy of the iliopsoas tendon complex. *Skeletal Radiol* 2008;37:55–58.

4. Wunderbaldinger P, Bremer C, Schellenberger E, et al. Imaging features of iliopsoas bursitis. *Eur Radiol* 2002;12:409–415.

5. Bianchi S, Martinoli C, Keller A, Bianchi-Zamorani MP. Giant iliopsoas bursitis: sonographic findings with magnetic resonance correlations. *J Clin Ultrasound* 2002;30:437–441.

6. Blankenbaker DG, De Smet AA, Keene JS. Sonography of the iliopsoas tendon and injection of the iliopsoas bursa for diagnosis and management of the painful snapping hip. *Skeletal Radiol* 2006;35:565–571.

7. Brew CJ, Stockley I, Grainger AJ, Stone MH. Iliopsoas tendonitis caused by overhang of a collared femoral prosthesis. *J Arthroplasty* 2011;26:504 e17–19.

8. Wank R, Miller TT, Shapiro JF. Sonographically guided injection of anesthetic for iliopsoas tendinopathy after total hip arthroplasty. *J Clin Ultrasound* 2004;32:354–357.

Henry A. Stiene, MD, FACSM

KEY POINTS

- High-frequency linear array transducer is preferred.
- A 21–22-gauge, 2–3-inch needle is desirable.
- The adductor longus is the most commonly injured adductor tendons

- The injection should use both long- and short-axis views to be most accurate.

Pertinent Anatomy

The hip adductors are a powerful group of muscles that consist of the adductor magnus/minimus, adductor longus, adductor brevis, and the gracilis and pectineus muscle groups. All of the muscles are innervated by the obturator nerve (L2–L4) with the exception of the pectineus, which is innervated by the femoral nerve (L2–L4). The adductor magnus also receives innervation from the posterior tibial nerve (L4–S3) (Figure 56-1).

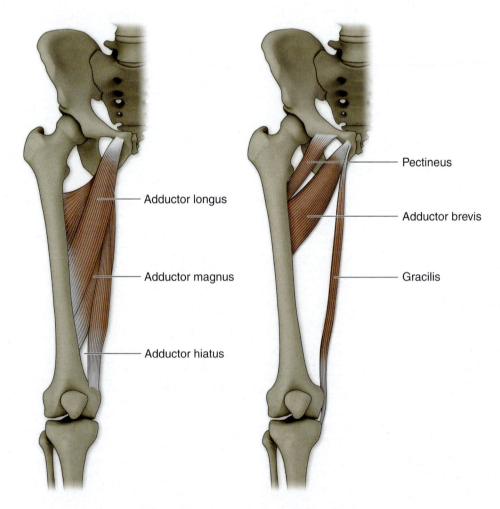

Adductor longus

Adductor magnus

Adductor hiatus

Pectineus

Adductor brevis

Gracilis

FIGURE 56-1 ■ Anatomy of the adductor tendons.

Common Pathology

Injuries to this muscle group are commonly known as "groin injuries" and can be simplified into two general categories: acute or chronic. Acute injuries occur frequently in athletes where a change of direction, push-off, or stop-and-go movements are common such as in soccer, football, hockey, lacrosse, basketball, or tennis, to name a few. The athlete usually feels a "pop" or "pull" at the time of injury and is often unable to continue to participate. Inflammation of the tendon sheath (tenosynovitis) is not very common in the adductor tendon group, but when it occurs, it most often involves the adductor longus tendon and is usually associated with acute overuse.

On the other extreme, chronic injuries occur in the setting of overuse or repetitive movements such as kicking a soccer ball where microtrauma leads to degeneration of the tendon and can result in chronic pain and dysfunction. Athletes often complain of a dull ache with these injuries, but sometimes are able to continue to play, despite the pain.

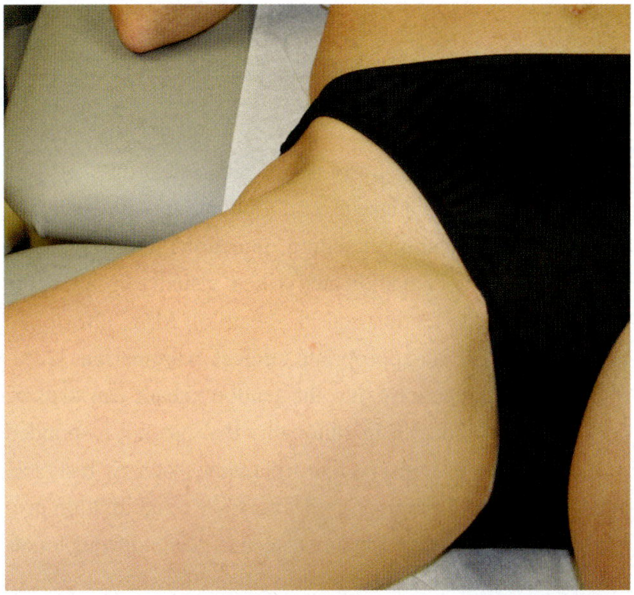

FIGURE 56-2 ■ Patient position: The patient is supine with the hip abducted, externally rotated, and the knee slightly flexed.

Ultrasound Imaging Findings

For musculoskeletal (MSK) ultrasound examination of the adductor muscle group, the patient is placed in the supine position with the hip slightly flexed, externally rotated, abducted, and the knee flexed. The examiner is then able to easily palpate the adductor longus tendon as it originates from the anterior aspect of the pubis (Figure 56-2).

By placing a high-frequency linear array transducer directly over the bulk of the muscle mass in the long axis, the examiner is able to identify the adductor longus muscle and tendon as it originates from the pubis. Deep to the adductor longus, the adductor brevis is identified, and deep and medial to the brevis lays the anterior muscle belly of adductor magnus. From there, the examiner can perform a linear slide medial and cephalad toward the pubic symphysis to identify the thin gracilis origin. Returning to the adductor longus tendon, the examiner then performs a linear slide lateral and cephalad to examine the pectineus. The adductor group can be examined in the short axis by palpating the adductor longus tendon and scanning from the pubis distal into the muscle belly to identify underlying pathology. To look for peritendinous inflammation, the anechoic fluid between the tendon and its sheath is best identified in this short-axis view.

It is important to document identification of all five muscle origins and any abnormalities that are noted (Figure 56-3).

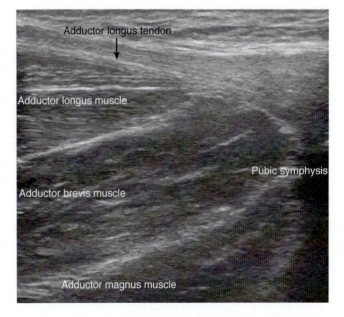

FIGURE 56-3 ■ Musculoskeletal ultrasound image of the adductor muscle group at the level of the bony pubis.

Indications for Ultrasound-Guided Procedures of the Adductor Muscles and Tendons

Different types of ultrasound-guided injections in and around the adductor muscles and tendons may be indicated in the appropriate clinical setting. Injections into the adductor tendon sheath are indicated when visualizing anechoic fluid between the tendon and its sheath on MSK ultrasound examination with an appropriate clinical examination. Ultrasound-guided injections into the tendon sheath can also be performed for adductor tendinopathy that has not responded to other forms of conservative treatment, such as rest, ice, nonsteroidal antiinflammatory drugs, and a rehabilitation program. Intratendinous procedures, such as percutaneous tenotomy or fenestration should be considered for these cases. In addition, placing a needle into the adductor muscles can be useful for treating acute muscle injuries, aspiration of cysts, hematomas, and other fluid-filled structures.

Equipment

■ Needle: 22–25-gauge, 1.5–2-inch needle
■ Injectate: 1 mL of local anesthesia and 1 mL of an injectable corticosteroid
■ High-frequency linear array transducer

Author's Preferred Peritendinous Technique

a. Patient position (see Figure 56-2)
    i. Supine with the hip externally rotated and abducted with the knee flexed
    ii. Patient's arms folded across the abdomen
b. Transducer position (Figures 56-4 and 56-5)
    i. Long axis to the adductor longus muscle/tendon as the orienting landmark
    ii. Turn transducer 90 degrees to short axis to best identify the tendon and its sheath
c. Needle orientation relative to the transducer
    i. Start out of plane and then rotate transducer 90 degrees so the needle becomes in plane

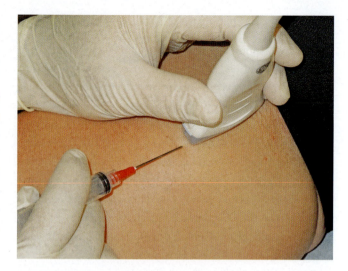

FIGURE 56-4 ■ Long-axis, in-plane approach from distal to proximal for an ultrasound-guided approach to the adductor longus tendon and its sheath.

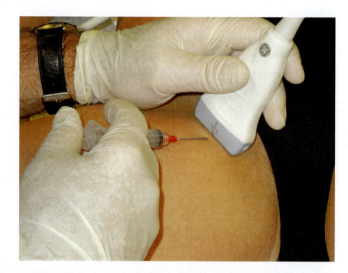

FIGURE 56-5 ■ Short-axis, out-of-plane approach from distal to proximal for an ultrasound-guided approach to the adductor longus tendon and its sheath.

d. Needle approach (Figure 56-6)
   i. Distal to proximal.
   ii. Use transducer to alternate between short and long axis to insure needle remains in the peritendinous space and tendon sheath as the needle advances.
e. Target
   i. The anechoic fluid space between the tendon and its surrounding sheath
f. Pearls and Pitfalls
   i. Anesthetic fluid alone can be injected initially when no anechogenic fluid is noted on ultrasound to insure good flow into the tendon sheath and avoid inadvertent injection of corticosteroid into the tendon itself.
   ii. Identify the adductor longus tendon by palpation and place the transducer over it in order to properly identify the entire group of tendons.
   iii. A distal-to-proximal approach for this injection makes the risk of intravascular injection low because the needle is moving away from the major neurovascular bundle in the area.

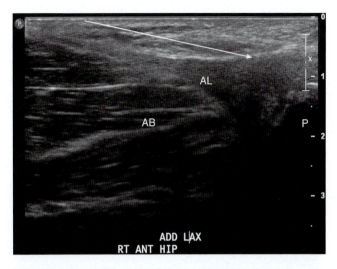

FIGURE 56-6 ■ Ultrasound image of peritendinous needle placement (*long arrow*) along the adductor longus tendon sheath (AL). View is long axis showing an in-plane approach. AB, adductor brevis muscle; P, pubic ramus.

Equipment

■ Needle
   • 25-gauge, 1.5-inch needle for local anesthesia
   • 18–20 gauge, 2–3 inch needle (or larger) for procedure
■ Injectate: limited amount of local anesthetic to allow for adequate pain control during needle fenestrations
■ High-frequency linear array transducer

Author's Preferred Intratendinous Technique

a. Patient position (see Figure 56-2)
   i. Supine with the hip externally rotated and abducted with the knee flexed
   ii. Patient's arms folded across the abdomen
b. Transducer position (see Figure 56-4)
   i. Long axis to the adductor longus tendon
c. Needle orientation relative to the transducer (Figure 56-7)
   i. In plane
d. Needle approach (see Figure 56-7)
   i. Distal to proximal
e. Target
   i. Adductor tendon where pathology is noted, most often at insertion to pubic symphysis

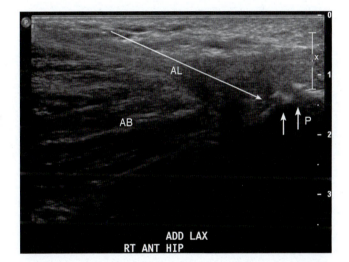

FIGURE 56-7 ■ Ultrasound image of adductor longus (AL) tendinosis with cortical irregularities (*small arrows*) seen at insertion to the pubic ramus. *Long arrow* indicates needle angle and position for tenotomy procedure with long axis, in-plane approach. AB, adductor brevis muscle; P, pubic ramus.

f. Pearls and Pitfalls
    i. Always rotate the transducer to short axis during the procedure to insure that the entire width of diseased tendon is treated (see Figure 56-5).
    ii. Identify the adductor longus tendon by palpation and place the transducer over it in order to properly identify the entire group of tendons.

iii. A distal-to-proximal approach for this injection makes the risk of intravascular injection low because the needle is moving away from the major neurovascular bundle in the area.

References

1. Bianchi S, Martinoli C, Abdelwahab IF, et al. *Ultrasound of the Musculoskeletal System*. Berlin: Springer; 2007.

2. Jacobson JA. *Fundamentals of Musculoskeletal Ultrasound*. 2nd ed. Philadelphia, PA: Saunders; 2012.

Robert Monaco, MD / Megan Groh Miller, MD

KEY POINTS

- Use a high frequency linear array transducer.
- The needle gauge and length depends on chronicity and the depth of the hematoma.
- Quadriceps hematomas are common in contact sports, most commonly seen involving the rectus femoris.

- Aspiration of significant hematomas allows improvement in range of motion and may result in faster return to play.
- Lavage may be needed in chronic hematomas.

Pertinent Anatomy

The quadriceps muscle group is made up of the rectus femoris, and three vastus muscles (medialis, lateralis, intermedius). The rectus crosses two joints and thus allows for hip flexion and knee extension along with the vasti (Figure 57-1).

Common Pathology

The quadriceps is commonly injured by direct trauma (contusion) to the thigh in contact sports such as football. It can also be injured by a muscle strain pattern during regulation of knee flexion and hip extension. The rectus femoris is the most commonly injured, as it is the most superficial and also crosses two joints.

Quadriceps contusions are graded mild, moderate, or severe based on the number of degrees present of active knee flexion. Pain and functional limitations vary based on the degree of injury, but in general the higher grade injuries are more painful and result in more functional limitations.

Ultrasound Imaging Findings

The optimal transducer for imaging is best determined by the size of the patient's quadriceps muscle and length of the injury. Superficial rectus femoris injuries can be investigated with a linear array probe scanning from 10–18 MHz. Many deeper contusions are better visualized by using a convex probe scanning at 4–6 MHz. Scans should be done in both long and short axis, and the sonographer should be careful to limit pressure to not decrease hematoma size (Figure 57-2).

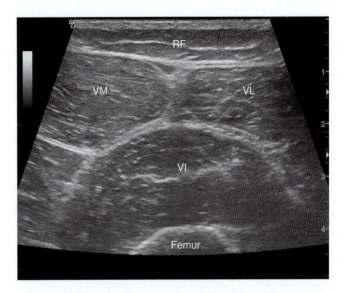

FIGURE 57-1 ■ Ultrasound convex view of mid-quadriceps anatomy. RF, rectus femoris; VI, vastus intermedius; VL, vastus lateralis; VM, vastus medialis.

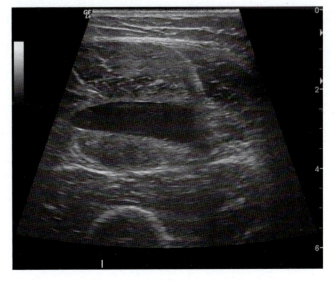

FIGURE 57-2 ■ Ultrasound image of quadriceps hematoma.

233

Using a panoramic view can be beneficial in determining the length and depth of injury (Figure 57-3).

The findings will vary on the type and chronicity of the injury and may include mixed echogenicity in the muscle of varying size and length. A hematoma formation will be hypoechoic acutely, with mixed echogenicity in the more chronic setting.

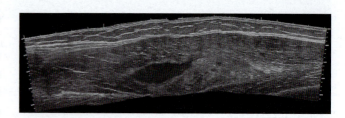

FIGURE 57-3 ■ Ultrasound panoramic view of hematoma.

Aspiration and Injection (Figure 57-4)

Aspiration of the hematoma may be indicated in those who have a significant reduction of active knee flexion (<90 degrees) and who are in need of returning to sports in an expedited fashion. Aspiration or injection is best done in the first 72 hours, as the hematoma is not yet solidified. These injections cannot be done without ultrasound guidance as the hematoma is often very deep (3–8 cm) and often unrecognizable without ultrasound. Clinical outcomes of aspiration versus traditional rehabilitation have not been done. Some clinicians may use a corticosteroid or platelet-rich plasma (PRP) post aspiration for hematoma or tears, although there is no evidence-based literature for or against this use.

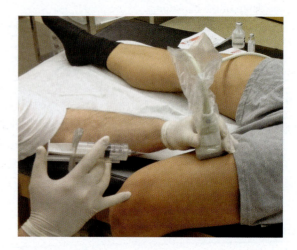

FIGURE 57-4 ■ Illustration of setup for ultrasound-guided aspiration on patient.

Equipment

- Needle
  - Depends on chronicity and depth of the hematoma: 22 gauge (larger gauge if more chronic); length between 2.5 and 6 inches (longer for a deeper hematoma)
- Injectate
  - Local anesthetic 1%; enough to anesthetize through subcutaneous tissues to cyst (~5 mL)
  - Optional: normal saline for lavage (see below)
- Transducer
  - Generally a high frequency linear array transducer; Low frequency curvilinear for deeper hematomas.

Author's Preferred Technique

a. Patient position

   i. Supine; knee slightly flexed if needed to increase size of the hematoma

b. Transducer position

   i. Longitudinal, over the hematoma

c. Needle orientation relative to the transducer

   i. In plane

d. Needle approach (Figure 57-5)

   i. Using a long-axis approach, enter the hematoma at its most distal aspect.

   ii. Enter distal to proximal.

e. Target

   i. Central portion of hematoma

f. Pearls and Pitfalls

   i. If aspiration is difficult, either use a larger gauge needle and/or lavage the area.

   ii. To lavage the area, use a syringe with 10 mL of a 50/50 mixture of normal saline and local anesthetic; then attempt reaspiration. It may also be useful to use a double-barreled syringe (such as an Avanca RPD syringe) to facilitate this. Lavaging is crucial to break up chronic partially solidified hematomas.

   iii. There may be multiple hematomas or it may be loculated requiring repositioning of the needle. Choose an entry point to maximize flexibility of needle manipulation.

   iv. Contraction of the quadriceps by the patient or manual pressure by an assistant may help facilitate hematoma mobilization.

   v. Strongly consider aspiration when you expect to yield a minimum of 5–10 cc of fluid.

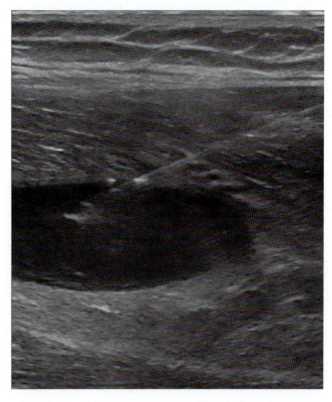

FIGURE 57-5 ■ Ultrasound visualization of needle entering hematoma.

References

1. Bencardino HT, Rosenberg ZS, Brown RR, et al. Traumatic musculotendinous injuries of the knee: diagnosis with MR imaging. *Radiographics* 2000 Oct;20 Spec No:S103–S120.

2. Cross TM, Gibbs N, Houang MT, et al. Acute quadriceps muscle strains: magnetic resonance features and prognosis. *Am J Sports Med* 2004 Apr;32:710–719.

3. Kary J. Diagnosis and management of quadriceps strains and contusions. *Curr Rev Musculoskelet Med* 2010 Oct;3(1-4): 26–31.

Joanne Borg Stein, MD

KEY POINTS

- A 22–25 gauge, 2- or 3-inch needle is recommended.
- A curvilinear array or linear array transducer may be used depending on patient body habitus.
- Use a lateral-to-medial approach.
- *Sciatic tunnel syndrome* refers to entrapment and neuralgia of the sciatic nerve in the gluteal triangle.
- Sciatic tunnel may result in chronic neuralgic pain in the posterior thigh.
- Be wary of intraneural or intravascular injection.
- With expertise, the circumferential hydrodissection technique should be attempted.

Pertinent Anatomy (Figure 58-1)

The anterior divisions of L4–S3 contribute to the sciatic nerve, which exits the greater sciatic foramen and passes below the piriformis and gluteus maximus muscle. It lies posterior to the quadratus femoris muscle just lateral to the ischial tuberosity at which position it is accessible to nerve block. The clinician may follow the course of the sciatic nerve distally in the posterior thigh in the plane anterior to the biceps femoris muscle before entering the popliteal triangle. The nerve may be accessed at any of these locations; however, a common site of entrapment is in the proximal subgluteal location.

Common Pathology

The sciatic nerve is vulnerable to injury, entrapment, and inflammation in the gluteal triangle. Piriformis or quadratus femoris muscle strain may result in scar tissue and sciatic neuralgia. Proximal hamstring injuries at the ischial tuberosity may result in local inflammation and traction with resultant sciatic neuralgia. Furthermore, the sciatic nerve is vulnerable with hamstring muscle strains of the posterior thigh.

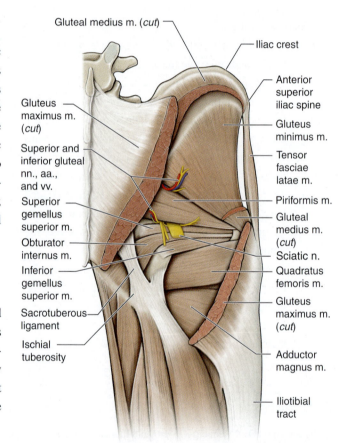

FIGURE 58-1 ■ Sciatic nerve in the subgluteal triangle: note position lateral to the ischial tuberosity and posterior to the quadratus femoris muscle. (Reproduced with permission from Morton DA, Foreman KB, Albertine KH, eds. *The Big Picture: Gross Anatomy.* New York: McGraw-Hill; 2011: figure 35-1C.)

Ultrasound Imaging Findings (Figure 58-2)

The sciatic nerve is best visualized with a linear array transducer at a medium frequency. In larger patients, a curvilinear array transducer at lower frequencies may be necessary. The patient may experience neuropathic pain with sonopalpation over the nerve. Adjacent muscle or tendon injury pattern or edema may be visualized.

Indications for Sciatic Nerve Block

Sciatic nerve blocks can be performed for patients with recalcitrant neuropathic pain that is unresponsive to resolution of the adjacent tendon or muscle injury, rest, icing, antiinflammatories, stretching and physical therapy. Perineural injection should not be attempted without guidance. Nerve stimulator guidance has been used in the past; however, ultrasound-guided injection allows the clinician direct visualization of the nerve and surrounding vasculature to maximize precision and avoid intravascular and intraneural injection.

Equipment

- Needle: 22–25-gauge, 2- or 3-inch needle depending on patient habitus
- Injectate: 2 mL local anesthetic ±1 mL of an injectable corticosteroid
- Medium frequency linear array or curvilinear array transducer, depending on body habitus

Author's Preferred Technique

a. Patient position (Figure 58-3)
   i. Prone
   ii. Alternate position: side-lying (with the hip in flexion, adduction and internal rotation)
b. Transducer position
   i. Anatomic axial plane transverse to the sciatic nerve
c. Needle orientation relative to the transducer
   i. In plane

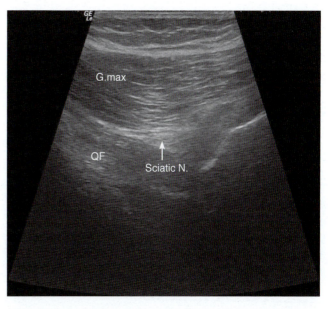

FIGURE 58-2 ▪ Ultrasound appearance of the sciatic nerve between the gluteus maximus and quadratus femoris muscles; lateral to the ischial tuberosity.

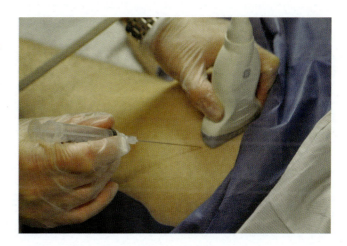

FIGURE 58-3 ▪ Prone position for sciatic nerve block.

d. Needle approach (Figure 58-4)
    i. Lateral to medial
e. Target
    i. Perineural circumferential spread injectate spread around the sciatic nerve
f. Pearls and Pitfalls
    i. The sciatic nerve block subgluteal approach in the lateral recumbent (semiprone) position may have the advantage of stretching the gluteal muscles and allow better access to the nerve in larger or obese patients.
    ii. The sciatic nerve lies on the medial side of the subgluteal region as well as the inferior gluteal artery; therefore, a lateral-to-medial approach may help avoid inadvertent intravascular injection.

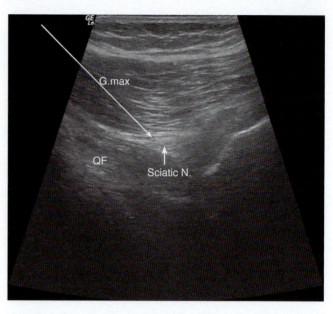

FIGURE 58-4 ▪ Needle orientation for sciatic nerve block.

References

1. Narouze SN, ed. *Atlas of Ultrasound-Guided Procedures in Interventional Pain Management.* New York: Springer; 2011.
2. Franklyn-Miller A, Falvey E, McCrory P. The gluteal triangle: a clinical patho-anatomical approach to the diagnosis of gluteal pain in athletes. *Br J Sports Med* Jun;43(6):460–406.
3. Bigelesisen P, Orebaugh S, Monyeri N, et al. eds. *Ultrasound-Guided Regional Anesthesia and Pain Medicine.* Philadelphia, PA: Lippincott Williams & Wilkins; 2010.

Danielle Aufiero, MD / Steven Sampson, DO

KEY POINTS

- A 22-gauge, 1.5–3-inch needle is used, depending on depth of femoral nerve.
- Use a high-frequency linear array transducer positioned with the nerve visualized in short axis and in-plane approach.
- The femoral nerve lies lateral to the femoral artery and vein in a neurovascular bundle and is encased in a fascia sheath.
- The femoral nerve is ideally localized at the level of the inguinal ligament to ensure no branches have occurred.
- The femoral nerve appears hyperechoic, triangular, and slightly flattened by the overlying fascia iliacus.

Pertinent Anatomy

The femoral nerve runs deep to the iliacus muscle and superficial to the psoas muscle and is encased in fascia. The femoral nerve is the most lateral component of the neurovascular bundle that lies in the anterior superior medial thigh, deep to the inguinal ligament. A common pneumonic applied to these structures in order from lateral to medial is NAVEL (nerve, artery, vein, empty space, and lymph node if present) (Figures 59-1 and 59-2).

Common Etiologies

The femoral nerve supplies the muscles and skin in front of the thigh, and the skin of the medial calf and foot.

Symptoms of femoral nerve dysfunction may include quadriceps weakness such as knee buckling or difficulty ascending stairs, and altered sensation in its skin distribution. Dysfunction of the femoral nerve can occur from several etiologies. There can be direct injury from traumatic catheter placement or pelvic fracture. Prolonged pressure from etiologies such as iliopsoas hematoma, abscess, or tumor has all been described. In addition, ischemia secondary to knee and hip flexed in supine position during intraoperative procedures can cause local compression. Lastly, systemic metabolic diseases such as diabetes mellitus (ie, diabetic amyotrophy with localized femoral neuropathy) or neurological conditions affecting peripheral nerves such as mononeuritis multiplex have been implicated.

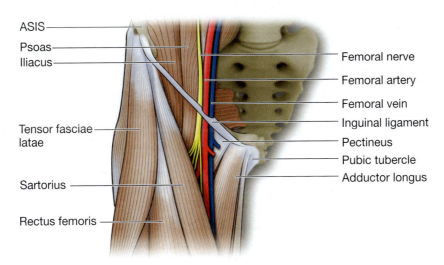

FIGURE 59-1 ■ Right hip anatomy: coronal view showing pertinent muscles and neurovascular structures as they course inferior to the inguinal ligament.

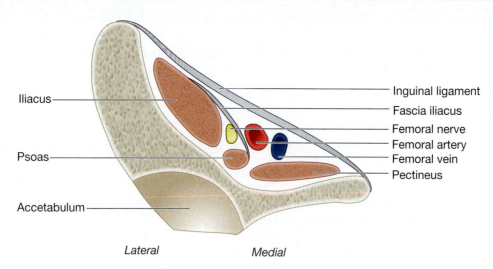

FIGURE 59-2 ■ Right hip anatomy: cross-section at the level of the inguinal ligament.

Ultrasound Imaging of the Femoral Nerve

The femoral nerve is best visualized in short axis using a high-frequency linear array transducer and a depth of less than 3 cm in the nonobese patient. If the nerve lies deeper than 4 cm, then a curvilinear probe or a medium-frequency linear array probe should be used. The femoral nerve shows up as a triangular hyperechoic region lateral to the femoral artery and up against the iliacus muscle, with a hyperechoic line superior to the nerve representing the fascia iliacus. Abnormal pathology of the nerve is not common and its absence does not necessarily equate to normal nerve function (Figure 59-3). Needle electromyogram testing is a helpful diagnostic tool, which can reveal abnormal spontaneous activity in the femoral nerve innervated muscles versus L2–L4 nerve roots, distinguishing femoral neuropathy from lumbar radiculopathy.

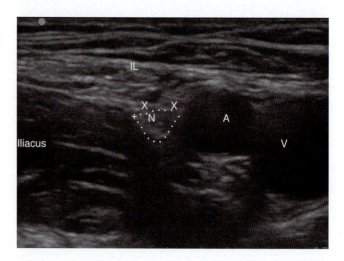

FIGURE 59-3 ■ Ultrasound of normal femoral nerve with nearby anatomy, right side. A, femoral artery; IL, inguinal ligament; N, femoral nerve; V, femoral vein; XX, iliacus fascia.

Indications for Femoral Nerve Injections

Injection of the femoral nerve can be performed for surgical, diagnostic, or therapeutic purposes. Intraoperative femoral nerve blocks can be used for surgeries of the anterior aspect of the thigh such as skin grafting, saphenous vein stripping, arthroscopic knee surgery, or medial ankle surgery. Postoperatively, femoral nerve catheters can be placed on the nerve for prolonged analgesia. Therapeutic injections can potentially reduce pain on a short-term basis for femoral neuropathy related to pressure, trauma, or mass. Diagnostic blocks can be performed for clinical presentations that raise suspicion of femoral neuropathy for confirmatory purposes. Therapeutic cortisone injections may be beneficial in femoral neuropathy secondary to inflammatory process or pressure induced dysfunction. The rate of vascular puncture in nerve-stimulation-guided femoral nerve catheters is 6% versus an unknown percentage in ultrasound-guided femoral nerve blocks.[1] However, studies that compared the timeliness of each guidance tool in general resulted in trends toward improved speed and efficiency with ultrasound guidance.[2]

Equipment

■ Needle: 22-gauge, 1.5–3-inch needle depending on depth of femoral nerve

■ Injectate

• Nerve block: 2 cc local anesthetic ± injectable corticosteroids

• Nerve hydrodissection and decompression: 5–10 mL total solution (combination of normal saline, local anesthetic, ± dextrose solution)

■ High-frequency linear array transducer

Author's Preferred Technique

a. Patient position

   i. The patient is supine with hip slightly abducted from midline.

   ii. If large body habitus, consider taping excess adipose in the abdominal region out of the way of the inguinal ligament for best visualization.

   iii. Placing leg in slight hip external rotation can further expose structures.

b. Transducer position (Figure 59-4)

   i. Anatomic coronal oblique plane where it intersects midpoint of inguinal crease in the upper anterior thigh

   ii. Femoral nerve located approximately one fingerbreadth lateral to the femoral artery at the mid-inguinal ligament

c. Needle orientation relative to the transducer (see Figure 59-4)

   i. In plane

d. Needle approach (Figure 59-5)

   i. Lateral to medial

e. Target (see Figure 59-5)

   i. Lateral border of femoral nerve sheath.

   ii. You will see hypoechoic injectate filling lateral aspect of sheath, which will push nerve more into view because of volume affect.

f. Pearls and Pitfalls

   i. Ensure the largest diameter of femoral nerve by locating it proximal to its branches just proximal to the inguinal crease.

   ii. If more than one artery is visualized, move the probe more proximal because this represents a point too far distal where branches have occurred.

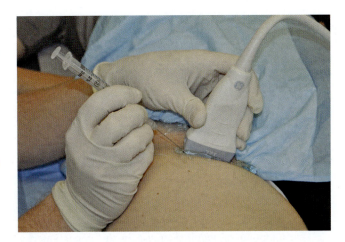

FIGURE 59-4 ■ Patient position with lateral-to-medial, in-plane technique to right femoral nerve using high-frequency linear array transducer.

   iii. Excessive pressure from the probe on the neurovascular bundle can obliterate femoral vein and can affect visualization of the target.

   iv. Specific complications include femoral neuritis, intraneural injection, prolonged block, and hematoma. Although direct injection into the nerve should be avoided, studies evaluating long term sequelae of intraneural injection have revealed no significant permanent nerve damage.[3,4]

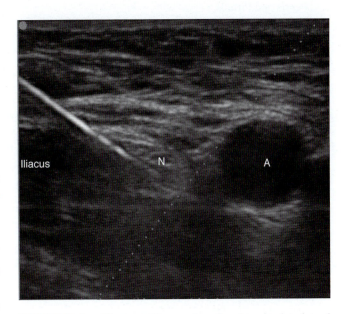

FIGURE 59-5 ■ Ultrasound image of needle advancing into lateral femoral sheath for femoral nerve block. A, femoral artery; N, femoral nerve. Note the use of beam steering on ultrasound image.

Alternate Technique

a. Patient position

   i. The patient is supine with hip slightly abducted from midline.

   ii. If patient has large body habitus, consider taping excess adipose in the abdominal region out of the way of the inguinal ligament for best visualization.

   iii. Placing leg in slight hip external rotation can further expose structures.

b. Transducer position (Figure 59-6)

   i. Anatomic coronal oblique plane where it intersects midpoint of inguinal crease in the upper anterior thigh

   ii. Femoral nerve located approximately one finger-breadth lateral to the femoral artery at the mid-inguinal ligament

c. Needle orientation relative to the transducer (see Figure 59-6)

   i. Out of plane

d. Needle approach (Figure 59-7)

   i. Distal to proximal

   ii. Use walk-down technique

e. Target (see Figure 59-7)

   i. Femoral nerve sheath inferior to fascia iliacus.

   ii. You will see hypoechoic injectate filling femoral sheath.

f. Pearls and Pitfalls

   i. See "Pearls and Pitfalls" under "Author's Preferred Technique."

   ii. Because the needle is visualized in cross-section and the exact needle tip may not be imaged, this technique is more concerning for intravascular or intraneural injection.

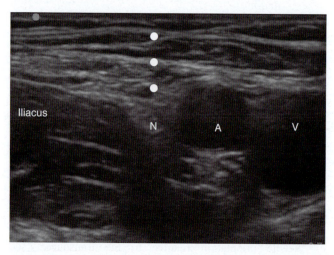

FIGURE 59-6 ▪ Patient position for distal-to-proximal, out-of-plane approach to femoral nerve.

FIGURE 59-7 ▪ Alternate technique for femoral nerve block using walk-down technique and out-of-plane needle approach. *Dots* represent needle tip with walk-down technique. A, femoral artery; N, femoral nerve; V, femoral vein.

References

1. Mariano ER, Loland VJ, Sandhu NS, et al. Ultrasound guidance versus electrical stimulation for femoral perineural catheter insertion. *J Ultrasound Med* 2009;28:1453–1460.

2. Brull R, Choi S. Is ultrasound guidance advantageous for interventional pain management? A review of acute pain outcomes. *Anesth Analg* 2011;10:1213.

3. Gruber H, Peer S, Kovacs P, et al. The ultrasonographic appearance of the femoral nerve and cases of iatrogenic impairment. *J Ultrasound Med* 2003;22:163–172.

4. Bigeleisen, P. Nerve puncture and apparent intraneural injection during ultrasound-guided axillary block does not invariably result in neurologic injury. *Anesthesiology* 2006;105:779–783.

Joanne Borg Stein, MD

KEY POINTS

- A medium-to high-frequency linear array transducer is often ideal. In larger patients, curvilinear array is recommended.
- A 22-gauge, 3.5-inch needle is recommended.
- Use an in-plane lateral-to-medial approach.

- Avoid intraneural or intravascular injection.
- Supplemental nerve stimulation is recommended located at cm lateral and distal to the pubic tubercle.

Pertinent Anatomy

The obturator nerve is mixed motor and sensory with contributions from spinal levels L2–L4.

The nerve reaches the inguinal region passing through the obturator foramen. The anterior branch passes between the adductor longus and brevis; supplying these muscles as well as the gracilis. It provides sensation to the medial thigh. The posterior branch passes between the adductor brevis and magnus and innervates the adductor magnus muscle (Figure 60-1).

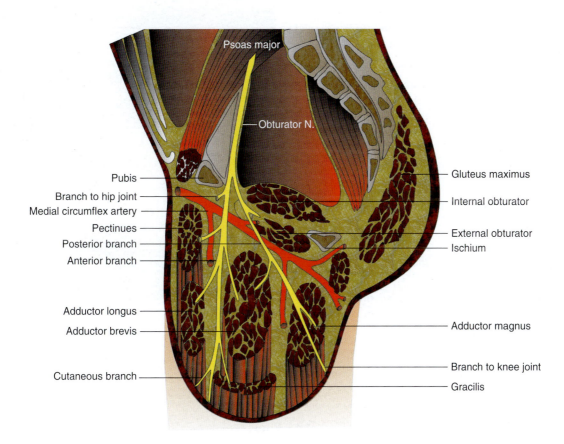

FIGURE 60-1 ■ Illustration of the obturator nerve and its terminal branches in relationship to the adductor muscles. (Reproduced with permission from Hadzic A, ed. *Hadzic's Peripheral Nerve Blocks and Anatomy for Ultrasound-Guided Regional Anesthesia.* 2nd ed. New York: McGraw-Hill; 2012: figure 37-4.)

Common Pathology

The obturator nerve is vulnerable to injury, entrapment, and inflammation in the obturator foramen in the setting of pelvis fracture. Injury to adjacent muscles may result in injury and pain, notably after adduction injuries ("groin pulls"). Adductor spasticity may accompany neurologic disorders and interfere with functional mobility, positioning, toileting and hygiene. Neurolysis is an effective treatment.

Ultrasound Imaging Findings

The obturator nerve is best visualized with a medium- to high-frequency linear array transducer. The patient may experience pain with sonopalpation over the nerve. Adjacent muscle or tendon injury pattern or edema may be visualized.[1]

Indications for Obturator Nerve Injection

Obturator nerve injections can be performed for patients with recalcitrant neuropathic pain and/or spasticity that is unresponsive to relative rest, ice, medication, stretching, and physical therapy. Perineural injection should not be attempted without guidance. Nerve stimulator guidance has been used in the past; however, the addition of ultrasound guidance allows the clinician direct visualization of the nerve and surrounding vasculature to maximize precision and avoid intravascular and intraneural injection.[2]

Equipment

- Needle: 22-gauge, 3.5-inch needle depending on patient habitus
- Injectate
  - Nerve block: 2 cc local anesthetic ±injectable corticosteroids
  - Nerve hydrodissection and decompression: 5–10 mL total solution (combination of normal saline, local anesthetic, ± dextrose solution)
- Medium- to high-frequency linear array transducer. Curvilinear array transducer may be needed in larger patient.

Author's Preferred Technique

a. Patient position (Figure 60-2)
   i. Supine with hip and knee flexed and hip in external rotation
b. Transducer position (Figure 60-3)
   i. Anatomic axial plane transverse to the obturator nerves parallel to the inguinal ligament and medial to the femoral neurovascular bundle

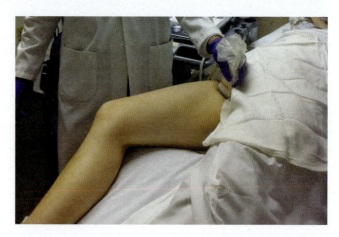

FIGURE 60-2 ■ Supine position for obturator nerve block. Hip and knee flexed. Hip is externally rotated.

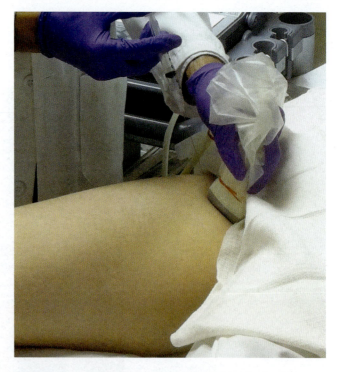

FIGURE 60-3 ■ Transducer and needle position for lateral to medial, in-plane approach to the obturator nerve.

c. Needle orientation relative to the transducer
  i. In plane
d. Needle approach (Figure 60-4)
  i. Lateral to medial
e. Target
  i. Perineural spread of injectate spread around the nerve in the plane between muscles
f. Pearls and Pitfalls
  i. Care must be taken to avoid the obturator artery.
  ii. Clinically, the practitioner may achieve best results by using nerve stimulation in addition to ultrasound guidance; especially for phenol neurolysis treatment of spasticity.
  iii. Injections can be performed to the anterior, posterior, or both branches as indicated clinically.

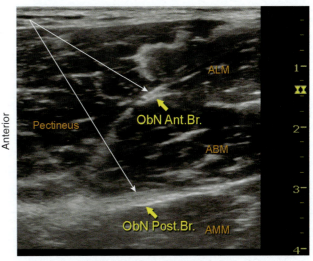

Obturator nerve-transverse view

FIGURE 60-4 ■ Ultrasound appearance of the obturator nerve in the medial inguinal region; anterior and posterior branches. *Long arrows* represent needle angle to anterior and posterior branches of obturator nerves. ABM, adductor brevis muscle; ALM, adductor longus muscle; AMM, adductor magnus muscle. (Reproduced with permission from Hadzic A, ed. *Hadzic's Peripheral Nerve Blocks and Anatomy for Ultrasound-Guided Regional Anesthesia*. 2nd ed. New York: McGraw-Hill; 2012: figure 37-3.)

References

1. Bodner G. High resolution sonography of the peripheral nervous system. Siegfreid Peer and Gerd Bodner: Springer; 2003.
2. Fukiwara Y, Komatsu T. Ultrasound-guided obturator nerve block. In: Bigelesisen P, Orebaugh S, Monyeri N, et al. ed. *Ultrasound-Guided Regional Anesthesia and Pain Medicine*. Philadelphia, PA: Lippincott Williams & Wilkins; 2010: 114–119.

Paul D. Tortland, DO, FAOASM

KEY POINTS

- Use a 25-gauge, 1.5–2-inch needle.
- A mid- to high-frequency linear array transducer is best.
- The lateral femoral cutaneous nerve (LFCN) is sensory only.
- The LFCN is best visualized just distal to the anterior superior iliac spine (ASIS).

- Probe short axis to body and nerve for visualization.
- Probe short axis and/or long axis to nerve for injection.
- Use injection for diagnostic purposed or attempt hydrodissection.

Anatomy

The lateral femoral cutaneous nerve (LFCN) arises directly from the lumbar plexus, with contributions from the L2–L3 nerve roots. Following the lateral border of the psoas muscle, the nerve courses through the pelvis toward the lateral aspect of the inguinal ligament. It deviates medially to the anterior superior iliac spine (ASIS) as it passes under the ligament (Figure 61-1). The nerve then traverses a superficial lacuna located between the sartorius and tensor fascia lata muscles.

The LFCN provides sensory innervation to the anterolateral aspect of the proximal and middle third of the thigh. It can become entrapped along its course, but the most common site is under the inguinal ligament or just distal to it.

Common Pathology

The most common pathology affecting the LFCN is an entrapment neuropathy resulting in paresthesias or anesthesia involving some or all of the distribution area of the nerve. This condition is known as *meralgia paresthetica*.

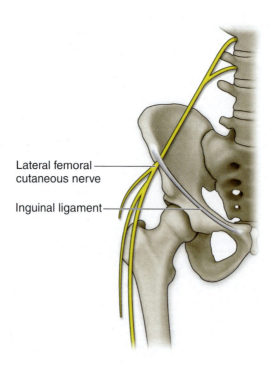

Lateral femoral cutaneous nerve

Inguinal ligament

FIGURE 61-1 ■ Anatomical course of lateral femoral cutaneous nerve (LFCN).

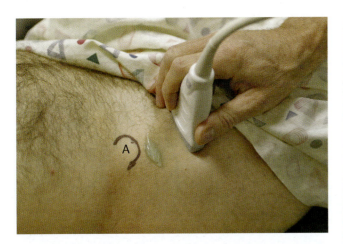

FIGURE 61-2 ■ Initial probe position to locate the lateral femoral cutaneous nerve (LFCN); short axis to body, several centimeters distal to the anterior superior iliac spine (ASIS [A]).

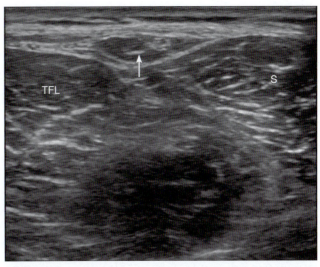

FIGURE 61-3 ■ Short-axis view distal to the anterior superior iliac spine indicating the lateral femoral cutaneous nerve (LFCN) (*arrow*) lying in a lacuna between the sartorius muscle (S) and the tensor fascia lata (TFL).

Ultrasound Imaging Findings

The LFCN is most easily located sonographically by placing the transducer short axis to the body (short axis to the nerve) several centimeters distal to the ASIS, as shown in Figure 61-2. Identify the sartorius (medial) and tensor fascia lata (lateral) muscles (Figure 61-3). Between the two muscles lies a small superficial triangular lacuna just deep to the overlying connective tissue. The nerve can be identified lying in this space (see Figure 61-3). The nerve can then be traced proximally to the inguinal ligament by performing a short-axis linear array slide.

Alternatively, the nerve may be found by placing the transducer long axis along the inguinal ligament with the heel of the probe resting on the ASIS (Figure 61-4A, B). The LFCN most commonly passes under the ligament roughly about 11 mm from the medial aspect of the ASIS, although it can traverse the ligament as far as 40 mm medial to the ASIS. An entrapped nerve will commonly appear enlarged or swollen (Figure 61-5).

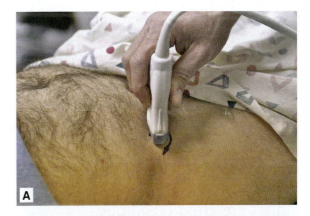

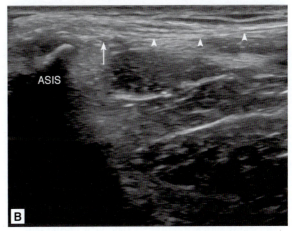

FIGURE 61-4 ■ **A.** Alternate probe position for locating the lateral femoral cutaneous nerve (LFCN): long axis to the inguinal ligament, with the heel of the transducer on the anterior superior iliac spine (ASIS). **B.** Short-axis view at the level the ASIS, indicating the LFCN (*arrow*) lying medial to the ASIS, just deep to the inguinal ligament (*arrowheads*).

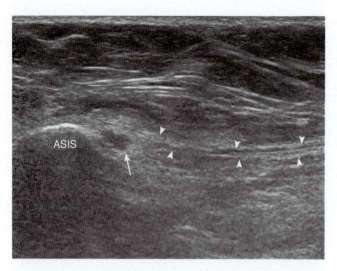

FIGURE 61-5 ■ Enlarged lateral femoral cutaneous nerve (LFCN) (*arrow*) lying medial to the anterior superior iliac spine (ASIS); inguinal ligament (*arrowheads*).

Equipment

- Needle: 25-gauge, 1.5–2-inch needle
- Injectate
  - Nerve block: 2 cc local anesthetic ± injectable corticosteroids
  - Nerve hydrodissection/decompression: 5–10 mL total solution (combination of normal saline, local anesthetic, ± dextrose solution)
- Mid- to high-frequency linear array transducer

Author's Preferred Technique

a. Patient position
   i. Patient lies supine.
   ii. The target area should be well exposed and free of restrictive clothing.
   iii. Physician stands on affected side.
b. Transducer position
   i. Nerve injection: Transverse to body and short axis to nerve.
   ii. Hydrodissection: Start short axis to nerve, then turn long axis to perform procedure.
c. Needle orientation
   i. Nerve block (Figures 61-6 and 61-7): In plane.
   ii. Nerve hydrodissection (Figure 61-8): Start out-of-plane. The probe is then repeatedly turned both in plane and out of plane to monitor progress.

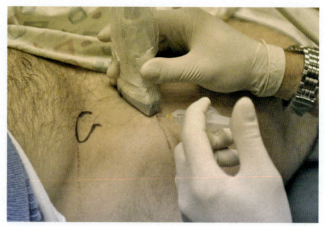

FIGURE 61-6 ■ Needle position for lateral femoral cutaneous nerve (LFCN) nerve block, in plane from lateral to medial.

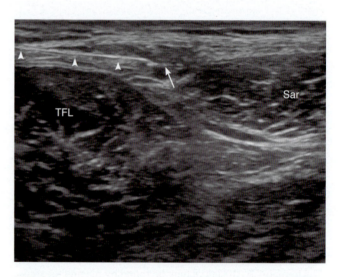

FIGURE 61-7 ■ Short-axis view indicating the needle (*arrowheads*) entering the lacuna containing the lateral femoral cutaneous nerve (LFCN) (*arrow*). Sar, sartorius; TFL, tensor fascia lata.

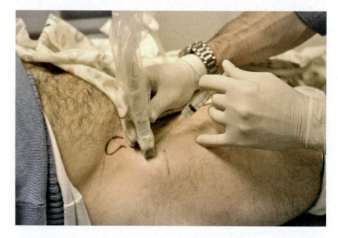

FIGURE 61-8 ■ Short-axis approach to lateral femoral cutaneous nerve (LFCN) nerve block.

d. Needle approach
    i. Nerve block: lateral to medial
    ii. Nerve hydrodissection: distal to proximal
e. Pearls and Pitfalls
    i. Given the very superficial nature of the course of the nerve at, and distal to, the ASIS, do not look for the nerve too deeply when performing a sonographic scan. Even in obese patients, the nerve lies just deep to the fascial plane separating the subcutaneous fat from the muscle layer.
    ii. Likewise, when performing the injection, be careful not to take too steep a needle approach initially.

References

1. Van Holsbeeck MT, Introcaso JH. *Musculoskeletal Ultrasound*, 2nd ed. St. Louis: Mosby; 2001.
2. Bianchi S, Martinoli C. *Ultrasound of the Musculoskeletal System.* Berlin: Springer; 2007.
3. Jacobson JA. *Fundamentals of Musculoskeletal Ultrasound.* Philadelphia, PA: Saunders; 2007:144–147.

Knee

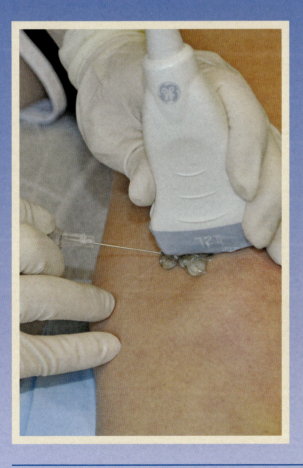

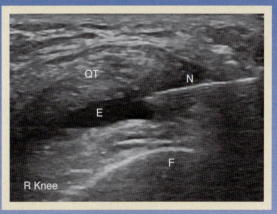

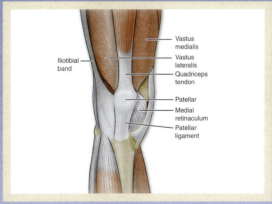

John C. Cianca, MD

Pertinent Anatomy

The knee joint is comprised of the distal femur and proximal tibia and fibula and the patella. There are three articulations within the knee joint: the femorotibial, the patellofemoral, and the tibiofibular. It is the first two articulations that are significant with respect to injections within the knee joint.

The knee joint is encased by a capsule like all other synovial joints and is stabilized by several ligaments. It is the most capacious joint capsule in the human body. The anterior and posterior cruciate ligaments are intraarticular, but extrasynovial. They lie in the center of the joint and, as such, may be encountered in a midline needle approach. The anterior medial and superior lateral aspects of the knee present the most accessible pathways to intraarticular needle penetration. The synovial lining of the joint capsule extends above the patella anteriorly as a pouch making it accessible to needle penetration from a superior lateral (Figure 62-1). The patellofemoral articulation is more accessible to penetration on the medial side, than laterally because of the more prominent

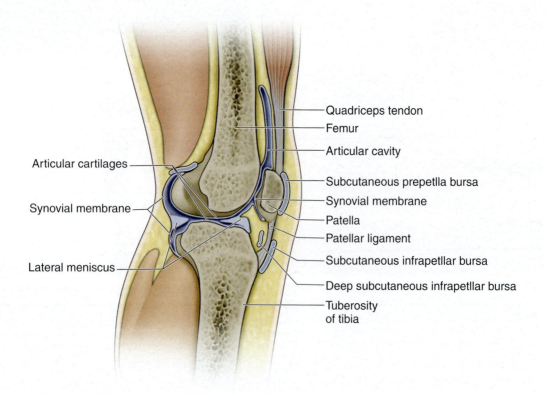

FIGURE 62-1 ■ Anatomy of knee joint with synovium and bursae.

anterior surface of the lateral femoral condyle. Inferiorly, the infrapatellar fat pad lies anterior to the synovial lining, thus it is extrasynovial. The thickness of the fat pad and the lack of a synovial pouch in this portion of the knee make needle penetration into the synovial space more difficult.

Common Pathology

The knee, like any other synovial joint, is susceptible to several arthritides. It is commonly affected by both osteoarthritis and rheumatoid arthritis. It may be affected by joint infection or gout. It is also vulnerable to intraarticular trauma particularly in athletes. As such, the knee is one of the most common sites of joint effusion. With the patient lying supine, a joint effusion is most noticeable in the superior lateral portion of the knee as the synovial pouch bulges superior laterally to the patellofemoral articulation. This can be seen in both long- and short-axis views with a linear array transducer placed over the quadriceps tendon using a 10–18 MHz setting, depending on the habitus of the patient (Figure 62-2). The effusion may be made to appear more prominent in this area by having patients press down on a towel roll placed under their posterior knee while in the supine position.

Degenerative changes within the knee may be seen in several views using ultrasound.

Osteophytes may be seen by placing a linear array transducer along the sagittal plane of the medial or lateral knee, bringing the joint lines into view. Meniscal extrusion and capsular deformity will also be seen with this view. The articular surface changes of the femur can be seen in long and short axis by having patients bend their knee to allow their foot to be flat on the examination table. The articular surface of the superior aspect of the femoral trochlea and the condylar heads is exposed and with the transducer placed over the region (long or short axis) is easily seen (Figure 62-3). Inferiorly, the articular surface of the inferior aspect of the femoral condyles can be seen using similar transducer positions.

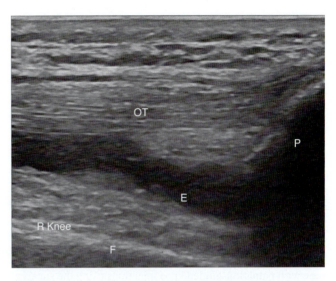

FIGURE 62-2 ■ Midline sagittal scan of the knee with an effusion. E, effusion; F, femur; P, patella; QT, quadriceps tendon.

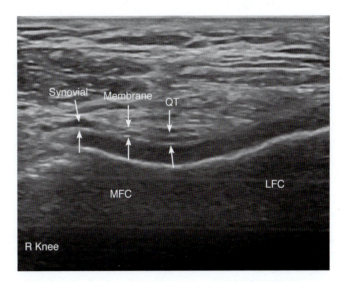

FIGURE 62-3 ■ Ultrasound image of the articular surface of the superior aspect of the femoral trochlea.

Indications for Knee Injection

The presence of an effusion may warrant needle aspiration. Even though the effusion may appear to be obvious, it is often intermingled with synovial tissue, which may become an unseen obstruction to a palpation-guided injection. Furthermore, depending on the technique used, a palpation-guided injection may encounter osteophytes, which if contacted could be painful or become an impediment to aspiration. Jackson et al. demonstrated a 71–93% accuracy rate in unguided injections of the knee without effusions depending on the injection portal used by one clinician.[1] Additionally, Curtiss et al. demonstrated 100% accuracy with ultrasound-guided injections as compared to 55% accuracy with palpation-guided knee injections using the superior lateral portal in cadavers when performed by inexperienced clinicians.[2] Jones et al. demonstrated only a 66% accuracy rate with unguided knee injection regardless of the level of clinical experience.[3] Therefore ultrasound-guided injection would provide more accuracy and may make the procedure less likely to be painful.

The treatment of knee arthritis with effusion often includes intraarticular corticosteroids or viscosupplements. The injection of steroids may be efficacious without accurate placement within the joint; but viscosupplementation efficacy is predicated on being intraarticular. In either case, an ultrasound-guided injection would promote more accuracy in a therapeutic injection of the knee.

Equipment

- Needle
  - 22-gauge, 1.5-inch needle with a 6–12-cc syringe for small-to-medium size effusions
  - 18–21-gauge, 1.5–2-inch needle with 12–25-cc syringe for large effusions
- Injectate
  - 2–3 mL of a local anesthetic and 1–2 mL of an injectable corticosteroid or 2–6 mL of hyaluronic acid
- High-frequency linear array transducer

Author's Preferred Technique

In the presence of an effusion, the superior lateral approach is both obvious and straightforward. This technique also allows the clinician ergonomic efficiency. If no effusion is present, local anesthetic may be used as a contrast medium as the needle is advanced and the joint capsule is hydrodissected from the overlying quadriceps tendon and the underlying prefemoral fat pad.

a. Procedure setup
   i. Patient: supine with a towel roll place under the affected knee.
   ii. The opposite knee should be adducted slightly from the midline to allow the clinician more room to maneuver with the syringe when injecting the knee.
b. Transducer position (Figure 62-4)
   i. Short axis to distal quadriceps tendon and effusion
c. Needle orientation relative to the transducer
   i. In plane
d. Needle approach
   i. Lateral to medial, angled slightly posteriorly, depending on point of entry, patient habitus, and effusion volume (Figure 62-5)
e. Target
   i. Suprapatellar synovial pouch of the synovial envelope
f. Pearls and Pitfalls
   i. The procedure is more difficult without an effusion because of isoechoity of the tissues in view. In this instance, advance the needle until it is underneath the quadriceps tendon to ensure that the needle has penetrated deep enough to be in the synovial envelope (Figure 62-5A)
   ii. Be careful to be in between the quadriceps tendon and the prefemoral fat pad with the needle. Care must be taken not to inject the quadriceps tendon in the absence of an effusion.

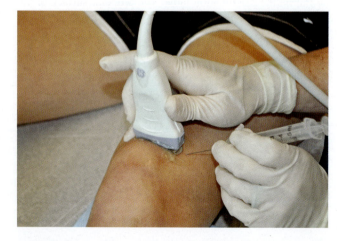

FIGURE 62-4 ■ Setup for the superior lateral injection technique. The transducer is positioned above the patella in short axis to the quadriceps tendon overlying the superior joint recess of the synovial lining of the knee.

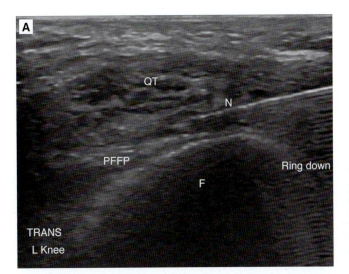

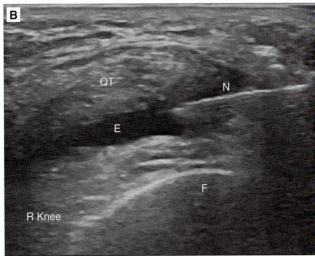

FIGURE 62-5 ■ **A.** Superior lateral injection of the knee without effusion. The needle is being advanced into the synovial envelope which is a potential space underneath the quadriceps tendon (QT) and above the prefemoral fat pad (PFFP) and the femur (F). Note the needle tip surrounded by lidocaine being injected as the needle is advanced. **B.** Superior lateral injection of the knee. The needle (N) is being advanced from lateral to medial into the effusion (E), which is in the synovial envelop of the knee underneath the quadriceps tendon (QT) and above the femur (F). Note the ring down artifact from the needle.

Alternate Technique

When there is no effusion present, the superior approach presents less obvious visibility to the joint space because the superior synovial pouch is not distended, and there is only a potential space that is difficult to see because of the isoechoity of the quadriceps tendon, the synovial membrane, and the underlying prefemoral fat pad. The medial midpatellar region presents an obvious window to the intraarticular penetration of the knee with or without effusion. A high-frequency linear array transducer is placed along the short-axis plane of the knee with the patella being the anatomic superior border and the medial femoral condyle being the inferior anatomic border. The medial patellar retinaculum will lie in between the two boney structures, and underneath it is the joint space (Figure 62-6). A similar view on the lateral side of the knee is more occluded because of the larger contour of the lateral femoral condyle.

a. Procedure setup
  i. Patient: supine with a towel roll place under the affected knee.
  ii. The opposite knee should be adducted slightly from the midline to allow the clinician more room to maneuver with the syringe when injecting the knee.

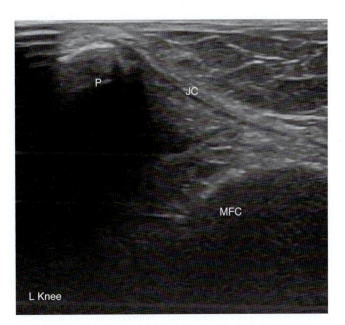

FIGURE 62-6 ■ Ultrasound image of the mid medial subpatellar injection technique. Note the patella (P) as the superior boundary and the medial femoral condyle (MFC) as the lower boundary with the joint capsule (JC) extending between the two structures as a hypoechoic line and representing the medial border of the synovial lining of the knee. The right side of the image is the medial aspect of the knee.

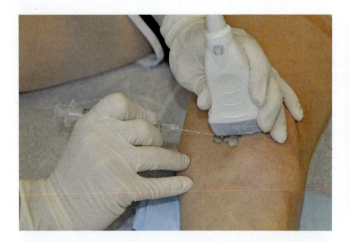

FIGURE 62-7 ■ Setup for the midmedial subpatellar injection technique. Note the position of the screen relative to the line of sight of the injection. The transducer is placed superior to the medial joint line overlying the patellar and the medial femoral condyle with the medial aspect of the synovial lining of the knee joint in between.

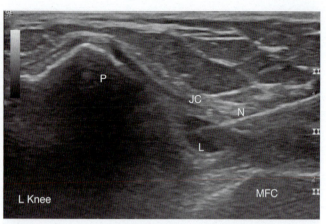

FIGURE 62-8 ■ Ultrasound image of the mid medial subpatellar knee injection. The needle (N) is being advanced medial to lateral angling deep to the transducer between the patella (p) and the medial femoral condyle (MFC) through the joint capsule (JC) in to the synovial envelope of the knee. Not the hypoechoic signal from the lidocaine pooling under the joint capsule serving as a confirmation of intraarticular penetration.

b. Transducer position (Figure 62-7)
    i. Overlying the midmedial patella and medial femoral condyle, in plane to the medial retinaculum
c. Needle orientation relative to the transducer
    i. In plane
d. Needle approach (Figures 62-8 and 62-9)
    i. Medial to lateral, angling slightly superiorly under the transducer. This will vary depending on the size and shape of the knee.
e. Target
    i. Synovial envelope underneath the patella, deep to the medial patellar retinaculum
f. Pearls and Pitfalls
    i. A local anesthetic can be used as an effective contrast agent with this technique. It will often cause the medial retinaculum to bulge outwardly from the joint when the needle is inside the joint space. It will also add contrast to the hyperechoic soft tissues of the knee joint.
    ii. Although more difficult to access, aspiration from this approach is possible with a large effusion.
    iii. This is generally a very safe technique because of the absence of any structures that would pose a danger, with the exception of osteophytes, which are often present in arthritic knees.

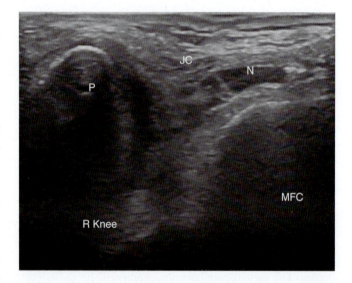

FIGURE 62-9 ■ An ultrasound image of a midmedial subpatellar injection in which the needle is shown beneath the joint capsule in the synovial envelop of the knee. The needle (N) has penetrated the joint capsule and injectate (hypoechoic signal) is distending the joint capsule. Note the needle tip in the left portion of the hypoechoic pool of injectate lying in between the patella (P) and the medial femoral condyle (MFC).

References

1. Jackson D, Evans N, Thomas B. Accuracy of needle placement into the intra-articular space of the knee. *J Bone Joint Surg Am* 2002;84:1522–1527.

2. Curtiss H, Finnoff J, Peck E. Accuracy of ultrasound-guided and palpation-guided knee injections by an experienced and less-experienced injector using a superolateral approach: a cadaveric study. PM R 2011;3:507–515.

3. Jones A, Regan M, Ledingham J, et al. Importance of placement of intra-articular steroid injections. *BMJ* 1993; 307:1329–1330.

4. Netter FH. *CIBA Collection of Medical Illustrations, Volume 8: Musculoskeletal System Part I.* Summit, NJ: CIBA–Geigy; 1987: 94–97.

5. Cailliet R. Chapters 1–4. In: *Knee Pain and Disability.* Philadelphia, PA: FA Davis; 1983.

6. Hamill J, Knutzen K. *Biomechanical Basis of Human Movement.* 3rd ed. Baltimore, MD: Lippincott, Williams & Wilkins; 2009: 208–219.

Brandon J. Messerli, DO / Garrett S. Hyman, MD, MPH / R. Amadeus Mason, MD

KEY POINTS

■ Use an 18–21 gauge, 1.5–2-inch needle for ease of aspiration.

■ Use a high- frequency linear array transducer.

■ The approach is typical from distal to proximal for easier avoidance of neurovascular structures.

■ A Baker's cyst, or popliteal cyst, is commonly believed to result from a ruptured knee-joint capsule that creates a communication to the gastrocnemius-semimembranosus (G-SM) bursa.

■ Distended bursae may connect to joint capsule via a communicating stalk.

■ Do not mistake a hypoechoic semimembranosus tendon (due to anisotropy) for a Baker's cyst.

Pertinent Anatomy

The gastrocnemius-semimembranosus (G-SM) bursa lies between the tendon of the medial head of the gastrocnemius and the tendon of the semimembranosus. It is located superficial to the medial femoral condyle and joint capsule (Figure 63-1).[1,2]

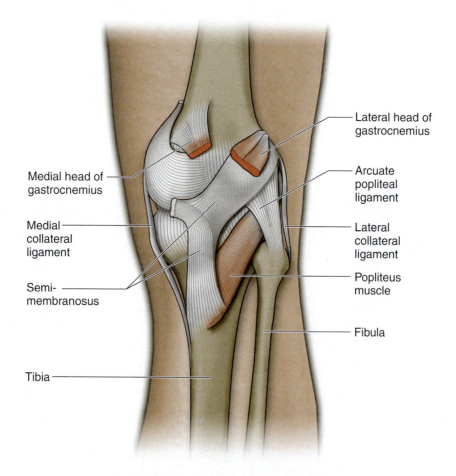

Medial head of gastrocnemius

Medial collateral ligament

Semi-membranosus

Tibia

Lateral head of gastrocnemius

Arcuate popliteal ligament

Lateral collateral ligament

Popliteus muscle

Fibula

FIGURE 63-1 ■ Structures of the posterior knee.

A cyst is a closed sac-like structure that is not a normal part of the tissue where it is found. When this cyst occurs in the popliteal fossa it is called a *popliteal* or *Baker's cyst*. Baker's cysts are usually found at or below the joint line usually located posteromedially, in plane between the gastrocnemius and underlying soleus or the overlaying semimembranosus (Figure 63-2).

Baker's cysts are commonly associated with pathology in the posterior third of the medial meniscus. Posterior horn meniscal tears that extend to the capsule may cause a defect that allows only unidirectional flow of fluid. The Baker's cyst is connected to the joint through a unidirectional valvular opening, so the presence of increased fluid pressure (eg, an effusion, or repetitive squatting) forces fluid through this valve into the cyst. Baker's cysts are located between the distal semimembranosus tendon and the medial head of gastrocnemius.

Baker's cysts can also be found in rheumatoid arthritis. This type of cyst usually results from the outflow of fluid through a normal bursal communication point, usually the semimembranosus or medial gastrocnemius bursa. Herniation of the synovial membrane through the joint capsule is another common mechanism.

Common Pathology

Bursitis can occur because of blunt trauma, repetitive stress, underlying osteophytes, or inflammation (ie, rheumatoid arthritis, synovial osteochondromatosis, pigmented villonodular synovitis). Any knee intraarticular pathology causing an effusion can result in a Baker's cyst, which involves a communication from the knee joint to the G-SM bursa.

Ultrasound Imaging Findings

The G-SM bursae are best visualized in both long and short axis using a high-frequency linear array transducer at a frequency and a depth suitable for the body habitus. The bursa, or cyst, should be described based on the echotexture, simple versus complex nature of the fluid, and size. Typically there is anechoic fluid, although septations and a complex fluid collection with hyperechoic foci may be seen.[3] The bursa can rupture, and then anechoic fluid may leak further distally in the calf. The bursa or cyst should be without Doppler flow.

A Baker's cyst may cause no symptoms or be associated with knee pain and/or tightness behind the knee and calf, especially when the knee is extended or fully flexed. Baker's cysts sometimes cause visible swelling in the posterior knee

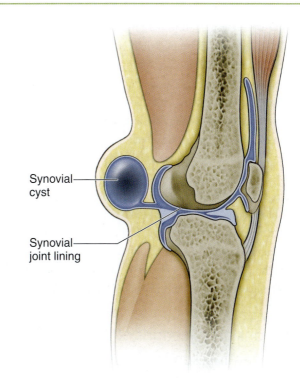

Synovial cyst

Synovial joint lining

FIGURE 63-2 ■ Baker's cyst.

especially when compared to the uninvolved knee. They are usually soft, somewhat compressible, and minimally tender.

Baker's cysts can sometimes rupture and the fluid can dissect down the inner leg cause bruising down to the inner ankle. Baker's cyst rupture and dissection can cause rapid-onset unilateral calf swelling that is often similar to the presentation of a deep venous thrombosis of the calf. Ultrasound evaluation for this is very important prior to considering an aspiration.

Findings of a Baker's cyst and intraarticular pathology, and the bursa should be assessed for a communication to the knee joint. Ultrasound may have 100% accuracy for detection of Baker's cysts if there is a homogenous anechoic and/or hypoechoic fluid signal between the tendons of the medial gastrocnemius and semimembranosus (Figure 63-3).

Indications for Injections of the Gastrocnemius-Semimembranosus Bursa

Note that the mere presence of a distended bursa does not support the need for an aspiration or injection procedure. We suggest an intervention only when posterior knee pain correlates with the physical examination and imaging findings. In addition, you can first try more conservative approaches such as relative rest, ice, nonsteroidal antiinflammatories, physical therapy, modalities, and/or orthotics. The reoccurrence of a distended bursa or cyst is common. Curative treatment may mean treating the intraarticular source of synovitis.

Equipment

- Needle: 18–21 gauge, 1.5–2-inch needle
  - A smaller gauge needle may be used first to provide a local anesthetic prior to using a larger gauge needle.
- Syringe: 10- or 20-cc syringe for aspiration
- Injectate
  - 1–2 mL of local anesthetic
  - 1 mL of an injectable corticosteroid
- High-frequency linear array transducer

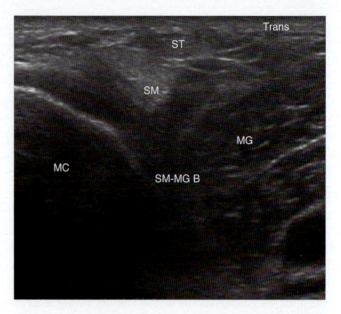

FIGURE 63-3 ▪ Short-axis view of the posteromedial popliteal fossa, demonstrating the relationship between the semimembranosus tendon (SM), medial gastrocnemius (MG), medial femoral condyle (MC), semitendinosus tendon (ST), and the expected location of a semimembranosus-gastrocnemius bursa (SM-MG B).

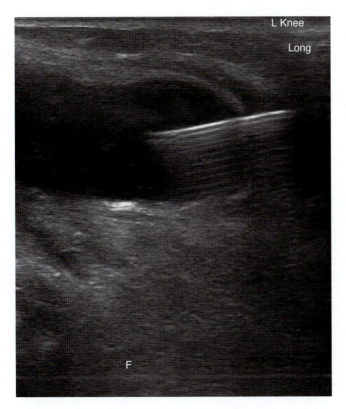

FIGURE 63-4 ■ Ultrasound image of needle position with a Baker's cyst from a distal-to-proximal, in-plane approach.

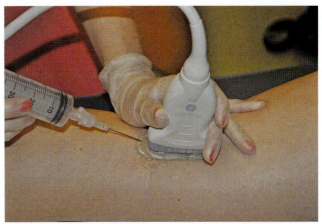

FIGURE 63-5 ■ Needle approach for a Baker's cyst with distal-to-proximal, in-plane approach.

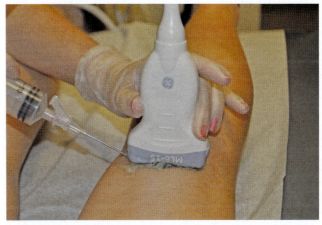

FIGURE 63-6 ■ Alternate needle approach for a Baker's cyst lateral-to-medial, in-plane approach.

Author's Preferred Injection Technique

a. Patient position
   i. Prone
b. Transducer position
   i. Preferred (in setting of larger bursae and cysts): long axis to the bursa, medial or lateral to the medial gastrocnemius tendon, distal to the semimembranosus tendon
   ii. Optional: Short axis to the bursa (Figure 63-6)
c. Needle orientation relative to the transducer
   i. In plane (Figure 63-4)
d. Needle approach (Figure 63-5)
   i. Preferred: distal to proximal when transducer is long axis relative to the bursa
   ii. Optional: medial to lateral when transducer is short axis relative to the bursa (Figure 63-6)
e. Target
   i. Middle of cyst cavity.
   ii. Under direct visualization, the needle can be redirected to break up any septations and aspirate any loculated fluid. After aspirating, keep the needle in the collapsed cyst, switch to the corticosteroid/lidocaine syringe and inject its full contents. The fluid should flow easily with little or no resistance.
f. Pearls and Pitfalls
   i. Identify all neurovascular structures in the popliteal fossa before the aspiration and injection. If the suspected Baker's cyst is in atypical location you need to rule out a tumor or vascular malformation.
   ii. In adults, intraarticular pathology is the most common cause for a Baker's cyst; the cyst will likely recur if the intraarticular pathology is not identified and address.
   iii. Do not mistake the semimembranosus tendon, which may appear hypoechoic due to anisotropy, for a Baker's cyst.

iv. The following may mimic the appearance of a distended G-SM bursa: (1) myxoid liposarcoma, which is distinguished by a lack of fluid directly between the medial gastrocnemius and semimembranosus tendons; (2) popliteal artery aneurysm, which should be assessed for Doppler flow and pulsations; (3) parameniscal cysts, which can also be distinguished by a lack of fluid directly between the medial gastrocnemius and semimembranosus tendons.

v. Evaluate the suspected Baker's cyst in the long-axis *and* short-axis planes, making sure to identify its connection to the joint if present.

vi. Localization and avoidance of the neurovascular structures is essential. Power Doppler should be used when initially assessing any cyst and to plan the needle approach.

vii. Rupture of a Baker's cyst can result in dissection of synovial fluid distally into the calf, which can mimic symptoms of a deep venous thrombosis.

viii. Baker's cysts are less common in children and are generally found in boys. They usually do not communicate with the joint and usually are not associated with intraarticular pathology and, as such, respond well to aspiration and injection. Before aspirating, it is essential to do a workup for soft tissue tumors such as lipomas, xanthomas, vascular tumors, and fibrosarcomas.

References

1. McCarthy CL, McNally EG. The MRI appearance of cystic lesions around the knee. *Skeletal Radiol* 2004:33:187–209.
2. Guerra J Jr, Newell JD, Resnick D, Danzig LA. Pictorial essay: gastrocnemio-semimembranosus bursal region of the knee. *AJR Am J Roentgenol* Mar 1981;136(3):593–596.
3. Ward EE, Jacobson JA, Fessell DP, et al. Sonographic detection of Baker's cysts: comparison with MR imaging. *Am J Radiol* 2001:176:373–380.

Jeffrey M. Payne, MD

KEY POINTS

- Use a 27-gauge, 1.25-inch needle for administration of local anesthetic and an 18–20 gauge, 1.5–2.0-inch needle for aspiration and subsequent injection of cyst.
- A high-frequency linear array transducer should be used to evaluate meniscal cysts.
- The majority of meniscal cysts are associated with tears of the adjacent meniscus.

- There are multiple different approaches for this procedure based on the location of the cyst.
- Meniscal cysts can be multilobulated, and it is important to drain all aspects of the cyst.
- The cystic material is often gelatinous, and lavage can be helpful in facilitating aspiration.

Pertinent Anatomy

The lateral and medial menisci are crescent-shaped, fibrocartilaginous structures that are located on the articular surface of the tibia and provide increased congruity for the articulating surface of the femoral condyles (Figure 64-1). The menisci are thick peripherally and thin centrally. The primary function of the menisci is to reduce the compressive stress at the tibiofemoral joint.

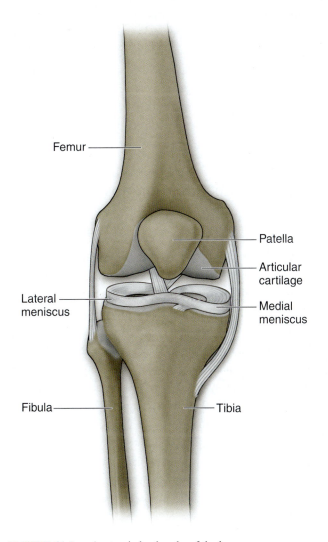

FIGURE 64-1 ■ Anatomic landmarks of the knee.

Common Pathology

A meniscal cyst is a focal collection of fluid located adjacent to (parameniscal) or within the meniscus (intrameniscal). Most meniscal cysts are located in the parameniscal soft tissues and are associated with horizontal cleavage tears of the adjacent meniscus, although there are several reports in the literature of cysts occurring without an associated meniscal tear. Several theories on the pathophysiology and etiology of meniscal cysts have been proposed. The most prevalent theory is that meniscal cysts result from the extravasation of synovial fluid into the parameniscal soft tissues through an adjacent meniscal tear.[1] An alternate theory is that meniscal cysts are the result of cystic degeneration of the meniscus, which may enlarge the meniscus (intrameniscal cyst) and subsequently be extruded into the parameniscal tissues (parameniscal cyst).[1] Meniscal cysts can be asymptomatic and incidentally found on magnetic resonance imaging or ultrasound examination. However, patients with meniscal cysts may present with localized pain, decreased knee range of motion, and a palpable, firm, soft-tissue swelling. Meniscal cysts can fluctuate in size. Large cysts can cause local pressure effects on adjacent structures, such as compression of the peroneal nerve or erosion of bone.

Ultrasound Imaging Findings

A meniscal cyst should be evaluated using a high-frequency linear array transducer at a frequency of 8–12 MHz. Depending on the position of the cyst, coronal or sagittal ultrasound images are typically the most useful to assess the cyst.[2] The sonographic appearance of meniscal cysts can range from a unilobulated, uniformly hypoechoic mass to a mass presenting with multiple hyperechoic septa and mixed echogenicity.[3] This variable echogenicity is likely related to the different composition of fluid that meniscal cysts may contain. This may include clear synovial-like fluid, gelatinous or bloody material, and solid inflammatory tissue.[3] The cardinal sonographic feature of a meniscal cyst is not the echogenicity, but rather a clear communication of the cyst to the adjacent meniscus.[3] This helps to differentiate a true meniscal cyst from other cysts or bursae about the knee as well as soft tissue tumors that may mimic a meniscal cyst.

Indications for Aspiration and Injection of a Parameniscal Cyst

The traditional surgical treatment for meniscal cysts is either open surgical excision or arthroscopic drainage of the cyst in combination with debridement or repair of any meniscal abnormality.[4] Percutaneous aspiration and injection of meniscal cysts can be performed as an alternative to operative intervention for symptomatic patients who may have a contraindication to surgery or who wish more conservative treatment. Aspiration of the meniscal cyst alone is felt to primarily be a temporizing measure because the underlying meniscal tear is unchanged.[4] Therefore, if surgery is not going to be performed, treatment of the underlying meniscal tear (ie, injection of the knee joint, physical therapy) could be considered along with aspiration and injection of the cyst. Aspiration and injection of meniscal cysts has been described based on palpation by Muddu et al.[5] Gelatinous material was able to be obtained from 12 of the 19 cysts (63%) that were aspirated, and all cysts were injected with 40 mg of methylprednisolone.[5] Ultrasound-guided aspiration and injection of meniscal cysts has been described by MacMahon et al., with thick gelatinous fluid aspirated from 18 of 18 cysts (100%).[4] All cysts were completely aspirated using ultrasound guidance, and each cyst was subsequently injected with 40 mg of methylprednisolone and 1 mL of 0.5% bupivacaine.[4] Clinical outcomes of ultrasound-guided meniscal cyst aspiration and injection versus palpation-guided meniscal cyst aspiration and injection have not been described.

Equipment

- Needle: 27-gauge, 1.25-inch needle for administration of local anesthetic; 18–20 gauge, 1.5–2.0 inch needle for aspiration and subsequent injection of cyst
- Injectate: 1 cc of 1% lidocaine (Xylocaine) and 1 cc of 40 mg methylprednisolone
- High-frequency linear array transducer

Author's Preferred Technique

a. Patient position
   i. Depending on the location of the cyst, the patient will be supine or side-lying.
b. Transducer position
   i. The transducer position will vary depending on the location of the cyst, but will most likely be in an anatomic coronal or sagittal plane.
c. Needle orientation relative to the transducer
   i. In plane (long axis)
d. Needle approach
   i. Lateral to medial or medial to lateral depending on the location of the cyst
e. Target (Figure 64-2 and Figure 64-3)
   i. The meniscal cyst
f. Pearls and Pitfalls
   i. Pre-procedure scanning should be performed to identify surrounding neurovascular structures prior to performing the procedure.
   ii. Applying too much pressure with the transducer may cause compression of the cyst, leading to suboptimal visualization and making the aspiration difficult.
   iii. Meniscal cysts can be multilobulated, and it is important to drain all aspects of the cyst.
   iv. The cystic material can be thick and gelatinous and difficult to aspirate. Therefore, lavage with lidocaine (Xylocaine), sterile water, or normal saline may be helpful for facilitating aspiration of the cyst.
   v. There are multiple different approaches for this procedure based on the location of the cyst. The specific technique taken should be one that would provide both optimal visualization of the meniscal cyst and a safe trajectory for the needle.

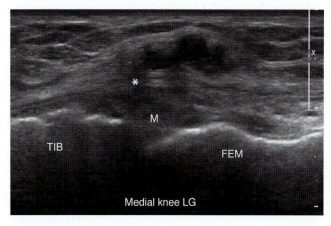

FIGURE 64-2 ■ Anatomic long-axis view of medial knee demonstrating a hypoechoic degenerative medial meniscus (M) with a communicative stalk (*asterisk*) extending through the medial collateral ligament into a multilobulated cyst. FEM, femur; LG, longitudinal; TIB, tibia. (Courtesy of Jay Smith, MD, Mayo Clinic, Rochester, MN.)

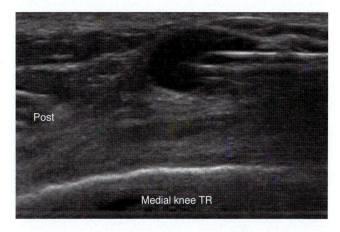

FIGURE 64-3 ■ Anatomic short-axis view of the same cyst during lavage and aspiration with a 19-gauge needle. POST, posterior; TR, transverse. (Courtesy of Jay Smith, MD, Mayo Clinic, Rochester, MN.)

References

1. Campbell SE, Sanders TG, Morrison WB. MR imaging of meniscal cysts: incidence, location, and clinical significance. *AJR Am J Roentgenol* 2001;177(2):409–413.
2. Martinoli C, Bianchi S. In: Bianchi S, Martinoli C, eds. *Ultrasound of the Musculoskeletal System.* Berlin Heidelberg: Springer-Verlag; 2007:729–732.
3. Seymour R, Lloyd DC. Sonographic appearances of meniscal cysts. *J Clin Ultrasound* 1998;26(1):15–20.
4. MacMahon PJ, Brennan DD, Duke D, Forde S, Eustace SJ. Ultrasound-guided percutaneous drainage of meniscal cysts: preliminary clinical experience. *Clin Radiol* 2007;62(7):683–687.
5. Muddu BN, Barrie JL, Morris MA. Aspiration and injection for meniscal cysts. *J Bone Joint Surg Br* 1992;74(4):627–628.

Jeffrey M. Payne, MD

KEY POINTS

- Use a 25-gauge, 1.5-inch needle.
- A high-frequency linear array transducer is used to visualize the proximal tibiofibular joint (PTFJ).
- There is significant variation in the angulation of the PTFJ.

- The transducer is oriented in the anatomic transverse oblique plane over the PTFJ.
- Needle orientation relative to the transducer is out of plane (short axis).
- The PTFJ injection is a small-volume injection (1.5–2.0 cc).

Pertinent Anatomy

The proximal tibiofibular joint (PTFJ) is a diarthrodial synovial joint consisting of the articulation of the medial fibular head with the posterolateral tibia (Figure 65-1). The joint is surrounded by a fibrous capsule which is thicker anteriorly and is reinforced by the anterior superior and posterior superior tibiofibular ligaments. There is significant variation in the shape, size, and angulation of the PTFJ and the joint has been classified into two types, horizontal and oblique.[1] The PTFJ has been reported to communicate with the knee joint in 10%-64% of adults.[2]

Common Pathology

The PTFJ is often overlooked as a cause of lateral knee pain because of a low index of suspicion and a variable clinical presentation. Significant translations and rotations occur within the PTFJ during normal knee and ankle movements that make the joint susceptible to repetitive stresses that can lead to osteoarthritis.[3] Degenerative osteoarthritis of the PTFJ can occur in isolation or concomitantly with knee osteoarthritis. Symptoms are often nonspecific and may include lateral knee pain that can radiate proximal or distal, an antalgic gait, difficulty climbing stairs, hamstring tightness, and symptoms of instability.[4] The PTFJ can also be injured by direct trauma. A less common disorder is a ganglion cyst arising from the PTFJ, but is important to recognize as it can be associated with compression of the common peroneal nerve.[5]

Ultrasound Imaging Findings

The PTFJ is best visualized in an anatomic transverse oblique plane using a high-frequency linear array transducer at a frequency of 8–12 MHz and a depth of less than 3 cm. Initial

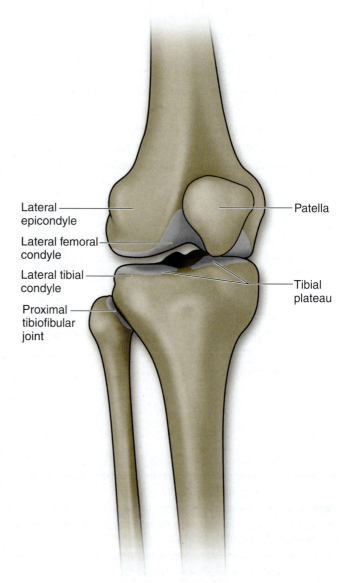

Lateral epicondyle

Lateral femoral condyle

Lateral tibial condyle

Proximal tibiofibular joint

Patella

Tibial plateau

FIGURE 65-1 ■ Normal anatomy of the proximal tibiofibular joint.

positioning of the transducer can be accomplished by placing the lateral end of the transducer over the fibular head. The medial end of the transducer is then oriented toward the inferior patellar pole, thus aligning the long axis of the transducer perpendicular to the usual orientation of the PTFJ.[3] There is large individual variation with respect to the orientation of the PTFJ. Therefore, the medial end of the transducer can then be rotated clockwise and counterclockwise, while the lateral end of the of the transducer is anchored to the fibular head, in order to produce the best visualization of the PTFJ.[3] Ultrasound findings can include cortical irregularities, joint effusions, and less commonly ganglion cysts arising from the PTFJ.

Indications for Injections of the Proximal Tibiofibular Joint

Injection of the PTFJ can be performed for patients with recalcitrant pain that is unresponsive to rest, icing, antiinflammatories, and physical therapy. Injection of the PTFJ has been described based on palpation (ie, unguided).[6] There have been no studies evaluating the success of the palpation-guided technique. Ultrasound-guided PTFJ injection has been described by Smith et al. with a success rate of 100% with ultrasound-guided injection versus 58% with palpation-guided injection performed on unembalmed cadavers.[3] Clinical outcomes of ultrasound-guided PTFJ injections versus palpation-guided injections have not been described.

Equipment

■ Needle: 25-gauge, 1.5-inch needle
■ Injectate
  • 1 cc local anesthetic
  • 1 cc corticosteroid (PTFJ will typically only hold 1.5–2.0 cc)
■ High-frequency linear array transducer

Author's Preferred Technique

a. Patient position
  i. Side-lying with the anterior PTFJ facing the ceiling and the knee flexed 20–30 degrees to widen the anterior PTFJ. This position can be maintained through rolled-up towels or bolsters.
b. Transducer position (Figure 65-2)
  i. Anatomic transverse oblique plane over the proximal tibiofibular joint

c. Needle orientation relative to the transducer
  i. Out of plane (short axis)
d. Needle approach (see Figure 65-2)
  i. Inferior to superior
  ii. Walk-down technique
e. Target (Figure 65-3)
  i. The PTFJ, deep to the anterior superior proximal tibiofibular ligament
f. Pearls and Pitfalls
  i. Pre-procedure scanning should be performed to identify the common, superficial, and deep peroneal nerves

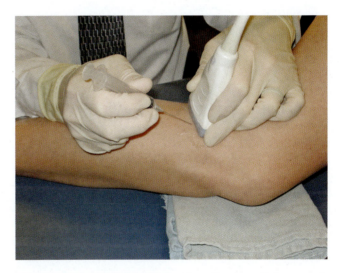

FIGURE 65-2 ■ Patient position and needle approach for a proximal tibiofibular joint injection.

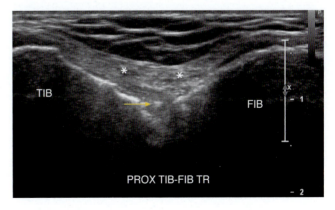

FIGURE 65-3 ■ Proximal tibiofibular joint injection using an out-of-plane (short-axis) approach. The needle tip is depicted by the *yellow arrow*, and the *asterisks* delineate the anterior superior tibiofibular ligament. Top is superficial; bottom, deep; left, medial; and right, lateral. (Courtesy of Jay Smith, MD, Mayo Clinic, Rochester, MN.)

References

1. Ogden JA. The anatomy and function of the proximal tibiofibular joint. *Clin Orthop Relat Res* 1974;101:186–191.
2. Bozkurt M, Yilmaz E, Atlihan D, et al. The proximal tibiofibular joint: an anatomic study. *Clin Orthop Relat Res* 2003;406:136–140.
3. Smith J, Finnoff J, Levy B, Lai J. Sonographically guided proximal tibiofibular joint injection: technique and accuracy. *J Ultrasound Med* 2010;29:783–789.
4. Bozkurt M, Yilmaz E, Akseki D, Havitcioglu H, Gunal I. The evaluation of the proximal tibiofibular joint for patients with lateral knee pain. *Knee* 2004;11:307–312.
5. Forster BB, Lee JS, Kelly S, et al. Proximal tibiofibular joint: an often-forgotten cause of lateral knee pain. *AJR Am J Roentgenol* 2007;188:W359–W366.
6. Saunders S, Longworth S. In: Saunders S, Longworth S. *Injection techniques in orthopaedic and sports medicine.* 2nd ed. London: Saunders; 2002:84–85.

Ronald W. Hanson Jr, MD, CAQSM

KEY POINTS

- Use an 18–22-gauge needle.
- Use a high-frequency linear array transducer.
- A longitudinal, in-plane approach is generally used.

- Percutaneous needle tenotomy (PNT) is indicated only in quadriceps tendinosis pain that is refractory to a comprehensive rehabilitation approach.
- Injection of a corticosteroid agent is not indicated with this procedure.

Introduction

This chapter deals with recalcitrant quadriceps tendon pathology that is felt to require either an injection or percutnaeous needle tenotomy (PNT) treatment prior to considering surgical intervention.

PNT is a procedure first described in detail by McShane for lateral epicondylosis in 2006.[1] In general terms, it describes using a needle to fenestrate (make micro-incisions or micro-damage) a degenerative tendon to transform the state of the tendon into an acute traumatic one and encourage a regenerative response. Although the technique has been described and validated for the common extensor tendons, PNT has been used in many other tendons with limited scientific evidence to date.

Anatomy (Figure 66-1)

The quadriceps tendon is a conjoined tendon of the knee extensor muscles (rectus femoris, vastus lateralis, vastus medialis, and vastus intermedius) and has its insertion on the proximal patella. The tendon has traditionally been thought to be arranged in a trilaminar configuration, with rectus femoris anterior, vastus intermedius posterior, and the vastus medialis and lateralis tendons central. Some authors cite quadrilaminar or bilaminar arrangement in cadaveric studies, making the anatomy notably variable.[1] As with most tendons, the quadriceps tendon is relatively hypovascular, being supplied by three vascular beds (medial, lateral, peripatellar). A watershed zone appears between 1 and 2 cm proximal to its insertion, making this a common area for degeneration and tears.

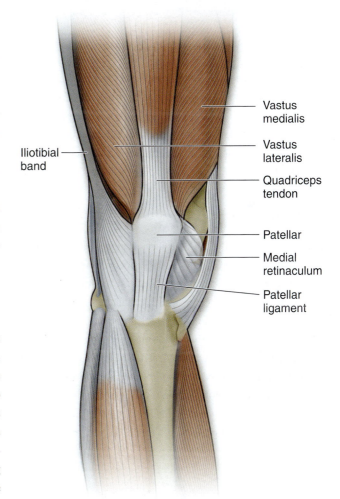

FIGURE 66-1 ■ Distal quadriceps anatomy.

Vastus medialis

Vastus lateralis

Iliotibial band

Quadriceps tendon

Patellar

Medial retinaculum

Patellar ligament

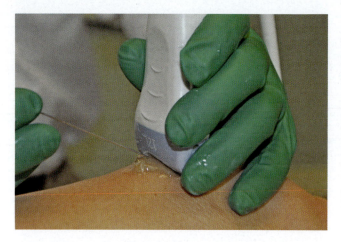

FIGURE 66-2 ■ Out-of-plane approach with transducer in the short axis to the distal quadriceps tendon.

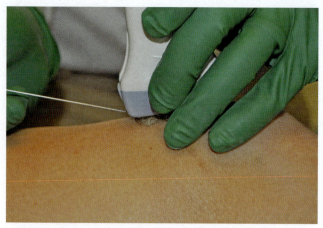

FIGURE 66-3 ■ In-plane approach with the transducer in the long axis to the distal quadriceps tendon.

Ultrasound Imaging Findings

The quadriceps tendon is visualized in both long (Figure 66-2) and short axis (Figure 66-3) at 1–4 cm with a high-frequency linear array transducer at 8–15 Hz. Findings similar to other tendinopathies are common and include thickening, hypoechogenicity, and loss of normal fibrillar pattern of the tendon (Figure 66-4).

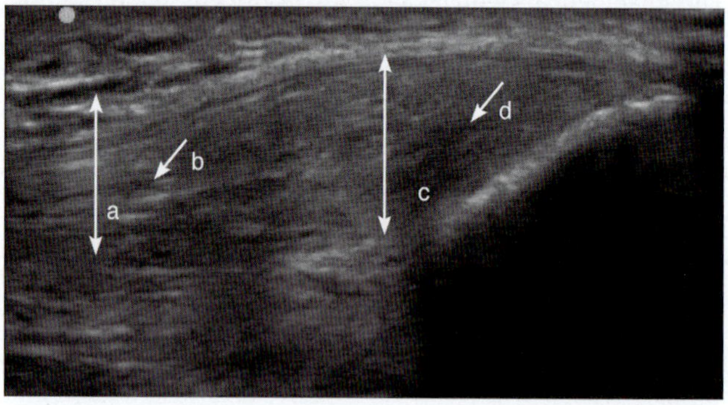

Injection Indications

Injection is indicated with the failure of appropriate conservative management that includes rest, anti-inflammatories and aggressive rehabilitation. Initial injection techniques should have been attempted before PNT, given the more invasive nature of the procedure. Further, a definitive certainty through exhaustive workup, examination, imaging, diagnostic injections, and patience is suggested. There is no evidence that corticosteroids should be used in tendon procedures.[2,3] Some physicians use autologous whole blood, platelet rich plasma, or stem cell solutions with the PNT procedure. There is limited evidence regarding the efficacy of these procedures.

FIGURE 66-4 ■ Quadriceps tendinosis: (a) normal thickness versus (c) thickened tendon; (b) normal brightness and fibrillar pattern versus (d) darker with loss of fibrillar pattern.

Equipment

- Needle: Usually a 22-gauge and up to an 18-gauge (per physician preference), 2–3.5-inch needle
- Injectate: anesthetic, saline, or regenerative agent only
- High-frequency linear array transducer

Author's Preferred Technique

a. Patient position
   i. Supine with knee flexed approximately 30–60 degrees with support under knee
b. Transducer position
   i. Suprapatellar region with quadriceps tendon in long axis
   ii. Alternate position 1: Probe in long-axis position to the tendon fibers with a short-axis
   iii. Alternate position 2: Probe in short-axis position with either a short- or long-axis needle. The short-axis position with the needle in long axis view is particularly helpful if the tendon is degenerative in a focal areal medially or laterally.
c. Needle orientation relative to the transducer
   i. In-plane approach (Figure 66-5)
   ii. Out-of-plane approach (Figure 66-6)
d. Needle approach
   i. Proximal to distal
e. Target
   i. Tendinotic area of the quadriceps tendon. Although there is no "standard" number of fenestrations, with subsequent needle passes, you will feel the tissue become less tough, or conversely, some tendinosis is very loose, and you will need to complete fewer passes with the needle
f. Pearls and Pitfalls
   i. Survey the tendon extensively to plan your starting point and to identify critical anatomic structures.
   ii. Avoid normal tendon if possible.
   iii. Visualize the tendinosis in whatever position allows you to approach the tissue in long-axis visualization with the least amount of additional strokes or repositioning of the needle. Needle length, type, and caliber are a matter of preference; the author prefers a 20-gauge, 2–3.5-inch Quincke tip needle depending on body habitus and location of tendinosis within the tendon.
   iv. The cutting edge of the needle can be useful to create more significant lesions where appropriate.
   v. Needling of the enthesis for insertional tendinosis is suggested by the author (as often there are cortical irregularities or enthesophytes) to encourage angiogenesis from the periosteum.

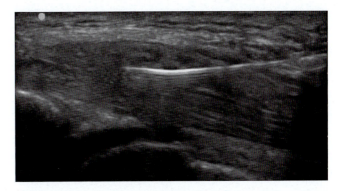

FIGURE 66-5 ■ Ultrasound image with 22-gauge needle within an area of tendinosis and performing fenestration.

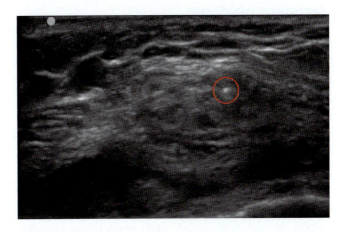

FIGURE 66-6 ■ Ultrasound image: short-axis view of needle tip (*dot center of red circle*) applied within the degenerative portion of the quadriceps tendon.

   vi. The author suggests creating a needle track with injectate to an area of established blood supply, usually to the muscle tendon junction, local visualized vessels, and/or the periosteum to encourage the formation of blood supply to the region.

References

1. McShane JM, Nazarian LN, Harwood MI. Sonographically guided percutaneous needle tenotomy for treatment of common extensor tendinosis in the elbow. *J Ultrasound Med* 2006;25:1281–1289.
2. McShane JM, Shah VN, Nazarian LN. Sonographically guided percutaneous needle tenotomy for treatment of common extensor tendinosis in the elbow: is a corticosteroid necessary? *J Ultrasound Med* 2008 Aug;27(8):1137–1144.
3. Speed CA. Fortnightly review: corticosteroid injections in tendon lesions. *BMJ* 2001;323(7309):382–386.

Joseph J. Albano, MD

Pertinent Anatomy

The patellar tendon lies just beneath the skin extending from the inferior pole of the patella to the tibial tuberosity.

Common Pathology

Tendinitis is an acute inflammatory condition characterized by the presence of white blood cells (WBCs) in the damaged tissue. Tendinosis is a chronic condition, with the absence of WBCs associated with mucoid degeneration of the tendon (Figure 67-1). A common concomitant finding is intrasubstance or interstitial (longitudinal) tears. Often, increased vascularity of the tendon and/or Hoffa's fat pad coexists.

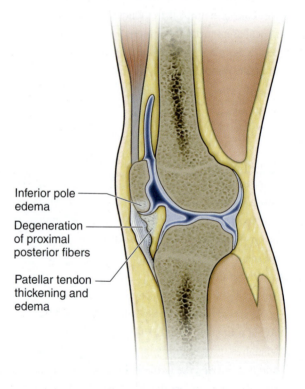

Inferior pole edema

Degeneration of proximal posterior fibers

Patellar tendon thickening and edema

FIGURE 67-1 ■ Patellar tendinosis is a chronic condition characterized by mucoid degeneration, typically involving the proximal posterior portion of the tendon. As the condition progresses, edema and increased vascularity occur in the tendon and in Hoffa's fat pad adjacent to the tendon.

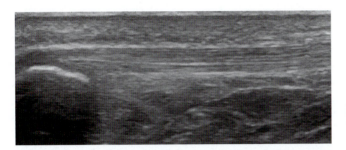

FIGURE 67-2 ■ Normal patellar tendon in the sagittal or long-axis plane. The normal patellar tendon is hyperechoic, fibrillar, of uniform thickness, and with undisrupted linear echogenic fibers.

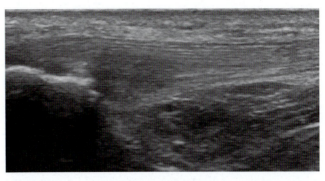

FIGURE 67-3 ■ Patellar tendinosis: hypoechoic thickening, most commonly found on the deep surface of the proximal portion of the patellar tendon.

Ultrasound Imaging Findings

Because of the proximity to the skin surface, a high-frequency linear array transducer at a frequency of 10–12 Hz and a depth of 2–3 cm is best with the transducer in the sagittal plane, long axis to the patellar tendon. Confirm the findings with a short-axis image. The normal patellar tendon is hyperechoic, fibrillar, of uniform thickness, and with undisrupted linear echogenic fibers (Figure 67-2). Tendinosis of the patellar tendon appears as hypoechoic thickening, which is most commonly found on the deep surface of the proximal portion of the patellar tendon (Figure 67-3). There may also be calcification of the degenerative tendon (Figure 67-4), intrasubstance tears (Figure 67-5), partial thickness tears (Figure 67-6A, B), and/or hyperemia (with color or power Doppler imaging) (Figure 67-7). The hyperemia can be found in the substance of the tendon or deep to the tendon, in Hoffa's fat pad.

Intrasubstance tears may be difficult to visualize on static diagnostic ultrasound images. Long-axis anechoic or hypoechoic areas in the substance of the tendon may hint at the presence of these intrasubstance tears. Confirm their presence with infiltration of local anesthetic or other fluid to expand the potential space.

Pathologic findings may also be found at the insertion of the tendon with or without involvement of the physis. For the skeletally immature patient, Osgood-Schlatter disease appears as distal tendon thickening, swelling of the nonossified cartilage, and possibly with fragmentation of the tibial tuberosity.

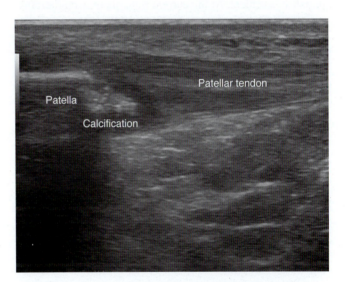

FIGURE 67-4 ■ Calcification within the degenerative tendon.

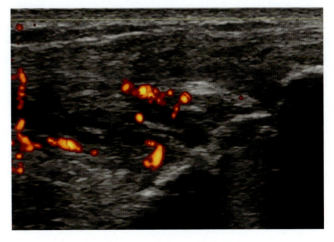

FIGURE 67-5 ■ Intrasubstance tears of the patellar tendon insertion. The anechoic areas to the left of the image are the tears. Hyperemia surrounds the tears.

Indications for Injection of the Patellar Tendon

Patellar tendinosis is a disabling and often chronic and refractory condition. Initial treatment may consist of relative rest, ice, taping, nonsteroidal antiinflammatory drugs, eccentric exercises, physical therapy, and extracorporeal shock-wave therapy. Injections may be considered after failure of these initial treatments or after failure of surgical treatment. Unguided injection of the patellar tendon is not advised because of the small target area, especially with intrasubstance tears. Needle placement must be precise in the medial-lateral and superficial-deep planes or the target may be missed. Thus, ultrasound guidance is critical. At the current time, there is no literature comparing guided versus unguided injections.

Equipment

- Needle: 18–22-gauge, 1.5-inch needle
  - For percutaneous needle tenotomy, especially with a calcified tendon, an 18-gauge needle is recommended.
- High-frequency linear array transducer
- Ethyl chloride spray may be used as a topical agent if desired.
- Injectate
  - Use 1–2 mL of a local anesthetic. For the tendon, use as small a dose as possible or none at all. Typically, sufficient anesthesia is achieved with a total of <2 mL. Because of the possible toxicity of anesthetic agents to the tendon, normal saline may be injected into the tendon to assist in visualizing intrasubstance tears. An alternative to local anesthesia is a block of the genicular nerves (medial superior and inferior, lateral superior and inferior).

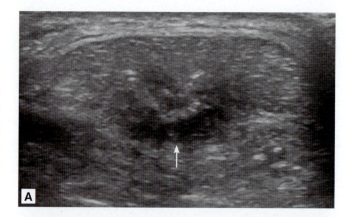

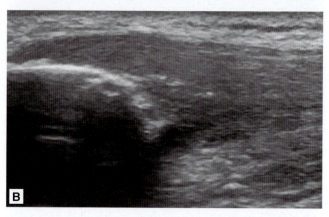

FIGURE 67-6 ■ **A.** Partial thickness tear of the patellar tendon, short-axis view, as identified by the *arrow*. **B.** Partial thickness tear of the patellar tendon, long-axis view. Note the thickened portion of the tendon overlying the inferior pole of the patella.

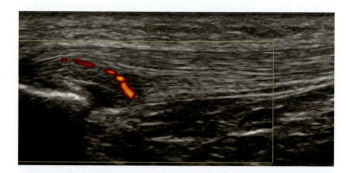

FIGURE 67-7 ■ Hyperemia of the patellar tendon identified with power Doppler imaging. The thickened hypoechoic tendon with hyperemia is just medial to the normal lateral portion of the tendon.

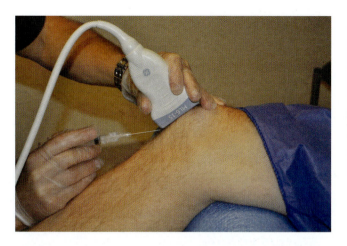

FIGURE 67-8 ▪ Patient position for patellar tendon injections. With the standard approach, the knee is slightly flexed and supported. The transducer is long axis to the tendon and needle approach is in plane from distal to proximal.

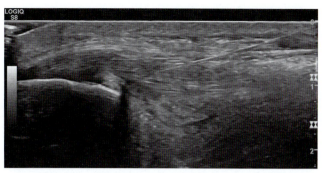

FIGURE 67-9 ▪ Ultrasound image of patellar tendon injection using an in-plane approach, long axis to the patellar tendon.

Author's Preferred Technique

a. Patient position
   i. Supine with a roll beneath the knees to obtain knee flexion of approximately 30 degrees to straighten the extensor mechanism and reduce anisotropy.
b. Transducer position
   i. Anatomic sagittal plane over the proximal patellar tendon (Figure 67-8)
c. Needle orientation relative to the transducer
   i. In plane (Figure 67-9)
d. Needle approach
   i. Inferior to superior
e. Target
   i. Hypoechoic region of the tendon

Alternate Technique

a. Patient position
   i. Supine with a roll beneath the knees to obtain knee flexion of approximately 30 degrees to straighten the extensor mechanism and reduce anisotropy.
b. Transducer position (Figure 67-10)
   i. Anatomic sagittal plane over the proximal patellar tendon (see Figure 67-8)
c. Needle orientation relative to the transducer (see Figures 67-10 and 67-11)
   i. Oblique and out of plane to enable contact with the periosteum of the inferior pole of the patella as well as the tendon. Needle repositioning through the same skin portal enables medial to lateral coverage of the tendon.

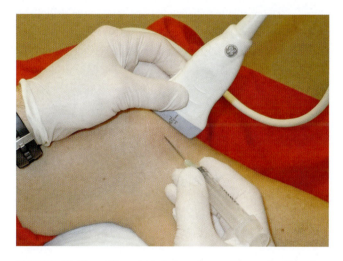

FIGURE 67-10 ▪ Alternate technique for patellar tendon injection. The knee is slightly flexed and supported. The transducer is long axis (but confirm with the short-axis view once the needle is positioned). The needle technique is oblique from the medial or lateral side.

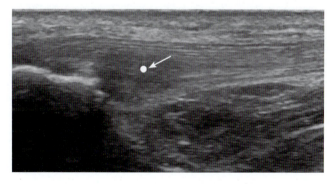

FIGURE 67-11 ▪ Ultrasound image of out of plane injection of the patella tendon with position of needle tip (*arrow*).

d. Needle approach
   i. Oblique from the medial or lateral aspect and con-firm with diagnostic ultrasound the location of the pathology (medial or lateral) and enter from the side of the pathology.
e. Target
   i. Hypoechoic region of the tendon (Typically, this is the medial and deep portion of the proximal patellar tendon.)
f. Pearls and Pitfalls
   i. Start with the transducer longitudinally with an oblique needle orientation. When the needle appears to be in the pathologic tissue, turn the transducer transversely. The needle may be medial or lateral to the pathology. Therefore, short-axis and long-axis views are essential to ensure precise placement of the needle within the pathologic area.

References

1. Housner JA, Jacobson JA, Morag Y, et al. Should ultrasound-guided needle fenestration be considered as a treatment option for recalcitrant patellar tendinopathy? A retrospective study of 47 cases. *Clin J Sport Med* 2010 Nov;20(6):488–490.
2. Finnoff JT, Fowler SP, Lai JK, et al. Treatment of chronic tendinopathy with ultrasound-guided needle tenotomy and platelet-rich plasma injection. *PMR* 2011 Oct;3(10):900–911.
3. Filardo G, Kon E, Della Villa S, et al. Use of platelet-rich plasma for the treatment of refractory jumper's knee. *Int Orthop* 2010;34:909–915.
4. Kon E, Filardo G, Delcogliano M, et al. Platelet rich plasma: new clinical application. A pilot study for treatment of jumper's knee. *Injury* 2009;40:598–603.
5. Albano JJ, Alexander RW. Autologous fat grafting as a mesenchymal stem cell source and living bioscaffold in a patellar tendon tear. *Clin J Sport Med* 2011;21:359–361.

Joseph J. Albano, MD

KEY POINTS

- Use an 18-gauge, 1.5-inch needle for aspiration.
- Use a high-frequency linear array transducer.
- Depth is less than 2–3 cm.

- The transducer is in the sagittal plane, long axis to the patellar tendon.
- Needle approach is long axis or short axis, from the lateral or medial knee.

Pertinent Anatomy (Figure 68-1)

The prepatellar bursa lies superficial to the patellar tendon.[1]

Common Pathology

The prepatellar bursa may be injured by repetitive micro-trauma, such as occurs with occupational kneeling in carpet layers and tilers. It may also occur in people who wash floors on their hands and knees, giving rise to the term *housemaid's knee*. There may or may not be bursal effusion associated with the clinical bursitis. It may also be acutely damaged by any direct blow to the patella, which commonly occurs with a fall onto the patella, resulting in a hemorrhagic bursitis. With acute trauma, a patellar fracture must be ruled out. A much less common etiology is a Morel-Lavallee lesion.[2]

Bursitis caused by an infectious etiology should always be entertained in the appropriate clinical scenario.

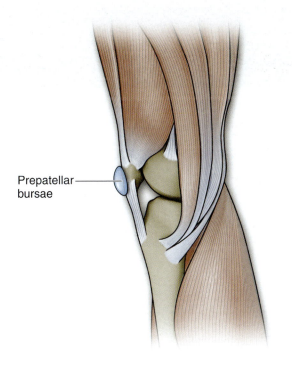
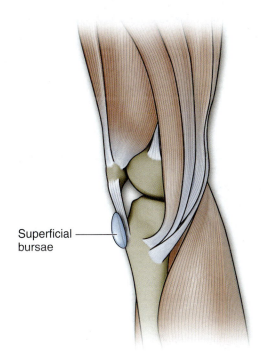

Prepatellar bursae

Superficial bursae

FIGURE 68-1 ■ Anatomy of the prepatellar bursa.

Ultrasound Imaging Findings

Because of the proximity to the skin surface, a high-frequency linear array transducer at a frequency of 10–12 Hz and a depth of 2–3 cm is best with the transducer in the sagittal plane, long axis to the patellar tendon. Confirmation with a short-axis image is helpful in determining the width of the bursal enlargement. The bursae may be distended (Figure 68-2) and the fluid may have variable echogenicity, ranging from anechoic to hypoechoic to mixed and complex echogenicity. In addition, hyperemia may exist with subcutaneous edema without overt bursal effusion (Figure 68-3).

Indications for Prepatellar Bursal Injections

Of all the bursae in the vicinity of the knee, the most common one to be involved is the prepatellar bursa. The reasons for this may be due to (1) the infrequent occurrence of symptomatic deep and infrapatellar bursitis; (2) the very small volume of fluid in these bursae; (3) these bursitises are a secondary result of another process, such as patellar tendinosis or Osgood-Schlatter disease.[3] Consider aspiration for the following reasons (1) to diminish the size of the bursae and lessen pain, (2) to evaluate for infectious etiology, (3) to evaluate for one of the other rare causes of bursitis, such as gout. Note that the bursal effusion may recur, especially with prepatellar bursitis.

Equipment

- ■ Needle
  - 27-gauge, 1.25-inch needle to anesthetize the skin and subcutaneous structures.
  - 18-gauge, 1.5-inch needle for aspiration of a large volume of fluid. Once the needle is in place and the fluid is aspirated, change the syringe without removing the needle.
- ■ Injectate
  - 0.5 mL of an injectable corticosteroid
  - 0.5 mL of a local anesthetic
- ■ High-frequency linear array transducer
- ■ Ethyl chloride spray may be used as a topical agent if desired.

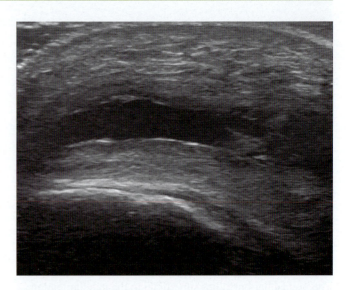

FIGURE 68-2 ■ Short-axis view, prepatellar bursa with bursal fluid. Note that the transducer is floated on a layer of gel with light application of pressure enabling adequate visualization of the bursal fluid.

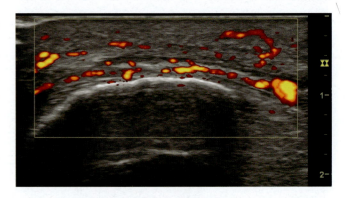

FIGURE 68-3 ■ Short-axis view, prepatellar bursitis without bursal fluid but with hyperemia.

Author's Preferred Technique

a.   Patient position (Figure 68-4)

    i.   Supine with a roll beneath the knees to obtain knee flexion of approximately 30 degrees. This will straighten the extensor mechanism and reduce anisotropy. It will also shift fluid to the suprapatellar recess from other parts of the knee. If there is only a small amount of fluid in the prepatellar bursae, full knee extension may allow better visualization of the fluid.

b.   Transducer position (see Figure 68-4)

    i.   Short axis to the patellar tendon, but confirm with a long-axis view. When evaluating the prepatellar bursa for fluid, ensure to place a layer of gel on the skin and float the transducer on this layer of gel while applying minimal pressure (see Figure 68-2). This will prevent displacement of the bursal fluid, which will occur with the slightest pressure (Figure 68-5).

c.   Needle orientation relative to the transducer (see Figure 68-4)

    i.   Long axis (LAX)

d.   Needle approach (Figures 68-4 and 68-6)

    i.   In plane

e.   Target (see Figure 68-1)

    i.   Prepatellar bursa

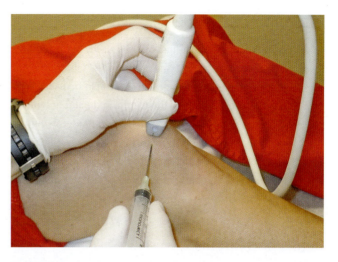

FIGURE 68-4 ■ Needle approach for the prepatellar bursa also demonstrating patient positioning for aspiration and injection. The knee is slightly flexed with a roll behind it. The transducer is short axis to the patella and the needle approach is long axis to the transducer.

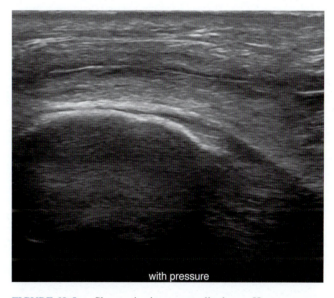

FIGURE 68-5 ■ Short-axis view, prepatellar bursa. Heavy pressure forces the bursal fluid away from the transducer.

Alternate Technique

- A medial knee approach may also be used, but it requires more of a reach by the examiner across the table.
  - A out of plane needle approach may also be used. With the transducer in LAX to the patella and patellar tendon, the needle is advanced from the lateral side of the patient. This technique is more difficult as the needle is not visualized along the entire path, but as only one specific "dot." The transducer can be used to follow this dot to ensure visualization of the needle.

Pearls and Pitfalls

- The most commonly treated bursa of the knee is the prepatellar bursa.
- With prepatellar bursitis secondary to acute trauma, always rule out a patellar fracture.
- Because of the superficial nature of the prepatellar bursa, use caution to avoid piercing the transducer with injection. Consider placing the needle into the desired location prior to placing the transducer on the skin.

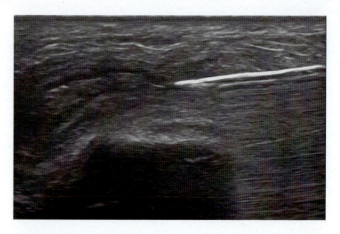

FIGURE 68-6 ▪ Short-axis view of the prepatellar bursa. In plane positioning of the needle.

- Applying too much transducer pressure will displace the bursal fluid causing a false negative examination.
- Post injection place a compression dressing, such as an ACE bandage or a knee sleeve, especially with prepatellar bursal aspiration. When the patient returns to an occupation that requires repetitive kneeling, a donut pad surrounding the bursa is helpful to minimize repetitive microtrauma.

References

1. Aguiar RO, Viegas FC, Fernandez RY, et al. The prepatellar bursa: cadaveric investigation of regional anatomy with MRI after sonographically guided bursography. *AJR Am J Roentgenol* 2007 Apr;188(4):W355–358.
2. Mathieu S, Prati C, Bossert M, et al. Acute prepatellar and olecranon bursitis. Retrospective observational study in 46 patients. *Joint Bone Spine* 2011 Jul;78(4):423–424. Epub May 6, 2011.
3. Aaron DL, Patel A, Kayiaros S, Calfee R. Four common types of bursitis: diagnosis and management. *J Am Acad Orthop Surg* 2011 Jun;19(6):359–367.

Beth M. Weinman, DO / Kate E. Temme, MD / Megan L. Noon, MD / Anne Z. Hoch, DO

KEY POINTS

- Use a 25-gauge, 1.5-inch needle.
- Use a high-frequency linear array transducer.
- Examine patients in slight knee flexion to reduce patellar tendon anisotropy.

- When visualizing the superficial infrapatellar bursa, use a thick layer of gel to prevent unintentional fluid dispersion.
- Avoid injecting into the patellar tendon.

Pertinent Anatomy

The distal patellar tendon separates the superficial and deep infrapatellar bursae. The superficial bursa lies between the patellar tendon and the subcutaneous tissue while the deep bursa lies between the patellar tendon and the proximal tibia. The deep infrapatellar bursa is further divided into anterior and posterior compartments by an apron-like projection from the retropatellar fat pad.[1] There is no communication between the deep infrapatellar bursa and the knee joint.[2,3] Location of the bursae are best determined by palpating the distal patellar tendon just proximal (1–2 cm) to the tibial tubercle (Figure 69-1).

Common Pathology

The infrapatellar bursae may be injured by direct trauma such as a fall or collision. More commonly, the bursae are inflamed as a result of microtrauma resulting from overuse injuries. Activities that may result in superficial infrapatellar bursitis include running, jumping, crawling, or kneeling in an erect position. The latter of these mechanisms is known as "clergyman's knee," which may or may not occur in conjunction with patellar tendinopathy. Gout and syphilis may cause inflammation of the superficial bursa.[4] Deep infrapatellar bursitis may be associated with Osgood-Schlatter disease, ankylosing spondylitis, juvenile idiopathic arthritis,[5] tight hamstrings

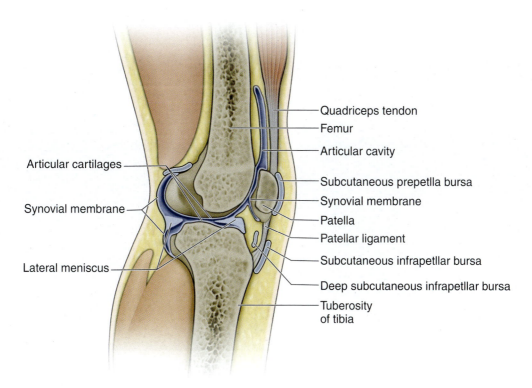

Articular cartilages

Synovial membrane

Lateral meniscus

Quadriceps tendon
Femur
Articular cavity
Subcutaneous prepetlla bursa
Synovial membrane
Patella
Patellar ligament
Subcutaneous infrapetllar bursa
Deep subcutaneous infrapetllar bursa
Tuberosity of tibia

FIGURE 69-1 ■ Anatomy of knee joint with synovium and bursae.

and/or distal patellar tendinopathy. The deep infrapatellar bursa is less susceptible to infection than the superficial bursa. Chronic inflammation may result in bursal calcification.[2]

Ultrasound Imaging Findings

The infrapatellar bursae are best visualized from the lateral aspect of the knee[5] in long axis using a high-frequency linear array transducer at a depth of 1–2 cm. A normal superficial infrapatellar bursa is difficult to visualize, but the deep infrapatellar bursa may be seen as a flat 2–3-mm anechoic structure just superficial to the tibial epiphysis.[7,8] Normal, minimal physiologic fluid collections are often present within the deep bursa. Therefore, ultrasound-guided diagnosis of deep infrapatellar bursitis requires the appropriate clinical setting, supported by the presence of larger amounts of bursal fluid compared to the contralateral, asymptomatic knee. The deep bursa will take on an hourglass appearance in the transverse plane or short-axis (SAX) view[2] (see Figure 69-2A and B).

Common ultrasonographic findings of acute bursitis include anechoic fluid collections and bursal wall thickening. Color or power Doppler will reveal areas of hyperemia consistent with inflammation, and the patient may report pain with transducer palpation. Deep infrapatellar bursitis is often associated with distal patellar tendinopathy, so examiners may also see marked effusion and a focally enlarged distal patellar tendon. Large effusions will cause the deep bursa to appear convex in shape. Bursal calcifications will appear as hyperechoic masses with posterior acoustic shadowing.

Indications for Injections of the Infrapatellar Bursae

Injection of the infrapatellar bursae may be performed in patients with persistent symptoms despite conservative management with rest, nonsteroidal antiinflammatory drugs, bracing, and physical therapy to address underlying biomechanical dysfunction. Additionally, ultrasound-guided injection may be done for diagnostic purposes as well as in patients who failed nonguided injection.

Equipment

▪ Needle: 25-gauge, 1.5-inch needle
  • Injectate
  • 1 mL of an injectable corticosteroid
  • 1 mL of a local anesthetic
▪ High-frequency linear array transducer

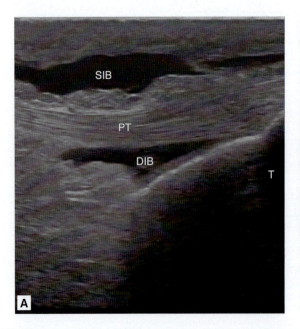
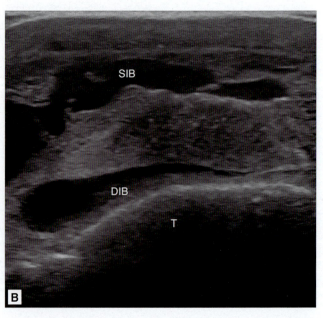

FIGURE 69-2 ▪ **A.** Longitudinal, long-axis (LAX) view. **B.** Transverse, short-axis (SAX) view. DIB, deep infrapatellar bursa; PT, patellar tendon; SIB, superficial infrapatellar bursa; T, tibia.

Superficial Infrapatellar Bursa

Longitudinal and Long Axis to the Patellar Tendon Technique

a. Patient position (Figure 69-3)

   i. Supine with a rolled towel underneath the knee to gently flex the joint to 20–30 degrees

b. Transducer position (Figure 69-4)

   i. Long axis (LAX) to the tendon with the proximal portion in contact with the patella

c. Needle orientation relative to the transducer

   i. In plane

d. Needle approach

   i. Cephalad to caudad

   ii. Needle insertion at the center of the lower pole of the patella

e. Target

   i. Superficial infrapatellar bursa

f. Pearls and Pitfalls

   i. Avoid injecting into the patellar tendon. Gentle injection should be easily accomplished. If resistance is met, the needle may be in the patellar tendon, and the needle should be withdrawn or advanced slightly until little resistance is encountered.

   ii. Fluid in the superficial bursa is easily compressed with probe pressure. Visualization with a thick layer of ultrasound gel will help to prevent unintentional dispersion of fluid.

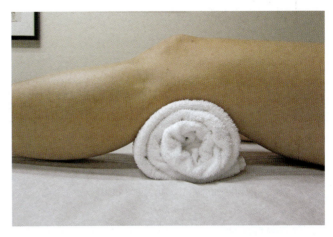

FIGURE 69-3 ■ Patient positioning for infrapatellar bursa ultrasound.

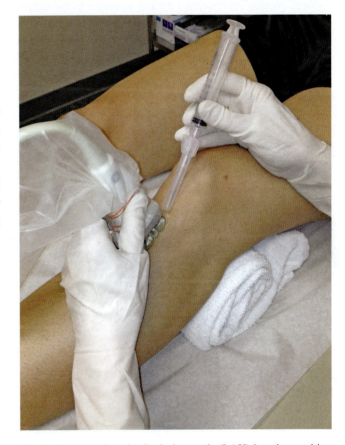

FIGURE 69-4 ■ Longitudinal, long-axis (LAX) imaging position showing transducer and needle placement.

Transverse Plane and Short Axis to the Patellar Tendon Technique

a. Patient position (see Figure 69-3)
    i. Supine position with a rolled towel underneath the knee to gently flex the joint to 20–30 degrees
b. Transducer position (Figure 69-5)
    i. Anatomic transverse plane (perpendicular to the patellar tendon) or SAX view, with the probe placed just distal to the patella
c. Needle orientation relative to the transducer
    i. In plane
d. Needle approach
    i. Lateral to medial
    ii. Medial to lateral
    iii. Needle insertion just medial or lateral to the center of the lower pole of the patella
e. Target
    i. Superficial infrapatellar bursa
f. Pearls and Pitfalls
    i. Avoid injecting into the patellar tendon. Gentle injection should be easily accomplished. If resistance is met, the needle may be in the patellar tendon, and the needle should be withdrawn or advanced slightly until little resistance is encountered.
    ii. Fluid in the superficial bursa is easily compressed with probe pressure. Visualization with a thick layer of ultrasound gel will help to prevent unintentional dispersion of fluid.

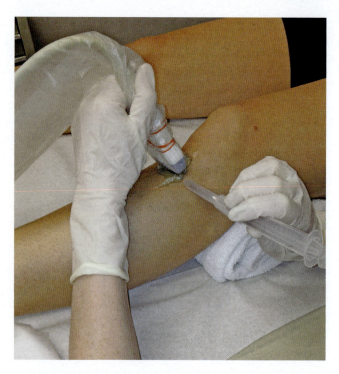

FIGURE 69-5 ■ Transverse, short-axis (SAX) imaging position showing transducer and needle placement.

Deep Infrapatellar Bursa

Transverse Plane and Short-Axis Injection Technique

a. Patient position (see Figure 69-3)
   i. Supine with a rolled towel underneath the knee to gently flex the joint to 20–30 degrees
b. Transducer position (see Figure 69-5)
   i. Anatomic transverse plane (perpendicular to the patellar tendon) or SAX view, just distal to the patella
c. Needle orientation relative to the transducer
   i. In plane
d. Needle approach
   i. Lateral to medial
   ii. Medial to lateral
   iii. The lateral-to-medial approach is preferred because of the anatomic location of the deep infrapatellar bursa, which commonly extends past the lateral border of the patellar tendon.[6] Under sterile technique, the needle is inserted just proximal to the tibial tubercle (Figure 69-6). The needle should slide beneath the patellar tendon into the deep infrapatellar bursa. Care should be taken not to inject into the patellar tendon.
   iv. Alternate needle approach: Under sterile technique, the needle is inserted just distal and lateral to the midline lower patellar margin. The needle is inserted at a right angle to the patella, passing inferiorly to the patellar tendon and into the deep infrapatellar bursa. If it strikes the patella, a more inferior trajectory should be attempted after slightly withdrawing the needle. Care should be taken not to inject into the patellar tendon.
e. Target
   i. Deep infrapatellar bursa
f. Pearls and Pitfalls
   i. Avoid injecting into the patellar tendon. Gentle injection should be easily accomplished. If resistance is met, the needle may be in the tendon and should be withdrawn or advanced slightly until little resistance is encountered.
   ii. Small, physiologic fluid collections should not be confused with bursitis of the deep infrapatellar bursa. The diagnosis of deep infrapatellar bursitis is supported by larger effusions (Figure 69-7), bilateral comparisons, and the appropriate clinical picture.

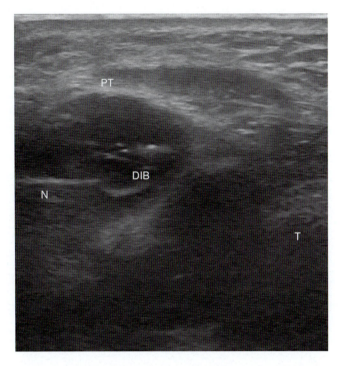

FIGURE 69-6 ■ Transverse, short-axis (SAX) view. DIB, deep infrapatellar bursa; N, needle; PT, patellar tendon; T, tibia.

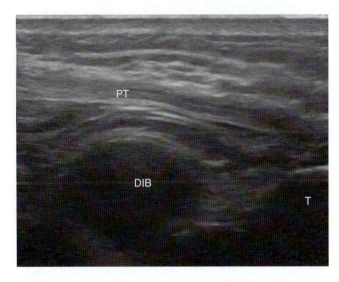

FIGURE 69-7 ■ Transverse, short-axis (SAX) view. DIB, deep infrapatellar bursa; PT, patellar tendon; T, tibia.

References

1. Saunders S, Longworth S. *Injection Techniques in Orthopaedics and Sports Medicine.* Philadelphia, PA: Elsevier; 2006:110–111.

2. LaPrade RF. The anatomy of the deep infrapatellar bursa of the knee. *Am J Sports Med* 1998;26:129–132.

3. Waldman SD. *Pain Review: Expert Consult.* Philadelphia, PA: Saunders; 2009:587–589.

4. Canale ST, Beaty JH. Tendinitis and bursitis. In: Canale, ST, Beaty JH. *Campbell's Operative Orthopedics.* 11th ed. Philadelphia, PA: Elsevier; 2008:972.

5. Alqanatish JT, Petty RE, Houghton KM, et al. Infrapatellar bursitis in children with juvenile idiopathic arthritis: a case series. *Clin Rheumatol* 2011:263-267.

6. Viegas FC, Aguiar RO, Gasparetto E, et al. Deep and superficial infrapatellar bursae: cadaveric investigation of regional anatomy using magnetic resonance after ultrasound-guided bursography. *Skeletal Radiol* 2007;36:42–46.

7. Bianchi S, Martinoli C. *Ultrasound of the Musculoskeletal System.* Heidelberg, Germany: Springer; 2007:683–684.

8. Carr JC, et al. Sonography of the patellar tendon and adjacent structures in pediatric and adult patients. *Am J Roentgenol* 2001;176:1535–1539.

Eugene Yousik Roh, MD / Michael Fredericson, MD

KEY POINTS

- Use a 25-gauge, 1.5-inch needle for a peritendinous approach to the bursa.
- Use an 18–22-gauge, 1.5–2-inch needle for a tenotomy procedure.
- Use a high-frequency linear array transducer.
- The iliotibial band (ITB) impinges on the lateral condyle of femur at approximately 30 degrees of knee flexion.

- Be sure to identify and avoid the common peroneal nerve prior to beginning the procedure.
- Be sure to target and fenestrate all areas of tendinopathy if an intratendinous technique is used.

Pertinent Anatomy (Figure 70-1)

The iliotibial band (ITB) is composed of a dense connective tissue with thickness of 1.9 mm,[1,2] formed by the tensor fascia lata and gluteus maximus proximally at the greater trochanter and runs superficial to the vastus lateralis and over the lateral femoral condyle until the ITB attaches to Gerdy's tubercle on the tibia. At Gerdy's tubercle, the ITB merges with the biceps femoris and the vastus lateralis.

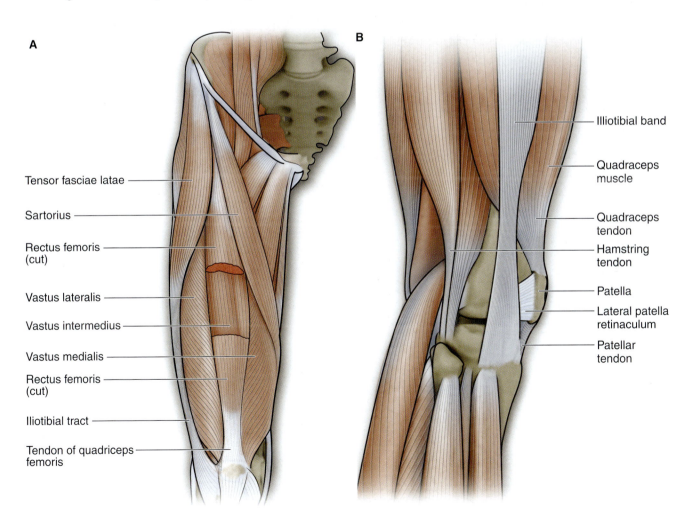

A

Tensor fasciae latae

Sartorius

Rectus femoris (cut)

Vastus lateralis

Vastus intermedius

Vastus medialis

Rectus femoris (cut)

Iliotibial tract

Tendon of quadriceps femoris

B

Illiotibial band

Quadraceps muscle

Quadraceps tendon

Hamstring tendon

Patella

Lateral patella retinaculum

Patellar tendon

FIGURE 70-1 ■ Anatomy of iliotibial band shown from (**A**) anterior and (**B**) lateral views.

Common Pathology

The ITB is located anterior to lateral femoral condyle with knee extension. It is generally thought that the ITB glides posteriorly with knee flexion, and it is located just superficial to lateral femoral condyle when knee is flexed approximately at 30 degrees. The ITB, ITB bursa, or a fat tissue between the ITB and lateral femoral condyle can be irritated during sporting activities such as long-distance running, cycling, and soccer by repetitive local friction of the ITB against the lateral femoral condyle.[3] This can produce a variety of changes in the area, including bursitis with inflammatory changes around the ITB, chronic tendinopathic changes in the ITB itself, or a combination of the two.

Ultrasound Imaging Findings

The ITB is best visualized in long axis using a high-frequency linear array transducer at a high frequency and depth of less than 3 cm. Common findings include thickening of the ITB, hypoechoic changes around the ITB, cortical irregularities at the lateral femoral condyle, and/or bursal distention, which starts deep but may also appear superficial to the ITB. Sono-palpation may illicit pain at the lateral femoral condyle.

Indications for Ultrasound-Guided Procedures of the Distal Iliotibial Band

Injection of the ITB bursa can be performed for patients who continue to have pain that is unresponsive to rest, icing, antiinflammatories, and physical therapy. An evaluation of a runner's technique or a cyclist's positioning on the bike is also important. Injection of the ITB "bursa" has been described based on palpation. With this palpation-guided technique, a needle is inserted until it contacts the bone. Then the needle is slightly withdrawn until an injectate can spread without a significant resistance. Clinical outcomes of ultrasound-guided versus palpation-guided injections have not been described.

Needle tenotomy of the ITB at the lateral femoral condyle should be considered when the above modalities have failed and the ultrasound findings support the diagnosis of tendinopathy. Although the percutaneous needle tenotomy can be done without any injectate, other injectates, such as autologous whole blood or platelet-rich plasma are used to enhance the healing process after tenotomy.[3,4]

Peritendinous Injection

Equipment

- Needle: 25-gauge, 1.5 inch needle
- Injectate
  - 1 mL of a local anesthetic
  - 1 mL of an injectable corticosteroid
- High-frequency linear array transducer

Author's Preferred Technique

a. Patient position (Figure 70-2)
    i.   Lateral decubitus.
    ii. Knee is flexed at 20–30 degrees. A pillow can be placed between knees.

b. Transducer position (see Figure 70-2)
    i.   Anatomic long-axis plane over the ITB visualizing the ITB and lateral femoral condyle

c. Needle orientation relative to the transducer (see Figure 70-2)
    i.   Out of plane

d. Needle approach (Figures 70-2 and 70-3)
    i.   Posterior to anterior.
    ii. Use walk-down technique.

e. Target (see Figure 70-3)
    i.   Between the ITB and lateral femoral condyle

f. Pearls and Pitfalls
    i.   Identify and avoid the common peroneal nerve.
    ii.   Identify and avoid lateral collateral ligament.
    iii. This technique will minimize risk of penetration of the ITB.

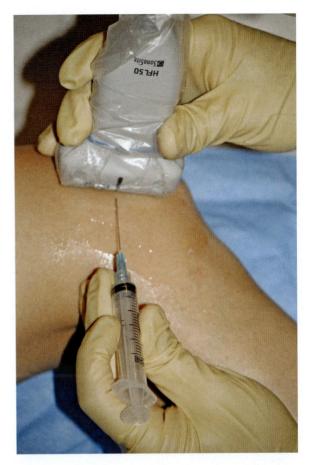

FIGURE 70-2 ■ Patient and transducer position for long-axis, out-of-plane injection into the bursa deep to the iliotibial band (ITB) at the lateral femoral condyle (LFC).

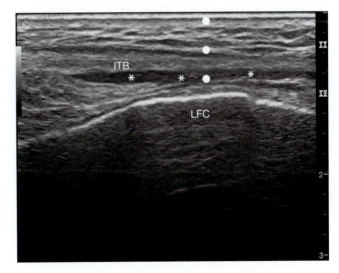

FIGURE 70-3 ■ Needle placement for long-axis, out-of-plane peritendinous approach from posterior to anterior. Dots represent walk-down technique to target. Asterisks indicate fluid under the ITB. ITB, iliotibial band; LFC, lateral femoral condyle.

Alternate Technique

a. Patient position (Figure 70-4)
   i. Lateral decubitus.
   ii. Knee is flexed at 20-30 degrees. A pillow can be placed between knees.
b. Transducer position (see Figure 70-4)
   i. Anatomic short-axis plane over the ITB visualizing the ITB and lateral femoral condyle
c. Needle orientation relative to the transducer (see Figure 70-4)
   i. In plane
d. Needle approach (Figures 70-4 and 70-5)
   i. Posterior to anterior
e. Target (see Figure 70-5)
   i. Between the ITB and lateral femoral condyle
f. Pearls and Pitfalls
   i. Identify and avoid the common peroneal nerve.

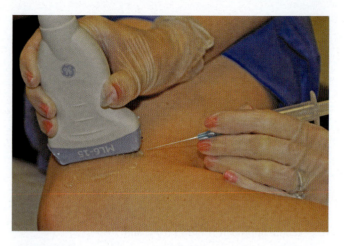

FIGURE 70-4 ■ Patient and transducer position for short-axis, in-plane injection from posterior to anterior into peritendinous and bursa region deep to the iliotibial band (ITB) at the lateral femoral condyle (LFC).

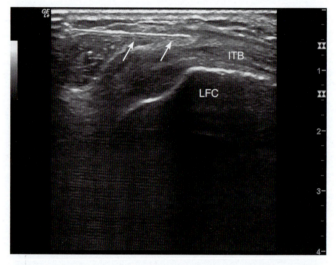

FIGURE 70-5 ■ Needle approach for short-axis, in-plane peritendinous approach. *Arrows* highlight needle entry from posterior to anterior. ITB, iliotibial band; LFC, lateral femoral condyle.

Percutaneous Tenotomy

Equipment

■ Needle
  • 25-gauge, 1.5-inch needle for local anesthesia
  • 18–22-gauge, 1.5–2-inch needle for procedure
■ Injectate: Limited amount of local anesthetic to allow for adequate pain control during needle fenestrations
■ High-frequency linear array transducer

Author's Preferred Technique

a. Patient position (Figure 70-6)
  i. Lateral decubitus.
  ii. Knee is flexed at 20-30 degrees. A pillow can be placed between knees.
b. Transducer position (see Figure 70-6)
  i. Anatomic long-axis plane over the ITB visualizing the ITB and lateral femoral condyle.
c. Needle orientation relative to the transducer (see Figure 70-6)
  i. In plane
d. Needle approach (Figures 70-6 and 70-7)
  i. Distal to proximal or proximal to distal
e. Target (see Figure 70-7)
  i. Tendonotic portion of tendon or area of maximal tenderness
f. Pearls and Pitfalls
  i. Identify and avoid the common peroneal nerve.
  ii. Identify and avoid lateral collateral ligament.
  iii. Repetitive fenestration should be performed until the needle passes through all abnormal tissue with ease.

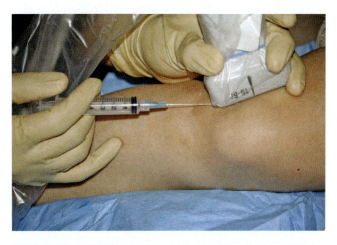

FIGURE 70-6 ■ Patient and transducer position for long-axis, in-plane tenotomy of the iliotibial band (ITB) at the lateral femoral condyle (LFC) from distal to proximal.

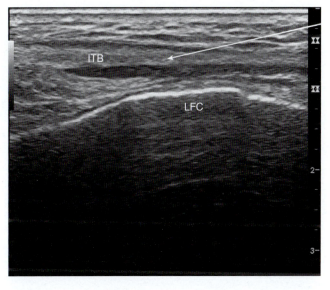

FIGURE 70-7 ■ Needle placement for tenotomy procedure, long axis, in plane, from distal to proximal. ITB, iliotibial band; LFC, lateral femoral condyle.

References

1. Goh LA, Chhem RK, Wang SC, Chee T. Iliotibial band thickness: sonographic measurements in asymptomatic volunteers. *J Clin Ultrasound* 2003 Jun;31(5):239–244.
2. Wang HK, Ting-Fang Shih T, Lin KH, Wang TG. Real-time morphologic changes of the iliotibial band during therapeutic stretching; an ultrasonographic study. *Man Ther* 2008 Aug;13(4):334–340.
3. Housner JA, Jacobson JA, Misko R. Sonographically guided percutaneous needle tenotomy for the treatment of chronic tendinosis. *J Ultrasound Med* 2009 Sep;28(9):1187–1192.
4. Finnoff JT, Fowler SP, Lai JK, et al. Treatment of chronic tendinopathy with ultrasound-guided needle tenotomy and platelet-rich plasma injection. *P M R* 2011 Oct;3(10):900–911.

Brandee L. Waite, MD

KEY POINTS

- Use a 20–25 gauge, 1.5-inch needle, depending on placement into sheath or for tenotomy of tendon.
- Use a high-frequency linear array transducer.
- The patient should be positioned in the contralateral, lateral decubitus position.
- The needle remains cephalad to common peroneal (fibular) nerve.

Pertinent Anatomy

The popliteus muscle originates at the posteromedial tibia and courses obliquely within the capsule of the knee to insert at the posterolateral femoral condyle. The primary insertion is in a fossa just distal to the lateral femoral epicondyle, deep and slightly anterior to the proximal end of the lateral fibular collateral ligament (FCL). Some fibers insert in close proximity to and into the posterior edge of the lateral meniscus (Figure 71-1).

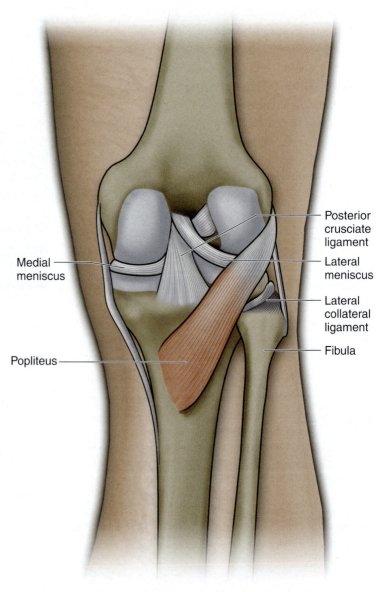

FIGURE 71-1 ■ Diagram of posterior knee showing orientation of popliteus muscle and tendon.

Common Pathology

The action of the popliteus is to "unlock" the knee as flexion is initiated from an extended position. It achieves this by rotating the femur laterally on the tibia (or medially rotating the tibia in relation to the femur, depending on perspective) while simultaneously assisting knee flexion. Additional popliteus fibers with meniscal insertion act to retract the posterior aspects of the lateral meniscus during knee flexion, thus avoiding compression damage to the meniscus between the femur and tibia.

Isolated popliteus injury is rare, but can occur with hyperextension injuries or twisting injuries. The muscle and tendon is also subject to overuse injury in runners and calcific tendinopathy.

Ultrasound Imaging Findings

The popliteus tendon can be visualized in long or short axis using a high-frequency linear array transducer and depth of less than 3 cm. Regions of hypoechoic signal within the tendon may indicate standard tendinopathy, whereas hyperechoic changes may be indicative of calcific tendinopathy.

Indications for Ultrasound-Guided Procedures of the Popliteus Tendon

Ultrasound-guided tenotomy of the popliteus tendon can be performed for patients with recalcitrant pain (at least 3–6 months), abnormal findings of tendinopathy or tendinosis with ultrasound imaging who are unresponsive to rest, icing, analgesics, physical therapy, and deep tissue massage or Active Release Techniques. Studies of ultrasound-guided tenotomy of the common extensor tendon in the elbow have shown up to 80% of patients with no pain at rest lasting over a year from the procedure.[1] Tenotomy in a variety of other tendons has shown to cause a statistically significant improvement in pain at 4 and 12 weeks post procedure.[2] Reported surgical tenotomy rates are variable and they tend to have longer healing time and potential for additional complications.[2]

Ultrasound-guided tendon sheath injections can be performed for diagnostic as well as therapeutic purposes.[3,4] It may be wise to consider a tendon sheath injection to confirm this as the pain source prior to pursuing a tenotomy or biologic injection into this region. Clinical outcomes of palpation- versus ultrasound-guided injections have not been described.

Tendon Sheath

Equipment

- Needle: 22–25 gauge, 1.5–2 inch needle
- Injectate
  - 1 mL of local anesthesia
  - 1 mL of an injectable corticosteroid
- High-frequency linear array transducer

Author's Preferred Technique

a. Patient position (Figure 71-2)
    i. Contralateral lateral decubitus position
    ii. Knee flexed 20–30 degrees and slightly internally rotated
b. Transducer position (see Figure 71-2)
    i. Locate the popliteus fossa and visualize tendon in short axis within fossa.
c. Needle orientation relative to the transducer (see Figure 71-2)
    i. In plane
d. Needle approach (Figures 71-2 and 71-3)
    i. Proximal to distal or distal to proximal
e. Target (see Figure 71-3)
    i. Popliteus tendon sheath.
    ii. Care should be taken to not inject into tendon itself.
f. Pearls and Pitfalls
    i. Locate and avoid common peroneal nerve in injection planning.
    ii. For a patient with lateral knee pain that is hard to diagnose, consider diagnostic injection into tendon sheath followed by provocation to see if pain is eliminated.

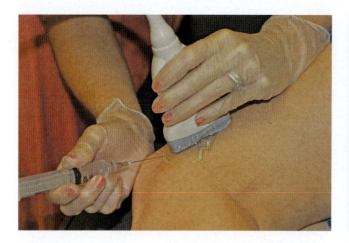

FIGURE 71-2 ■ Transducer position for tendon sheath injection with needle approach in plane from distal to proximal.

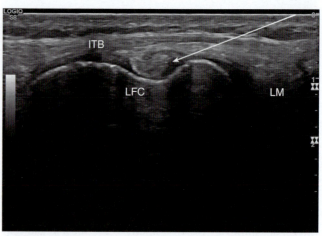

FIGURE 71-3 ■ Needle placement for peritendinous approach (*white arrow*). ITB, iliotibial band; LFC, lateral femoral condyle; LM, lateral meniscus.

Tenotomy

Equipment

- Needle
  - 25-gauge, 1.5-inch needle for local anesthesia
  - 20–22-gauge, 1.5–2-inch needle for procedure
- Injectate
  - Limited amount of local anesthetic to allow for adequate pain control during needle fenestration
- High-frequency linear array transducer

Author's Preferred Technique

a. Patient position (Figure 71-4)
    i.   Contralateral lateral decubitus position
    ii. Knee flexed 20–30 degrees and slightly internally rotated
b. Transducer position (see Figure 71-4)
    i.   Long axis to the popliteus tendon within the popliteus fossa.
    ii. If you have trouble visualizing the tendon, return to a long-axis view of the proximal FCL, then rotate transducer to be short axis (perpendicular) to the axis of the popliteus tendon to view the tendon in cross section. Toggle transducer and the cross-sectional ovular appearance of the popliteus tendon will alternate between hyper- and hypoechoic signal because of anisotropy. Once located in this manner, spin the transducer on the tendon and watch fibers transition into long-axis view.

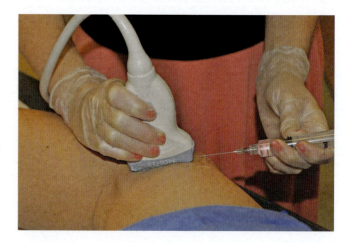

FIGURE 71-4 ■ Transducer position for tenotomy with probe long axis to tendon and needle oriented in plane from anterior to posterior.

c. Needle orientation relative to the transducer (see Figure 71-4)
   i. In plane
d. Needle approach (see Figure 71-4)
   i. Oblique, from anterior to posterior
e. Target (Figure 71-5)
   i. Popliteus intratendinous needle placement
f. Pearls and Pitfalls
   i. The needle remains cephalad and proximal to the common peroneal (fibular) nerve.
   ii. If injecting biological agent, perform fenestration first, then deposit injectate at separate regions within the fenestrated tendon.
   iii. Post procedure, patient physical activity should be restricted with gradual return to activity as symptoms improve.
   iv. It is important to note the angle of the popliteus muscle and tendon and position the probe with the posterior portion more inferior than the lateral portion (see Figure 71-4).

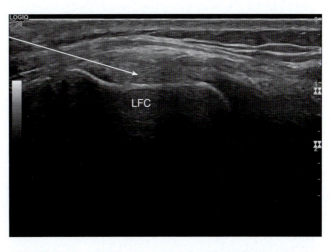

FIGURE 71-5 ■ Needle placement for intratendinous procedure (*white arrow*) from anterior to posterior. LFC, lateral femoral condyle.

References

1. McShane J, Shah V, Nazarian L. Sonographically guided percutaneous needle tenotomy for treatment of common extensor tendinosis in the elbow. *J Ultrasound Med* 2008;27:1137–1144.
2. Housner J, Jacobsen J, Misko R. Sonographically guided needle tenotomy for the treatment of chronic tendinosis. *J Ultrasound Med* 2009;28:1187–1192.
3. Smith J, Finoff J, Santaella-Sante B, Henning T, et al. Sonographically guided popliteus tendon sheath injection. *J Ultrasound Med* 2010; 29:775–782.
4. Petsche T, Selesnick F. Popliteus tendinitis: tips for diagnosis and management. *Phys Sportsmed* 2002 Aug;30(8):27–31.

Robert Monaco, MD / Megan Groh Miller, MD

KEY POINTS

- Use a 22–25-gauge, 1.5–2.5-inch needle, depending on the site.
- Use a high-frequency linear array transducer.
- The anatomy of the distal biceps femoris region is extremely complex.
- The distal biceps femoris is one of the more common sites of hamstring injuries.
- Ultrasound can be used to assess both the location and the severity of the injury and assist in narrowing the differential diagnosis.
- Extreme care must be taken to avoid iatrogenic injury to the tendon or collateral ligament, particularly with fenestration procedures or corticosteroid injections.

Pertinent Anatomy

The distal biceps femoris tendon complex is part of the hamstring muscle group and is made up of the long and short heads. It assists in flexion of the leg and adds stability to the lateral knee. The long head originates at the ischium and the short head originates primarily off the linea aspera of the femur. The muscle blends with its tendon approximately 3–4 inches above the knee joint line. It is important to realize that part of the biceps femoris complex remains muscular as it passes over the knee joint posteriorly.

The insertions of the tendons are fanlike with multiple attachments. The primary attachment is the fibula head, but other multiple attachments exist on the tibia and fibula and are variable. The tendon bifurcates into two arms, (superficial and deep), which envelope the distal fibular collateral ligament at the level of the fibula (Figure 72-1). A small bursa exists between the superficial component and the fibular collateral ligament.

The short head sends its attachments primarily to the long head muscle, and the fibular head, as well as multiple other areas of the lateral knee complex. The posterior lateral geniculate artery underlies the biceps femoris and fibular collateral ligament at the tibiofemoral joint line. The peroneal nerve also lies posterior.

Common Pathology

Diagnosis of pathology to the posterior lateral knee can be challenging because of the complexity of the anatomy. One needs to consider the following in the differential diagnosis: lateral meniscal disorders, iliotibial band syndrome, fibular collateral ligament sprains, bursopathy (fibular collateral

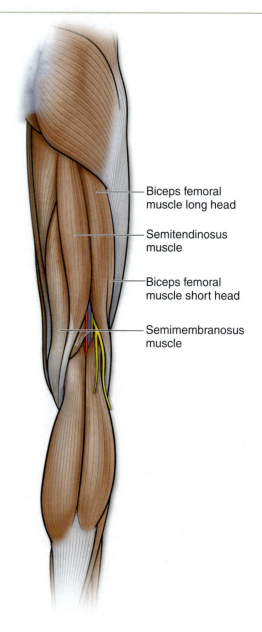

Biceps femoral muscle long head

Semitendinosus muscle

Biceps femoral muscle short head

Semimembranosus muscle

FIGURE 72-1 ■ Distal hamstring anatomy.

ligament at the biceps femoris), popliteus tendinopathy, proximal tibia-fibula joint problems, common peroneal neuropathy, complex posterior lateral corner injures, and biceps femoris pathology. Often, advanced imaging (ultrasound, magnetic resonance) is needed to supplement the history and physical in making a specific diagnosis.

Injuries to the distal biceps femoris tendon are one of the more common sites of hamstring injury. Injuries can range from a low-grade strain, to a complete rupture (rare). Most injuries occur along the muscle tendon junction, which begins approximately 3–4 inches above the knee joint. Injuries can also occur at varied insertion sites. Tendinosis and fibrosis of the region may also be noted, and presents similar to other tendon pathology in the body.

Ultrasound Image Findings

The optimal transducer for scanning this region is a high-frequency linear array transducer with the leg in extension or slight 10 degrees of flexion. Scans should be done in both long and short axis. On long axis, the biceps femoris muscle tendon junction is localized posteriorly at the knee joint. The short head of the biceps can be seen joining the long head at the musculotendinous junction.

The sonographer should then use a long-axis view to trace the biceps femoris complex distally looking for the bifurcation of the tendon around the fibular collateral ligament, which occurs at the level of the fibular head (Figure 72-2A).[1] It can be challenging to decipher the short head of the biceps insertion, and the clinician may best treat it as a complex. The sonographer needs to be careful, as the divergence of the tendons makes it appear as tendonitis, when it is likely due to resultant tendon thickening and anisotropy (Figure 72-2B).[2]

Thus the superficial and deep heads should also be visualized in an oblique short-axis orientation by lining up on the fibular collateral ligament. The superficial and deep head of the tendon are noted just proximal to its fibular insertion. The superficial head tends to be the larger of the two.[3]

Dynamic testing by firing of the hamstrings may be helpful in elucidating subtle findings and help correlate with clinical pain. Occasionally a snapping biceps femoris may be noted as the cause of pain.

Findings on ultrasound may include tendon thickening, and/or hypoechoic areas within the tendon consistent with tendinosis. Doppler findings may suggest tendinosis as well. Anechoic areas may represent partial injury. Occasionally, fluid around the tendon sheath is noted suggestive of tenosynovitis or bursitis, although this is less common. In addition,

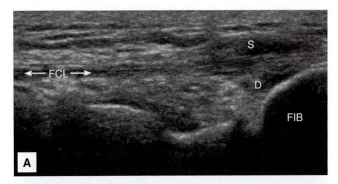

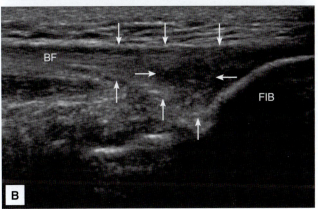

FIGURE 72-2 ■ **A.** Long-axis view demonstrating the superficial and deep heads of the bifurcating distal biceps femoris tendon, visualized above and below the distal fibular collateral ligament, just proximal to its fibular insertion. Left is cephalad, right caudad, top lateral, and bottom medial. D, deep bicep femoris tendon layer; FCL, fibular collateral ligament; FIB, fibular head; S, superficial bicep femoris tendon layer. **B.** Long-axis view of biceps femoris tendon in a patient without clinical or radiographic evidence of tendinosis. The distal biceps femoris tendon appears thickened and hypoechoic (*vertical arrows*), with a more central region of anechogenicity (*horizontal arrows*) representing the fibular collateral ligament within the tendon. The ligament is anechoic due to anisotropy. Left is cephalad, right caudad, top lateral, bottom medial. BF, biceps femoris; FIB, fibular head.

small avulsions off the insertion into fibular head may be noted. In acute settings, a hematoma may be noted. Rarely a complete avulsion may be noted but is usually associated with significant other injuries.

Injection

Injection of the complex may be indicated in those who have failed a significant course of rehabilitation and continue to have pain and dysfunction isolated to the biceps femoris muscle–tendon complex. The success rate of these injections is unclear. All injections in this region are highly encouraged to be ultrasound-guided secondarily to the complex anatomy with close proximity to the peroneal nerve and arterial structures. Clinicians may elect to inject either growth factors, such as platelet-rich plasma (PRP), to potentially enhance healing or a corticosteroid to potentially decrease fibrosis, although no evidence-based clinical studies are available to directly guide treatment for injuries at this site. Fenestration or tenotomy may be indicated in rare occasions for isolated tendinosis. However, one must be highly aware of potential iatrogenic damage to the lateral collateral ligament secondarily to the complex bifurcating anatomy of the biceps and the high prevalence of anisotropy in the region of the tendon insertion.

Equipment

- Needle: 22–25-gauge, 1.5–2.5-inch needle, depending on site
- Injectate: a local anesthetic agent—enough to anesthetize from subcutaneous tissue through the injury site—or other proliferant type of injectate
- High-frequency linear array transducer

Author's Preferred Technique

a. Patient position
   i. The patient is positioned lying prone or side-lying, with the knee slightly flexed (10 degrees).
b. Transducer position
   i. The transducer is placed longitudinal, over the tendon complex locating the primary attachment at the fibular head, and then moved to the pathologic area.
c. Needle orientation relative to the transducer
   i. In plane
d. Needle approach
   i. For insertional injury injections, the needle needs to be directed proximal to distal (Figure 72-3A, B). Myotendinous junction injuries are usually done in a similar fashion depending on site of injury.

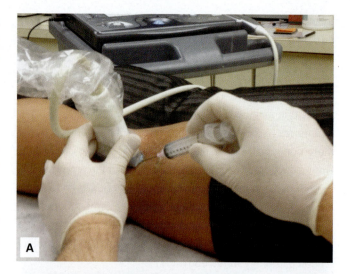

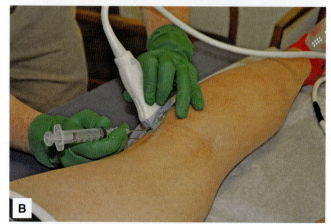

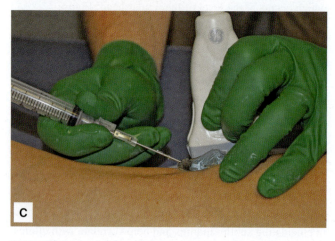

FIGURE 72-3 ■ **A** through **C.** Photographs of injection setup.

e. Target
   i. Distal insertion of the biceps femoris at the fibular head (Figure 72-4)
f. Fenestration or tenotomy
   i. For chronic tendinosis, the clinician may elect to fenestrate the tendon to promote healing. This is done by repeatedly moving the needle through the pathologic area of tendinitis multiple times. The amount will depend on the significance of the pathology as well as the needle gauge and clinician's experience, as there is no literature to guide treatment. More fenestrations may be needed for more significant pathology (although there has been no literature validating this technique) and when a smaller gauge needle is used.
   ii. The attachment may also be needled multiple times to break up calcifications, if present, and to promote a new healing cascade.
   iii. Many clinicians may also then inject PRP (2–3 mL) into the area to promote tendon healing.
g. Peritendinous injection
   i. The clinician may also inject around the tendon sheath, particularly if the tenosynovium is focally swollen. This occurs more commonly approximately 5–10 cm above the attachment at the muscle tendon junction. Either PRP or a corticosteroid may be considered, depending on the clinical scenario.
h. Pearls and Pitfalls
   i. When corticosteroids are used, exquisite care must be taken to ensure injection into the sheath and not directly into the tendon or fibular collateral ligament.
   ii. The diagnosis of *isolated* biceps femoris tendinosis should be approached with caution, as it must be distinguished from anisotropy, which is extremely common because of the anatomy. Clinical examination, multiple views, sonopalpation, and magnetic resonance imaging correlation may be helpful if no other pathology is noted. Fenestration or tenotomy should only be done by experienced hands with high-frequency probes.
   iii. To minimize the risk of injuring the peroneal nerve when performing insertional injections, map out and locate the nerve and use a limited volume of anesthetic fluid (~2 cc).
   iv. The clinician should be aware of anisotropy in this area mimicking tendinosis as well as the complex bifurcation of the biceps complex. It is advised that only experienced users using high-frequency probes consider tenotomy in this location.

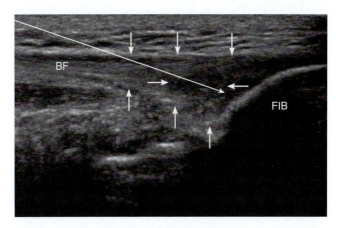

FIGURE 72-4 ▪ Ultrasound image with position of needle (*arrow*) into target. BF, biceps femoris; FIB, fibular head.

References

1. Sekiya J, Swaringen JC, Wojtys EM, et al. Diagnostic ultrasound evaluation of posterolateral corner knee injuries. *Arthroscopy* 2010 April;26(4):494–499.
2. Smith J, Sayeed YA, Finnoff DO, et al. The bifurcating distal biceps femoris tendon: potential pitfall in musculoskeletal sonography. *J Ultrasound Med* 2011;30:1156–1166.
3. Tubbs RS, Caycedo FJ, Oakes WJ, et al. Descriptive anatomy of the insertion of the biceps femoris muscle. *Clin Anat* 2006;19:517–521.

Brandon J. Messerli, DO / Garrett S. Hyman, MD, MPH

KEY POINTS

- A high-frequency linear array transducer is ideal.
- Use a long-axis, in-plane approach.
- Use a smaller gauge (22–25) needle for peritendinous injection.
- Use a larger gauge (18–20) needle for percutaneous tenotomy.
- Identify the pes anserine tendons (ie, semitendinosus, gracilis, and sartorius) pass posterior and then medial to the semimembranosus tendon.

Pertinent Anatomy

The semimembranosus muscle has a fusiform configuration with the muscle belly ending just above the knee joint. The distal tendon has five to six insertion sites. The "direct" or "main" insertion is at the infraglenoid tubercle of the posteromedial tibial plateau, immediately posterior to the medial collateral ligament (MCL) (Figure 73-1). The "pars reflexa" insertion turns 90 degrees anteriorly and passes deep to the MCL before attaching below the joint line. There are superficial fibers that attach directly to the MCL and deep fibers that insert at the posteromedial joint capsule. A broad "inferior" insertion occurs at the oblique popliteal ligament, posterior oblique ligament, and fascia of the popliteal muscle. Of note, 43% of cadaveric knees revealed an insertion at the posterior horn of the lateral meniscus, which likely functions to pull the meniscus posteriorly during deep knee flexion. The semimembranosus muscle functions primarily as a knee flexor and secondarily as a hip extensor and internal rotator of the tibia. The semimembranosus tendon may be involved in injuries affecting the posteromedial corner of the knee.

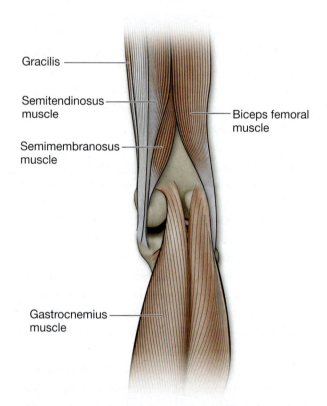

FIGURE 73-1 ■ Illustration of the posterior knee demonstrating muscles and tendons of the posterior medial knee. Note the semimembranosus tendon insertion onto the posterior tibial plateau of the knee.

Common Pathology

Acute injuries include strains, tears, avulsions, and contusions. Strains typically occur at the myotendinous junction because of excessive stretch and/or eccentric activation. First-degree tendon injuries reveal minor fiber disruption with interstitial edema and hemorrhage. Second-degree tendon injury involves a partial tear with perifascial fluid collection and hematoma. Third-degree tendon injury involves a complete tear with fiber contraction. Tendon avulsions are frequently caused by a valgus knee injury with associated tears of the anterior cruciate ligament, medial meniscus, and medial head of the gastrocnemius.

Chronic conditions involve overuse and repetitive stress mechanisms. Tendon injury can occur from friction over the joint capsule, medial femoral condyle, medial tibial plateau, joint line osteophytes, prosthetic components, or from the overlying semitendinosus tendon. Risk factors may include female sex, increased Q angle, and overpronation.

Ultrasound Imaging Findings

The semimembranosus tendon is best visualized in both long- (see Figure 73-1) and short-axis views using a medium- to high-frequency linear array transducer at a depth suitable for the body habitus.

Normal tendon architecture, as elsewhere, appears as a fibrillar pattern with tightly packed alternating hyperechoic and hypoechoic lines. Standards for tendon thickness have not been described. The semimembranosus tendon is not invested by a synovial sheath. The most common abnormal findings are that of tendinosis, which includes tendon thickening, hypoechogenicity, and an indistinct loosely packed fibrillar pattern. A tendon tear appears as a hypoechoic or anechoic region anteriorly (articular surface), posteriorly, or within the body of the tendon (intrasubstance).

Indications for Ultrasound-Guided Procedures of the Semimembranosus Tendon

Inadequate response with other conservative therapy including relative rest, ice, nonsteroidal antiinflammatories, physical therapy, modalities, and/or orthotics are the indications for an ultrasound-guided injection to the semimembranosus tendon. There is limited published evidence on the efficacy of tenotomy or injections for semimembranosus tendinopathy. One case report by Weiser in 1978 followed 100 subjects for 10 weeks after a non-ultrasound-guided lidocaine and triamcinolone injection for clinically diagnosed tendinopathy; all subjects had immediate pain relief, 58 subjects had long-lasting relief (not quantified), and 30 subjects had repeat injections in 3 to 5 months. There are no published data regarding the success of ultrasound-guided versus palpation-guided injections of the semimembranosus muscle or tendon.

Equipment

- Needle: 22- to 25-gauge, 1.5- to 2-inch needle
- Injectate: 1 mL of local anesthesia and 1 mL of an injectable corticosteroid
- Medium- to high-frequency linear array transducer

Peritendinous Technique

a. Patient position
    i. Prone or lateral decubitus positioning

FIGURE 73-2 ▪ Transducer and needle positioning for short-axis, in-plane injection to the peritendinous region of the semimembranosus.

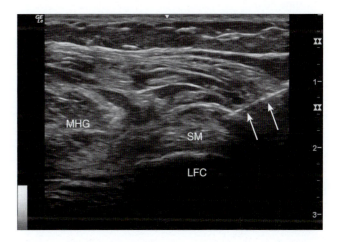

FIGURE 73-3 ▪ Short-axis ultrasound view of the distal semimembranosus tendon at the posterior medial knee. Arrows highlight the needle as it enters the semimembranosus peritendinous region, in plane, from medial to lateral.

b. Transducer position (Figure 73-2)
    i. Short axis to the semimembranosus tendon
c. Needle orientation relative to the transducer (see Figure 73-2)
    i. In plane
d. Needle approach (Figure 73-3; see Figure 73-2)
    i. Medial to lateral
e. Target (see Figure 73-3)
    i. Peritendinous region of semimembranosus

f. Pearls and Pitfalls

    i. Distinguishing injury to the semimembranosus tendon versus the MCL or the pes anserine tendons may be difficult. The MCL is immediately adjacent anteriorly, and the pes anserine tendons cross from posterior to anterior on the diagonal across the medial femoral condyle.

    ii. In the short-axis view of semimembranosus tendon, it is important not to mistake the tendon for a Baker's cyst as it can appear hypoechoic in this area if not imaged at the correct angle.

Equipment

■ Needle
- Use a 25-gauge, 1.5-inch needle for local anesthesia.
- Use an 18- to 20-gauge, 1.5- to 2-inch needle for the procedure.

■ Injectate
- Use a limited amount of local anesthetic to allow for adequate pain control during needle fenestrations.
- Use a medium- to high-frequency linear array transducer.

Tenotomy Technique

a. Patient position

    i. Prone or lateral decubitus positioning

b. Transducer position (Figure 73-4)

    i. Long axis over the medial or posterior aspect of the tendon

c. Needle orientation relative to the transducer (see Figure 73-4)

    i. In plane

d. Needle approach (Figure 73-5; see Figure 73-4)

    i. Proximal to distal

e. Target (see Figure 73-5)

    i. Regions of abnormal tendon pathology

f. Pearls and Pitfalls

    i. Distinguishing injury to the semimembranosus tendon versus the MCL or the pes anserine tendons may be difficult. The MCL is immediately adjacent anteriorly, and the pes anserine tendons cross from posterior to anterior on the diagonal across the medial femoral condyle.

    ii. In the long-axis view, be sure to note the semitendinosus superficial to the semimembranosus and not to inadvertently target the wrong tendon for this procedure.

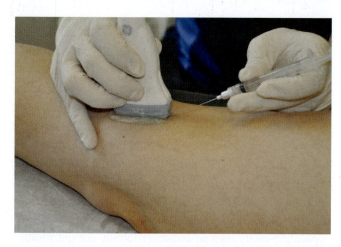

FIGURE 73-4 ■ Transducer and needle positioning for a long-axis, in-plane injection to the semimembranosus tendon.

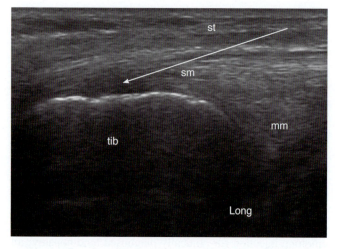

FIGURE 73-5 ■ Ultrasound view of long-axis distal semimembranosus (sm) tendon insertion onto the proximal posteromedial tibia (tib). The medial meniscus (mm) and joint line are just cephalad, and the semitendinosus tendon (st) passes dorsal to the semimembranosus. Note the arrow, which indicates the needle approach to perform tenotomy.

References

1. Bylund WE, Weber K. Semimembranosus tendinopathy: one cause of chronic posteromedial knee pain. *Primary Care* 2010 Sept;2(5):380–384.

2. Bencardino JT, Rosenberg ZS, Brown RR, et al. Traumatic musculotendinous injuries of the knee: diagnosis with MR imaging. *Radiographics* 2000 Oct:20:S103–S120.

3. Weiser HI. Semimembranosus insertion syndrome: a treatable and frequent cause of persistent knee pain. *Arch Phys Med Rehabil* 1979 July;60:317–319.

Jacob L. Sellon, MD / Jay Smith, MD

KEY POINTS

- High-frequency linear array transducers can be used to image and inject the bursa.
- The transducer can be oriented short or long axis relative to the pes anserine tendons.
- The pes anserine bursa is located between the medial collateral ligament and the pes anserine conjoint tendon.
- Tilting the transducer will increase pes anserine tendon conspicuity by creating anisotropy.
- Avoid nearby neurovascular structures (eg, inferior medial geniculate artery).

Pertinent Anatomy (Figure 74-1)

The pes anserinus is a tendinous confluence formed by the sartorius, gracilis, and semitendinosus tendons as they insert at a common point on the proximal anteromedial tibia. The pes anserine bursa lies in the potential space between these conjoint tendons and the underlying medial collateral ligament (MCL) and medial tibia.

Common Pathology

Pes anserinus pain usually results from bursitis or tendinitis and may be caused by repetitive overuse or direct trauma. Pain in this region has been associated with knee osteoarthritis, rheumatoid arthritis, diabetes mellitus, and obesity.[1] The diagnosis is usually based on clinical findings. Symptoms may be triggered by ambulation, and in particular, rising from a seated position or climbing stairs. The key finding on physical examination is tenderness in the region of the pes anserinus. Swelling in this area may also be present.

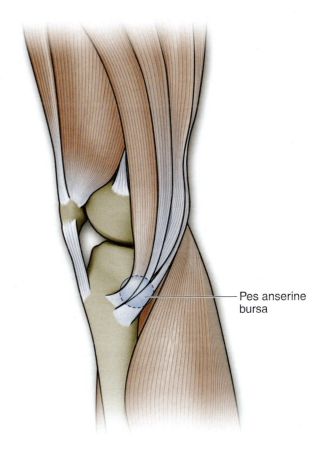

Pes anserine bursa

FIGURE 74-1 ■ Anatomy of the pes anserine bursa.

Ultrasound Imaging Findings

The pes anserine tendons and bursa are usually best visualized using a high-frequency linear array transducer. However, a lower frequency probe may be preferable for patients with large or edematous legs. The pes anserinus can be scanned in both short (Figure 74-2) and long axes (Figure 74-3) relative to the tendons. Tilting the transducer to introduce tendon anisotropy may increase the conspicuity of the pes anserine tendons and facilitate differentiation of the tendons from the underlying MCL (Figure 74-4). Although the sonographic appearance of the pes anserine region is often normal in patients presenting with clinical pes anserine tendinitis or bursitis, one may occasionally visualize bursal fluid and/or tendon hypoechogenicity, either of which may be accompanied by increased Doppler flow. The inferior medial geniculate artery lies deep to the MCL and should not be misinterpreted as bursal fluid or hypervascularity.

Indications for Pes Anserine Bursa Injection

Injection of the pes anserine bursa may be considered for patients with recalcitrant pain unresponsive to rest, icing, nonsteroidal antiinflammatory drugs, and physical therapy. Using a cadaveric model, Finnoff and colleagues documented a diagnostic accuracy rate (ie, injectate only located in bursa) of 92% following sonographically guided pes anserine bursa injections, compared to a 17% accuracy using a palpation-guided technique. In comparison, the therapeutic accuracy rates (ie, at least some injectate in the bursa) were 100% and 50%, respectively.[2] Regarding clinical efficacy, Yoon and colleagues reported that ultrasound-guided pes anserine bursa injections improved knee pain and function in patients with knee osteoarthritis and concomitant pes anserine tendinitis/bursitis.[3] However, to date, no studies have directly compared clinical outcomes of ultrasound-guided versus unguided injections.

Equipment

- ■ Needle: 25-gauge, 1.5-inch needle
  - • Injectate
  - • 1–2 cc 1% lidocaine
  - • 1 cc corticosteroid
- ■ High-frequency linear array transducer

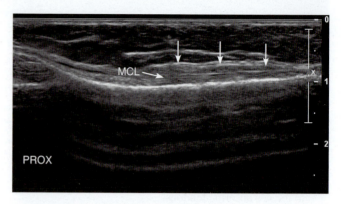

FIGURE 74-2 ■ Short-axis ultrasound image of pes anserine tendons (*downward arrows*) crossing superficial to the medial collateral ligament (MCL with *diagonal arrow*). The pes anserine bursa lies in the potential space between the pes anserine tendons and the MCL. Left, proximal; right, distal; top, superficial; bottom, deep.

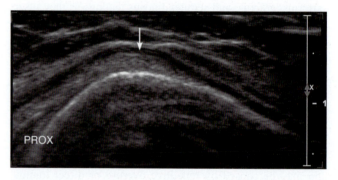

FIGURE 74-3 ■ Long-axis ultrasound image of the gracilis tendon (*downward arrow*) crossing the underlying medial collateral ligament. The tendon appears dark due to anisotropy. Left, proximal; right, distal; top, superficial; bottom, deep.

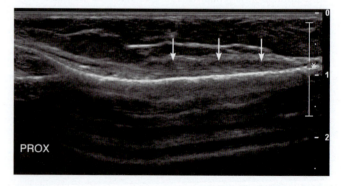

FIGURE 74-4 ■ Same ultrasound image as Figure 74-2 after tilting transducer. Pes anserine tendons (*downward arrows*) are now anisotropic, increasing conspicuity.

Author's Preferred Technique (Figures 74-5, 74-6, and 74-7)

a. Patient position
    i. Supine
    ii. Hip externally rotated and knee slightly flexed (rolled towel under knee)
b. Transducer position
    i. Anatomic coronal plane (same plane as the MCL) over the anterior fibers of the MCL
    ii. Pes anserine tendons should be seen in an oblique short-axis view as they cross the MCL
c. Needle orientation relative to the transducer
    i. In plane (long axis/longitudinal)
d. Needle approach
    i. Distal (inferior) to proximal (superior)
e. Target
    i. Deep to the pes anserine tendons (central tendon if multiple tendons are seen) and superficial to the MCL
    ii. If fluid is seen within the bursa, this can be targeted appropriately
f. Pearls and Pitfalls
    i. Tilt the transducer to increase tendon conspicuity as described above.
    ii. The angle of needle approach is shallow unless patient's leg is large.
    iii. Avoid injecting into the pes anserine tendons or MCL.
    iv. Doppler may help identify vessels (inferior medial geniculate artery, saphenous vein).
    v. The branches of the saphenous nerve may be located in this region.

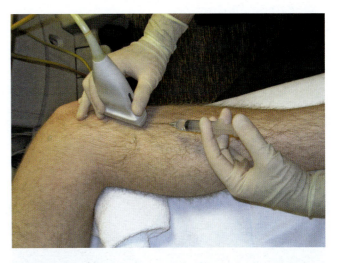

FIGURE 74-5 ■ Setup for pes anserine bursa injection using short-axis view of the pes anserine tendons.

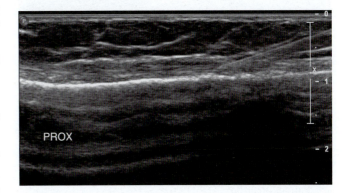

FIGURE 74-6 ■ Same ultrasound image as Figures 74-2 and 74-4, demonstrating needle advancing in plane, distal to proximal, into the region of the pes anserine bursa.

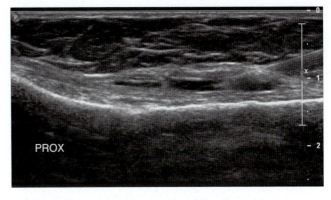

FIGURE 74-7 ■ Pes anserine "bursogram" following injection using setup and approach shown in Figures 74-5 and 74-6.

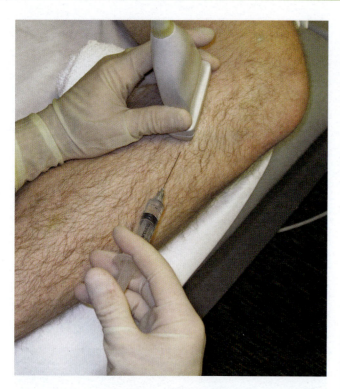

FIGURE 74-8 ▪ Setup for pes anserine bursa injection using a long-axis view of the pes anserine tendons.

Alternate Technique (Figures 74-8, 74-9, and 74-10)

a. Patient position
   i. Supine
   ii. Hip externally rotated and knee slightly flexed (rolled towel under knee)
b. Transducer position
   i. Start by finding the short-axis view of pes anserine tendons as described above, and center gracilis tendon on the screen.
   ii. Then rotate into long-axis view of central (gracilis) portion of conjoint tendon in anatomic coronal oblique plane.
c. Needle orientation relative to the transducer
   i. In plane (long axis/longitudinal)
d. Needle approach
   i. Distal (inferior) to proximal (superior)
e. Target
   i. Deep to the pes anserine tendons (central tendon if multiple tendons are seen) and superficial to the MCL.
   ii. If fluid is seen within the bursa, this can be targeted appropriately.

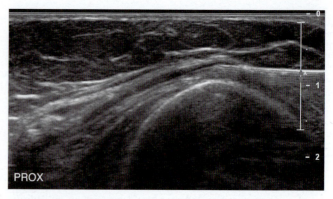

FIGURE 74-9 ▪ Same ultrasound image as Figure 74-3, demonstrating needle advancing in plane, distal to proximal, into the region of the pes anserine bursa.

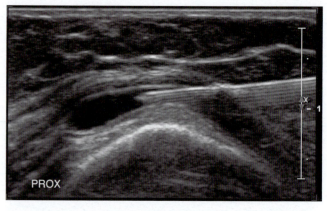

FIGURE 74-10 ▪ Pes anserine "bursogram" following injection using setup and approach shown in Figures 74-8 and 74-9.

f. Pearls and Pitfalls
   i. See "Pearls and Pitfalls" under "Author's Preferred Technique"

References

1. Handy JR. Anserine bursitis: a brief review. *South Med J* 1997;90:376–377.
2. Finnoff JT, Nutz DJ, Henning PT, Hollman JH, Smith J. Accuracy of ultrasound-guided versus unguided pes anserinus bursa injections. *PM R* 2010;2:732–739.
3. Yoon HS, Kim SE, Suh YR, Seo YI, Kim HA. Correlation between ultrasonographic findings and the response to corticosteroid injection in pes anserinus tendinobursitis syndrome in knee osteoarthritis patients. *J Korean Med Sci* 2005;20:109–112.

Troy Henning, DO

KEY POINTS

- An 18-gauge needle is needed for aspiration, a 25-gauge needle for injection.
- High-frequency linear array transducers are preferred.
- The bursa is found between the superficial and deep layers of the medial collateral ligament (MCL).
- The ligamentous and bursa structures should be interrogated in their long and short axis.

- Inadvertent saphenous nerve blockade or knee joint entrance is possible if strict needle visualization is not used.
- Gentle transducer pressure and/or use of standoff transducer gel technique improves visualization of the bursal effusion.

Pertinent Anatomy

The tibial collateral ligament bursa was originally described by Voshell et al. in 1944.[1] Throughout the literature, the bursa has also been referred to as the *medial collateral ligament bursa*, *no name bursa*, and *Voshell's bursa*.[1–3] The medial aspect of the knee is formed by three distinct fascial planes. The second and third planes correlate with the superficial and deep portions of the medial collateral ligament (MCL), respectively[2,4] (Figure 75-1). The tibial collateral ligament bursa is a constant bursa (congenital) found between the two layers of the MCL.[2,4]

Common Pathology

Effusions within the bursa develop from direct trauma or irritation (friction between two layers of MCL) of the bursa. One should note that fluid accumulations can develop between the superficial and deep layers of the MCL because of a variety of other causes, such as MCL sprains, perimeniscal cysts, ganglion cysts and effusions within nearby bursa (pes anserine and semimembranosus tibial collateral bursae).[3,5]

Ultrasound Imaging Findings

The tibial collateral ligament bursa is best visualized in long axis using a high-frequency linear array transducer at a frequency of 8–12 Hz and depth of less than 3 cm. Common findings include hypoechoic to anechoic fluid with the bursa. The bursa may or may not demonstrate septations. When interrogating the fluid collection, care should be taken to ensure effusion is isolated to the bursa. Fluid extension from an adjacent meniscal tear or obvious MCL injury suggests an alternate diagnosis.

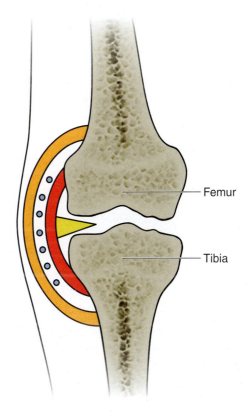

Femur

Tibia

FIGURE 75-1 ■ Coronal illustration of the knee. The superficial and deep portions of the tibial collateral ligament are depicted in *orange* and *red*, respectively. The *grey circles* represent location of the tibial collateral bursa. The *yellow triangle* represents the medial meniscus.

Indications for Injections of the Tibial Collateral Ligament Bursa

Injection of the tibial collateral ligament bursa can be performed for patients with recalcitrant pain that is unresponsive to rest, icing, antiinflammatories and bracing. Nonguided injection or aspiration of the bursa have been described and are based on palpation of the bursal effusion.[1] Jose et al. recently described a sonographic-guided injection approach.[4] To this author's knowledge there are no comparative studies assessing the accuracy and effectiveness of the nonguided versus guided aspiration or injection of this bursa.

Equipment

■ Needle
  • 25-gauge, 1.5-2-inch needle for injection
  • 18-gauge, 1.5-inch needle for aspiration
■ Injectate: 1 mL of a local anesthetic with or without an injectable corticosteroid
■ High-frequency linear array transducer

Author's Preferred Technique

a. Patient position (Figure 75-2)
  i. Supine with hip in neutral to external rotation, knee slightly flexed to patient comfort
b. Transducer position (see Figure 75-2)
  i. Slightly oblique coronal plane over the medial aspect of the femoral tibial joint. The distal aspect of the transducer is rotated anteriorly to visualize the anterior edge of the superficial tibial collateral ligament. This will allow the needle to pass deep to the superficial portion of ligament without piercing the ligament.
c. Needle orientation relative to the transducer (see Figure 75-2)
  i. In plane
d. Needle approach (Figure 75-3)
  i. Anterior to posterior parallel to long axis and in plane with transducer
  ii. Direct visualization of needle moving from superficial position down into bursa
e. Target
  i. Tibial collateral ligament bursa and between superficial and deep MCL layers (Figure 75-4)

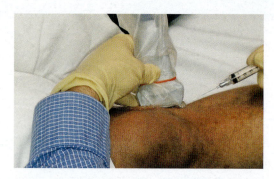

FIGURE 75-2 ■ Patient positioning on table: The leg can be slightly externally rotated, knee can be slightly flexed for patient comfort. Transducer orientation for in-plane technique: The transducer is placed in a slightly oblique coronal plane directly overlying the tibial collateral ligament bursa; distal aspect of transducer is rotated anteriorly to visualize the anterior edge of the superficial tibial collateral ligament allowing needle to pass deep to superficial portion of ligament without piercing the ligament.

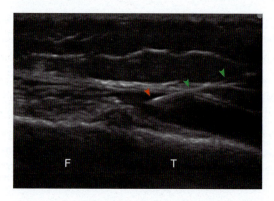

FIGURE 75-3 ■ Sonographic image of in-plane technique. A 25-gauge, 2-inch needle is visualized entering from a superficial anterior position to a deep posterior position into the bursa. Green arrow heads, shaft of needle; red arrow head, needle tip; top, superficial; bottom, deep; left, lateral; right, medial.

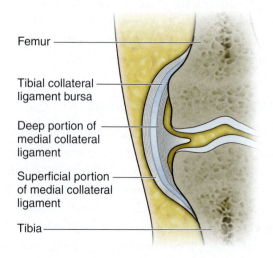

FIGURE 75-4 ■ The medial and tibial collateral ligament bursa and surrounding soft tissue structures.

f. Pearls and Pitfalls

  i. The use of the standoff technique with sterile ultrasound gel and light transducer pressure may allow for better visualization of the needle and bursa.

  ii. Poor visualization of the needle tip may lead to inadvertent placement of the needle or injectate within the knee joint or cause injury to the underlying medial meniscus.

  iii. Fluid extravasation outside of the bursa may anesthetize the traversing saphenous nerve.

Alternate Technique

a. Patient position (see Figure 75-2)

  i. Supine with hip in neutral to external rotation, knee slightly flexed to patient comfort

b. Transducer position (Figure 75-5)

  i. Anatomic coronal plane (same plane as femur and tibia) over the medial aspect of the femoral-tibial joint

c. Needle orientation relative to transducer (see Figure 75-5)

  i. Out of plane

d. Needle approach (Figures 75-6 and 75-7)

  i. The needle is progressively moved from a superficial position to the bursa using a walk-down technique.

e. Target

  i. Tibial collateral ligament bursa

f. Pearls and Pitfalls

  i. The use of the standoff technique with sterile ultrasound gel and light transducer pressure may allow for better visualization of the needle and bursa.

  ii. Poor visualization of the needle tip may lead to inadvertent placement of the needle or injectate within the knee joint or cause injury to underlying medial meniscus.

  iii. Fluid extravasation outside of the bursa may anesthetize the traversing saphenous nerve.

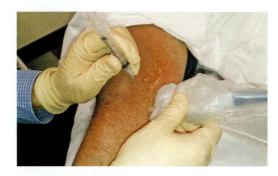

FIGURE 75-5 ■ Transducer orientation for out-of-plane technique. The transducer is placed in the coronal plane directly overlying the tibial collateral ligament bursa.

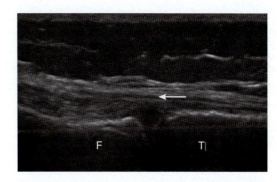

FIGURE 75-6 ■ Sonographic image of out-of-plane technique. A 25-gauge, 2-inch needle is directly visualized entering into the tibial collateral ligament bursa using a walk-down technique *arrow*. Top, superficial; bottom, deep; left, proximal; right, distal.

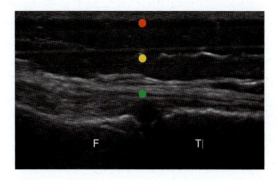

FIGURE 75-7 ■ Sonographic image of a walk-down technique. Red dot, initial superficial needle pass; yellow dot, second deeper needle pass; green dot, last needle pass at target level; top, superficial; bottom, deep; left, proximal; right, distal.

References

1. Voshell A, Brantigan O. Bursitis in the region of the tibial collateral ligament. *J Bone Joint Surg* 1944;4:793–798.
2. Maeseneer M, Van Roy F, Lenchik L, et al. Three layers of the medial capsular and supporting structures of the knee: MR imaging-anatomic correlation. *Radiographics* 2000;20:83–89.
3. Stuttle F. The no name and no fame bursa. *Clin Orthop* 1959;15:197–199.
4. Jose J, Schallert E, Lesniak B. Sonographically guided therapeutic injection for primary medial (tibial) collateral ligament bursitis. *J Ultrasound Med* 2011;30:257–261.
5. Rothstein C, Laorr A, Helms C, Tirman P. Semimembranosus-tibial collateral ligament bursitis: MR imaging findings. *AJR Am J Roentgenol* 1996;166:875–877.

John L. Lin, MD

KEY POINTS

- Use a 22–25-gauge, 2-inch needle.
- Use a high-frequency, linear array transducer.
- Use an in-plane medial-to-lateral approach to avoid peroneal nerve injury.

Pertinent Anatomy

The tibial nerve is the larger branch of the sciatic nerve following its medial-ward bifurcation from the peroneal nerve at the superior portion of the popliteal fossa (Figures 76-1 and 76-2). The tibial nerve then sends off the medial sural cutaneous nerve within the popliteal fossa, prior to branching off into multiple motor divisions. The medial sural cutaneous nerve ultimately joins the lateral sural cutaneous nerve from the common peroneal nerve to form the sural nerve.

The popliteal artery traverses antero-medial to the tibial nerve superior to the knee joint line, anterior, that is, deep, to the tibial nerve at the joint line, and antero-lateral when inferior to the joint line (see Figure 76-2).

Common Pathology

Although posterior tibial nerve entrapment at the tarsal tunnel is well known, tibial nerve pathology, such as entrapment superior to the tunnel, requiring ultrasonographic intervention is otherwise unusual. Occasionally, injection and infusion of pharmacological agents to the tibial nerve can be performed for lower extremity procedures or in the treatment of complex regional pain syndrome of the lower extremity.

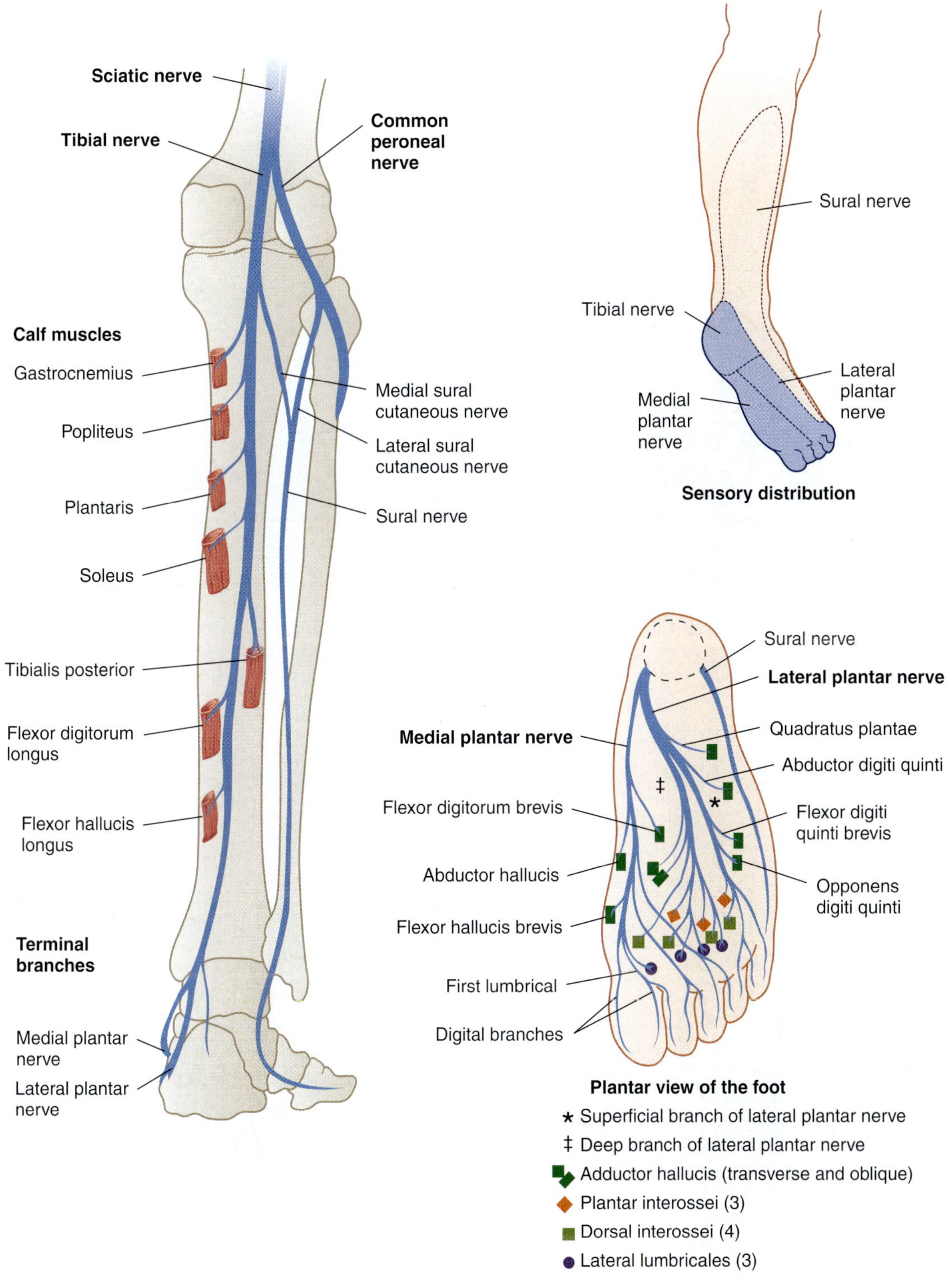

FIGURE 76-1 ■ Branches of tibial nerve. (Reproduced with permission from Waxman S. *Clinical Neuroanatomy*, 26th ed. New York: McGraw-Hill Medical; 2009: figure C-17.)

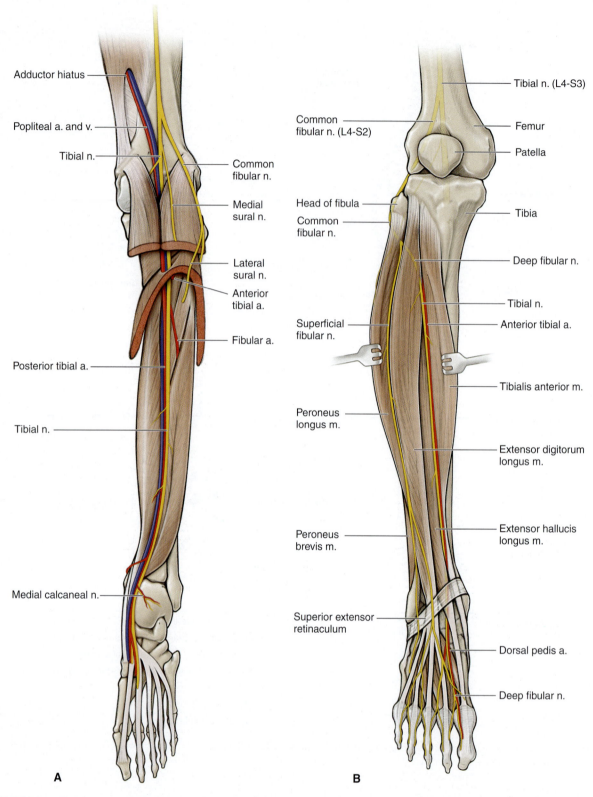

Adductor hiatus

Popliteal a. and v.

Tibial n.

Common fibular n.

Medial sural n.

Lateral sural n.

Anterior tibial a.

Fibular a.

Posterior tibial a.

Tibial n.

Medial calcaneal n.

A

Tibial n. (L4-S3)

Common fibular n. (L4-S2)

Femur

Patella

Head of fibula

Common fibular n.

Tibia

Deep fibular n.

Tibial n.

Anterior tibial a.

Superficial fibular n.

Tibialis anterior m.

Peroneus longus m.

Extensor digitorum longus m.

Peroneus brevis m.

Extensor hallucis longus m.

Superior extensor retinaculum

Dorsal pedis a.

Deep fibular n.

B

FIGURE 76-2 ■ Tibial nerve and the associated anatomy. (Reproduced with permission from Morton DA, Foreman KB, Albertine KH, eds. *The Big Picture: Gross Anatomy.* New York: McGraw-Hill; 2011: figure 37-4A.)

Ultrasound Imaging Findings

The tibial nerve is best visualized after its bifurcation with the common peroneal nerve from the sciatic nerve in short axis using a high-frequency linear array transducer at a frequency and a depth of 3–4 cm.[1,2] The axial imaging of the nerve resembles that of the cross section of salami (Figure 76-3). Below the nerve, the popliteal vein and artery can be visualized (Figure 76-4).

Indications for Injection of the Tibial Nerve

Primary indications for injection of the tibial nerve include: temporary anesthetic and motor block for distal leg interventions, for example, joint manipulation for ankle dislocation reduction, and occasionally in distinguishing of Achilles contracture versus hypertonicity in a spastic limb.

Equipment

- Needle: 22-gauge, 2-inch needle
- Injectate: 5–10 mL of a local anesthetic (long- or short-acting depending on the duration of block required)
- High-frequency linear array transducer
- Electromyographic stimulator, if needed for confirmation

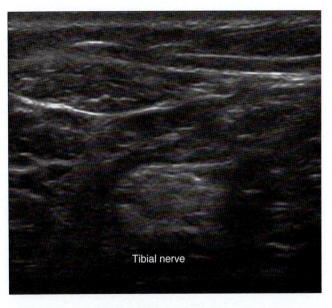

Tibial nerve

FIGURE 76-3 ■ Tibial nerve at the posterior knee.

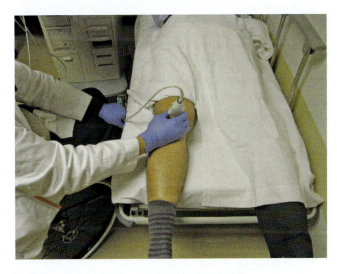

FIGURE 76-4 ■ Patient and ultrasound positioning.

Author's Preferred Technique

a. Patient position (see Figure 76-4)
   i. Prone
b. Transducer position (Figure 76-5)
   i. Short axis across the knee joint posteriorly, middle of the popliteal fossa.
   ii. Scan the popliteal fossa supero-inferiorly, from the superior bifurcation of the common peroneal nerve to the inferior bifurcation of the medial sural cutaneous nerve.
c. Needle orientation relative to the transducer (Figure 76-6)
   i. In plane
d. Needle approach (Figure 76-7)
   i. Medial to lateral
e. Target
   i. Perineural sheath of the tibial nerve
f. Pearls and Pitfalls
   i. Because of the proximity of the neurovascular structure, the entire needle needs to be visualized at all times throughout the injection, from skin entry to infusion.
   ii. An approach that is too superior can affect the peroneal nerve prior to the bifurcation.
   iii. An out-of-plane approach poses risk of piercing the nerve.
   iv. Avoid encroachment of the injectate laterally to affect the peroneal nerve unintentionally by injecting the tibial nerve further distally or by limiting injectate along the medial aspect of the tibial perineural sheath.
   v. When approaching the nerve superficial to deep, direct the needle bevel down to minimize piercing of the nerve.
   vi. A lateral approach may pose risk to piercing the common peroneal nerve on the way to target area and thus should be avoided.

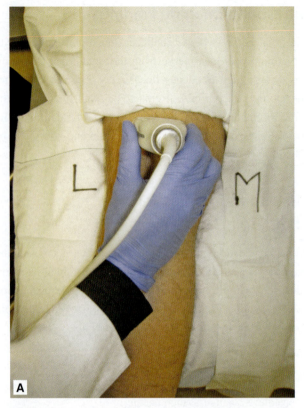

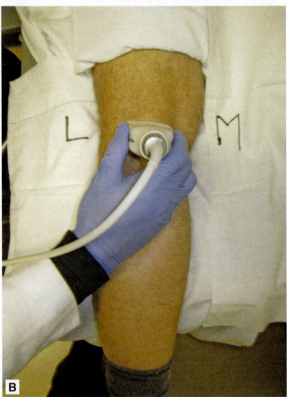

FIGURE 76-5 ▪ Popliteal fossa of the left knee with ultrasonographic probe in position, scanning from superior (**A**) to inferior (**B**). L, lateral; M, medial.

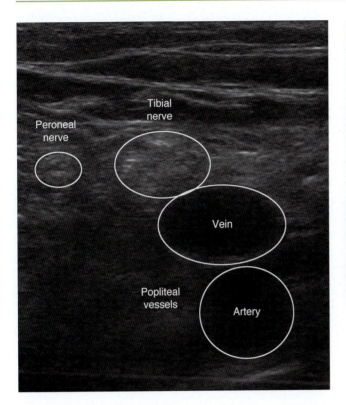

FIGURE 76-6 ■ Ultrasound image of the tibial nerve with respect to the peroneal nerve and popliteal vessels, just distal to the bifurcation of the sciatic nerve within the inferior half of the popliteal fossa.

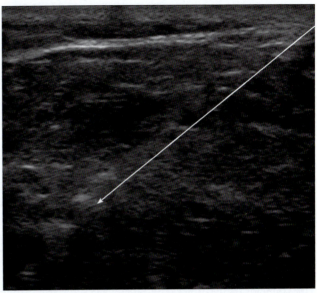

FIGURE 76-7 ■ In-plane needle approach of the tibial nerve at the popliteal fossa with the needle underlined.

Alternate Technique

The use of neurostimulator in conjunction may be helpful for confirmation for the novice injectors; however, monopolar needle stimulation may be attenuated by stimulation of a nerve very deep from the skin, because of the insulating property of the soft tissue, in particular adipose tissue. A current greater than 5 mA, commonly seen in the commercially available stimulators, may be necessary to evoke a motor response, especially for large nerves with thick perineural sheath.

References

1. Gruber H, Kovacs P. Sonographic anatomy of the peripheral nervous system. In: Baert AL, Knauth M, Sartor K, eds. *High-Resolution Sonography of the Peripheral Nervous System.* 2nd rev. ed. Berlin: Springer-Verlag; 2008:37–39, 52–54.
2. Jacobson JA. Chapter 9: the knee and Chapter 10: the leg. In: O'Neill J, ed. *Musculoskeletal Ultrasound: Anatomy and Technique.* New York: Springer Science and Business Media; 2008: 200–224.

John L. Lin, MD

KEY POINTS

- Use a 25-gauge, 1.5-inch needle.
- Use a high-frequency linear array transducer.
- Use an in-plane approach to avoid nerve injury.
- Major pitfall: An approach too superior will affect the tibial nerve prior to the bifurcation.
- Major pearl: Avoid an approach too distal after the bifurcation of the lateral sural cutaneous nerve to achieve an effective afferent block.

Pertinent Anatomy

The common peroneal nerve bifurcates laterally away from the sciatic and tibial nerves then branches off the lateral sural cutaneous nerve, prior to coursing toward the fibular head for further bifurcation and ultimately innervating the muscles of the anterior compartment through the deep peroneal nerve and lateral compartment through the superficial peroneal nerve (Figure 77-1).

Common Pathology

Common pathology involving the common peroneal nerve typically is compression between the fibula and an external object, for example, a bedrail of a hospital bed.

Ultrasound Imaging Findings (Figure 77-2)

The common peroneal nerve is best visualized after its bifurcation with the tibial nerve from the sciatic nerve in short axis using a high-frequency linear array transducer at a depth of 1–3 cm.

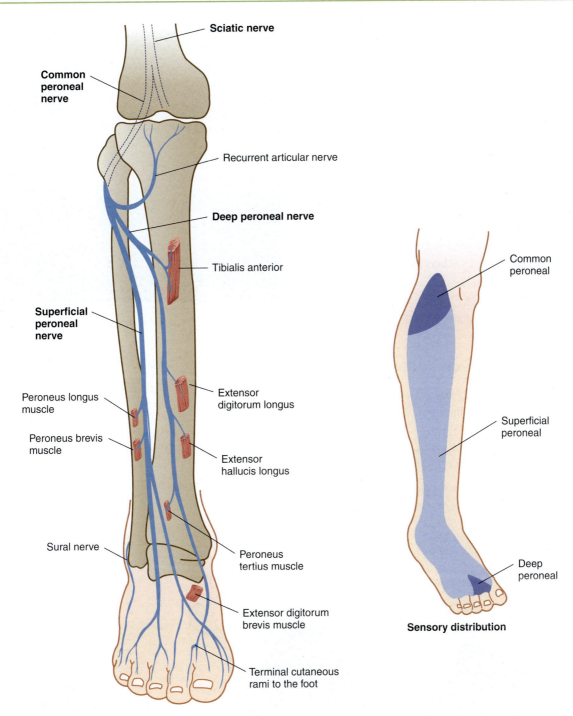

FIGURE 77-1 ■ Common peroneal nerve. (Reproduced with permission from Waxman S. *Clinical Neuroanatomy.* 26th ed. New York: McGraw-Hill Medical; 2009: figure C-16.)

Indications for Injection of the Tibial Nerve

The primary indication for the injection of the common peroneal nerve is temporary anesthetic and motor denervation block for distal leg manipulations or interventions, for example, invasive ankle procedures. Injection for compressive common peroneal neuropathy is not known to lead to improvement over alleviation of the compressive force.

Equipment

- Needle: 25-gauge, 2-inch Teflon-coated needle
- Injectate: 5–10 mL of a short-acting local anesthetic with or without a long-acting local anesthetic (depending on the duration of anesthesia desired)
- High-frequency linear array transducer
- Electromyographic stimulator, if needed for confirmation

Author's Preferred Technique

a. Patient position (Figure 77-3)
   i. Lateral decubitus of the contra-lateral side
b. Transducer position (see Figure 77-3)
   i. Short axis across the knee joint posteriorly, middle of the popliteal fossa.
   ii. Scan from the superior aspect of the popliteal fossa toward the fibular head.

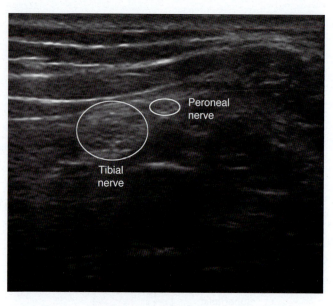

FIGURE 77-2 ■ Tibial and peroneal nerves at the posterior knee.

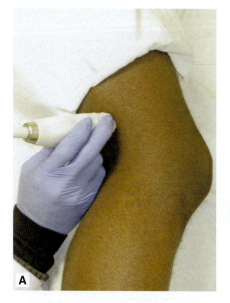
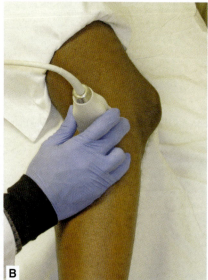
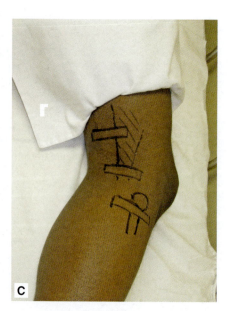

FIGURE 77-3 ■ A through C. Transducer positions for scanning the common peroneal nerve, from superior to inferior.

c. Needle orientation relative to the transducer
   i. In plane
d. Target
   i. Perineural sheath of the common peroneal nerve
e. Pearls and Pitfalls
   i. Avoid injury to the neurovascular bundle by visualizing the needle tip at all times in the long axis.
   ii. A short-axis approach poses risk of piercing the nerve when the needle tip is out of plane.
   iii. Avoid encroachment of the injectate medially to affect the tibial nerve unintentionally by injecting the common peroneal nerve further distally or by limiting injectate along the lateral aspect of the common peroneal perineural sheath.
   iv. When approaching the nerve superficial to deep, direct the needle bevel down to minimize piercing of the nerve.
   v. The use of a neurostimulator in conjunction may be useful for confirmation for novice injectors. Look for stimulation of the anterior and lateral compartment leg muscles with functional ankle dorsiflexion and eversion.
   vi. Because of the proximity of the neurovascular structure, the entire needle needs to be visualized at all times throughout the injection, from skin entry to infusion.

References

1. Gruber H, Kovacs P. Sonographic anatomy of the peripheral nervous system. In: Baert AL, Knauth M, Sartor K, eds. *High-Resolution Sonography of the Peripheral Nervous System*. 2nd rev. ed. Berlin: Springer-Verlag; 2008:34–37.
2. Jacobson JJ. Chapter 9: the knee and Chapter 10: the leg. O'Neill J, ed. *Musculoskeletal Ultrasound: Anatomy and Technique*. New York: Springer Science and Business Media; 2008:200–224.

Joanne Borg Stein, MD

KEY POINTS

- A 25-gauge, 2–3-inch needle is recommended.
- A high-frequency linear array transducer may be used, depending on the patient's body habitus.
- Use an in-plane, medial-to-lateral or lateral-to-medial approach.
- Position the patient supine with hip, thigh, and leg externally rotated.

Pertinent Anatomy (Figures 78-1 and 78-2)

The saphenous nerve is a pure sensory branch of the femoral nerve with contributions from L3–L4 dermatomes and splits from the femoral nerve just distal to the inguinal ligament. It travels distally with the superficial femoral artery and vein. Approximately two-thirds of the distance down the thigh, this neurovascular bundle passes through the adductor canal. The canal is triangular in configuration. The lateral border is the vastus medialis muscle; the medial border, the sartorius muscle; and inferior border, the adductor longus. Distal to the adductor canal, the nerve courses in a posterior and medial direction and is positioned in a fascial plane between the vastus medialis and sartorius. The nerve then branches. The infrapatellar division pierces the sartorius muscle, where it is vulnerable to injury against the prominence of the medial femoral condyle. Cutaneous saphenous nerve branches continue distally to supply the anterior tibia, medial leg, and foot to the medial side of the hallux.

Common Pathology

The saphenous nerve is vulnerable to injury, entrapment, and inflammation anywhere along its long course. That said, sports injuries involving direct impact, stretch, or muscle and tendon pathology of the adductor and medial thigh musculature is a common site of injury. This is especially true in the region of the adductor canal. The infrapatellar nerve is vulnerable to iatrogenic injury at the time of knee surgery or arthroscopy. The infrapatellar branch courses through the sartorius muscle and sharply around the prominence of the medial femoral condyle where it is susceptible to injury. Medial parameniscal cysts of the knee may also entrap the nerve. Distally, in the

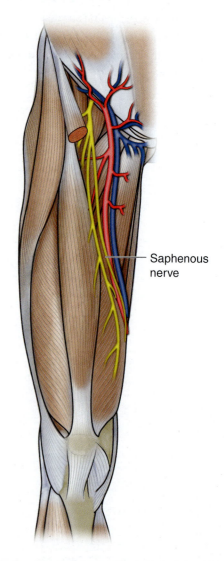

FIGURE 78-1 ■ Saphenous nerve in the distal third of the thigh. Note the position adjacent to the femoral vessels and deep to the adductor membrane.

leg, the saphenous nerve may be affected during saphenous vein surgery or after medial or high ankle injury.

Saphenous nerve syndrome refers to entrapment and neuralgia of the saphenous nerve as it courses through the adductor (Hunter's) canal in the medial thigh or distally at the medial knee (infrapatellar branches).

Patients may note pain and paresthesia at the medial distal thigh, knee, or leg.

Ultrasound Imaging Findings

The saphenous nerve is best visualized with a linear array 8–12 MHz transducer. The patient may experience neuropathic pain with sonopalpation over the nerve. Adjacent muscle or tendon injury pattern or edema may be visualized. One author reports visualization of a small stump neuroma or edematous enlargement of the nerve compared to the contralateral side.[1]

Indications for Saphenous Nerve Injection

Saphenous nerve injection can be performed for patients with recalcitrant neuropathic pain that is unresponsive to resolution of the adjacent scar tissue, tendon, muscle, or meniscal injury; rest, icing, medication, stretching, and physical therapy. Perineural injection should not be attempted without guidance. Nerve stimulator guidance has been used in the past; however, ultrasound-guided injection allows the clinician direct visualization of the nerve and surrounding vasculature to maximize precision and avoid intravascular and intraneural injection.[2]

Equipment

- Needle: 25-gauge, 2- or 3-inch needle depending on patient habitus
- Injectate
  - 2–3 mL of a local anesthetic
  - 1 mL of an injectable corticosteroid
- High-frequency linear array transducer

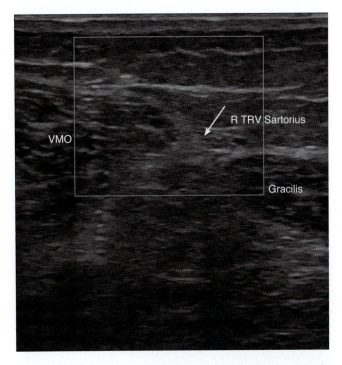

FIGURE 78-2 ■ Ultrasound appearance of the saphenous nerve in the distal thigh between the vastus medialis and sartorius muscles, adjacent to the femoral artery.

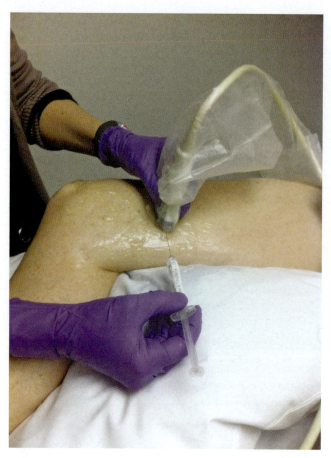

FIGURE 78-3 ■ Supine position for saphenous nerve injection using an posterior to anterior approach.

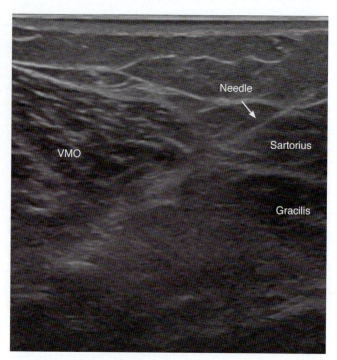

FIGURE 78-4 ■ Ultrasound image of saphenous nerve injection using a posterior to anterior approach.

Author's Preferred Technique

a. Patient position (Figure 78-3)
    i. Supine
b. Transducer position
    i. Anatomic axial plane short axis to the saphenous nerve
c. Needle orientation relative to the transducer
    i. In plane
d. Needle approach (mediodorsal positioning and ultrasound appearance)
    i. Posterior to anterior (Figures 78-3 and 78-4)
    ii. Alternate approach: Anterior to posterior (Figures 78-5 and 78-6)
e. Target
    i. Perineural circumferential spread of injectate spread around the saphenous nerve

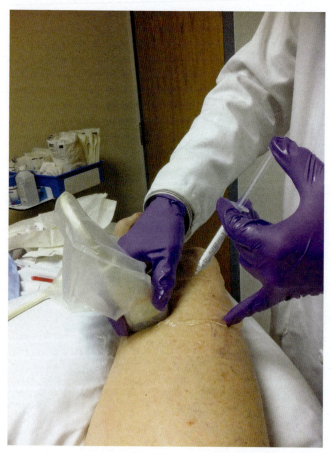

FIGURE 78-5 ■ Supine position for saphenous nerve injection using an anterior to posterior appraoch.

f. Pearls and Pitfalls

   i. If the nerve is difficult to visualize, the practitioner may inject in the fascial plane adjacent to the nerve.

   ii. Clinically, the practitioner may achieve best results by injecting at the location of a positive Tinel's sign or area of focal tenderness over the nerve that reproduces the patient's pain.

   iii. The practitioner may have difficulty locating this small nerve. In that case, the femoral vessels in the midthigh may serve as an easier landmark to identify. The nerve will be in a perivascular location.

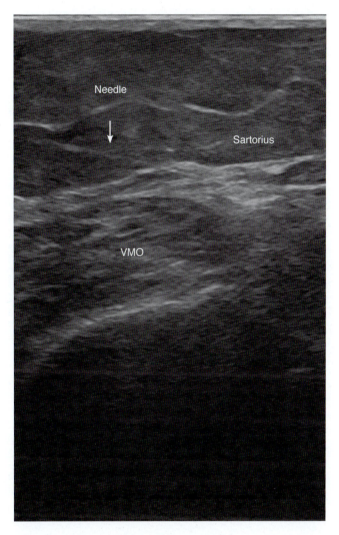

FIGURE 78-6 ■ Ultrasound image of saphenous nerve injection using an anterior to posterior approach.

References

1. Peer S, Bodner G. *High Resolution Ultrasonography of the Peripheral Nervous System*. Medical Radiology: Diagnostic Imaging and Radiation Oncology Series. Berlin: Springer-Verlag; 2010:106–108.

2. Bigeleisen P, Orebaugh S, Moayeri N, et al. *Ultrasound-Guided Regional Anesthesia and Pain Medicine*. Baltimore: Lippincott Williams & Wilkins; 2010:108–113.

Foot and Ankle

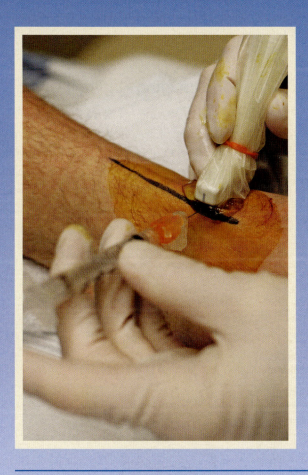

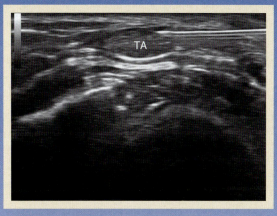

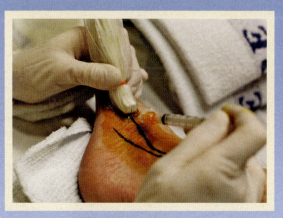

Charles E. Garten II, MD

KEY POINTS

- A 25-gauge, 1.5-inch needle, out-of-plane approach is preferred.
- Use a high-frequency linear array transducer in the long-axis position.

- Bending the needle prior to the injection will provide a better angle to operate the syringe during the procedure.

Pertinent Anatomy

The inferior or distal tibiofibular joint is a syndesmotic articulation of the concave surface of the distal tibia and the convex surface of the distal fibula. The anterior inferior tibiofibular ligament is a flat, strong ligament that courses superior and medial from the distal fibula to the tibia. The posterior inferior tibiofibular ligament is a broad, strong ligament that originates off the posterior tibia and courses obliquely and laterally to the distal fibula (Figure 79-1). The interosseus membrane is situated between the inferior anterior and posterior tibiofibular ligaments.

Common Pathology

An external rotation force to the foot can injure the distal tibiofibular joint. The injury is commonly referred to as a *high ankle sprain*. The injury may occur when a player's foot is planted on the ground and a lateral force internally rotates the tibia. One or both of the inferior tibiofibular ligaments may be involved. Because the inferior tibiofibular ligaments have a great effect on the stability of the ankle, an injury to the ligaments takes a longer time to heal than a typical lateral ligament ankle sprain.

Ultrasound Imaging Findings

The inferior tibiofibular joint is best visualized in long axis using a high-frequency linear array transducer at a frequency of 8–12 Hz and a depth of less than 3 cm. Common findings with an acute injury include ligament disruption, hematoma formation, and dynamic instability with stress views of the joint.[1] Chronic injuries to the ligaments may have thickening of the ligaments with calcification of the ligament and syndesmosis.

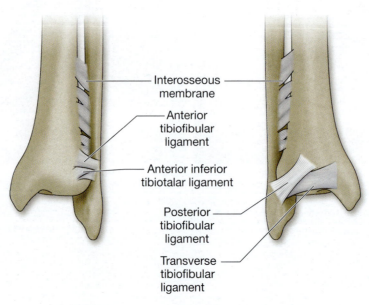

Interosseous membrane

Anterior tibiofibular ligament

Anterior inferior tibiotalar ligament

Posterior tibiofibular ligament

Transverse tibiofibular ligament

FIGURE 79-1 ■ Anatomy of the tibiofibular joint.

Indications for Injections of the Distal Tibiofibular Joint

Injection of the inferior anterior tibiofibular joint may be performed in patients with symptoms that are not responding to rest, bracing, ice, antiinflammatories, and physical therapy. There have been reports of high-level athletes receiving platelet-rich plasma (PRP) or corticosteroid injections for inferior tibiofibular joint injuries.[2] Theoretically, PRP injections have been used in some athletes to expedite the healing time on injuries to the anterior tibiofibular ligament; however, there are currently no well-designed studies to support, or refute, this practice.

Equipment

■ Needle: 25-gauge, 1.5-inch needle
■ Injectate: 1 mL of a local anesthetic
■ High-frequency linear array transducer

Author's Preferred Technique

a. Patient position (Figure 79-2)
    i. Supine
    ii. Leg extended, pillow beneath knee if needed for comfort
b. Transducer position (Figure 79-3)
    i. Anatomical short-axis plane over the anterior aspect of the distal tibia and fibula
c. Needle orientation relative to the transducer
    i. Out of plane approach
d. Needle approach (Figure 79-4)
    i. Superior to inferior, out-of-plane approach.
    ii. Use walk-down technique.
    iii. If available, use the center marker on transducer head to center the target on the screen and guide the needle in the appropriate plane.

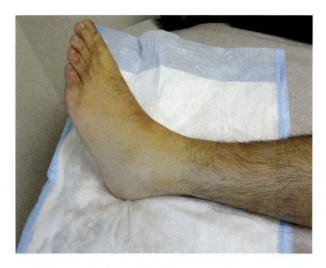

FIGURE 79-2 ■ Supine patient position.

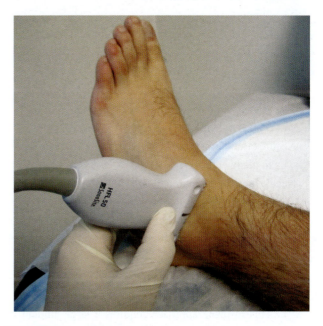

FIGURE 79-3 ■ Short-axis transducer position.

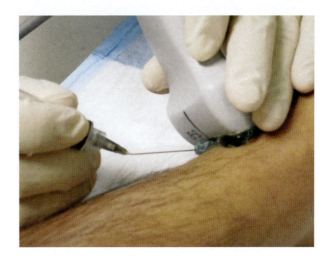

FIGURE 79-4 ■ Out-of-plane needle approach.

e. Target (Figure 79-5)
   i. Anterior tibiofibular ligament
f. Pearls and Pitfalls
   i. The anterior ligament is superficial (<5 mm beneath skin surface). Bending the needle approximately 40 degrees when uncapping it will allow provide a better angle to operate the syringe.
   ii. The local anesthetic may be injected prior to the PRP injection to allow for a less painful procedure.
   iii. The superior-to-inferior approach gives more room to operate the transducer and needle.

Alternate Technique

a. Patient position (see Figure 79-2)
   i. Supine
   ii. Leg extended, pillow beneath knee if needed for comfort
b. Transducer position (Figure 79-6)
   i. Anatomical sagittal plane centered over the anterior aspect of the distal tibia and fibula
   ii. Short-axis view of ligament
c. Needle orientation relative to the transducer
   i. In plane approach
d. Needle approach (Figure 79-7)
   i. Superior-to-inferior, in-plane approach.
   ii. For an easier needle approach, use a large amount of sterile gel to obliquely off-set transducer.
e. Target
   i. Anterior tibiofibular ligament
f. Pearls and Pitfalls
   i. This in-plane approach requires a large amount of sterile gel to obliquely set off the transducer face in order for the needle to reach the target.

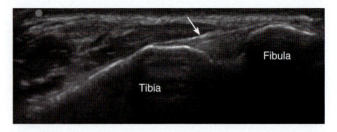

FIGURE 79-5 ■ Long-axis view of the anterior tibiofibular ligament (*white arrow* indicates the ligament).

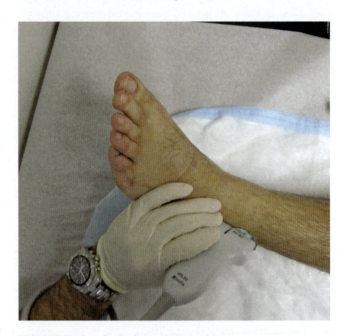

FIGURE 79-6 ■ Sagittal transducer position.

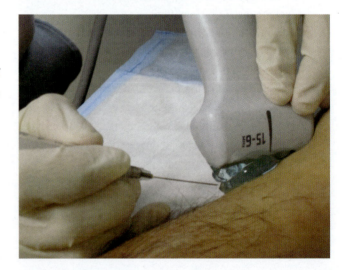

FIGURE 79-7 ■ In-plane needle approach.

References

1. Mei-Dan O, Kots E, Barchilon V, et al. A dynamic ultrasound examination for the diagnosis of ankle syndesmotic injury in professional athletes. *Am J Sports Med* 2009;37(5):1009–1016.

2. Doughtie M. Syndesmotic ankle sprains in football: a survey of National Football League athletic trainers. *J Athl Train* 1999;34(1):15–18.

Kevin deWeber, MD, FAAFP, FACSM

KEY POINTS

- Use a 22- to 25-gauge, 1.5-inch needle.
- Use a high-frequency linear array transducer.
- Orient the transducer long-axis to the plantar flexed foot anteriorly just medial to the tibialis anterior tendon; make sure no tendons or neurovascular structures overlie the joint space.
- Insert the needle long axis, distal to proximal at about a 30-degree angle, passing just over the talar dome.
- Insert the needle tip just deep to anterior recess joint capsule.
- The accuracy of the ultrasound-guided technique was 100% versus only 85% in the palpation-guided technique in a cadaveric study.

Pertinent Anatomy

The ankle joint proper is formed by the tibia, fibula, and talus. The distal tibia and fibula are joined tightly together and form the proximal roof or "plafond" of the joint, and they articulate with the talus distally. The tibiotalar joint comprises the majority of the joint's surface area, forming its superior and superomedial aspects; whereas the fibulotalar portion comprises the superolateral aspect. These aspects of the joint are continuous. Motion at the ankle joint occurs as the distal aspect of the talus tilts either downward or upward, allowing plantarflexion and dorsiflexion of the foot, respectively.

The anterior tibiotalar joint line is the most pertinent location for injections and is overlain with several structures. Starting from the medial malleolus and moving laterally, these include the tibialis anterior tendon, flexor hallucis longus tendon, the neurovascular bundle containing the dorsalis pedis artery and deep peroneal nerve, and the extensor digitorum longus muscle and tendon. The medial aspect of the joint line is ideal for its reliable lack of overlying tendons, nerves, or blood vessels.

Common Pathology

The tibiotalar joint is a common site of acute trauma, which can produce fractures, chondral lesions, and synovitis, all leading to effusion or hemarthrosis. It is a common site for inflammatory arthritides including rheumatoid arthritis and gout, and rarely infections. Osteoarthritis is uncommon but not rare. Pigmented villonodular synovitis (PVNS), a rare non-malignant synovial neoplasm, can also affect the joint.

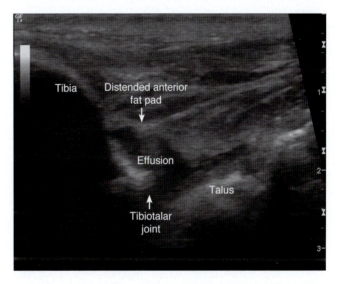

FIGURE 80-1 ■ Ultrasound view of anterior tibiotalar joint, which has a large effusion displacing the anterior fat pad.

Ultrasound Imaging Findings

Ultrasound of the anterior joint line should clearly identify the tibiotalar joint space. The entire anterior joint space from medial malleolus to lateral malleolus should be imaged as segments of the joint line can appear different. The ideal location for injection and aspiration should be free of any overlying tendons, nerves, or blood vessels. Ultrasound can easily identify joint effusion as the anterior capsule and fat pad are seen to be displaced anteriorly (Figure 80-1). An anteroposterior thickness of joint fluid up to 1.8 mm is normal (not including the 1–2 mm of hypoechoic hyaline cartilage overlying the talar dome); more than that is likely abnormal.[1] Defects in the cortical surface of the head of the talus may signify fractures. Synovium may be thickened in inflamma-tory arthritis or with PVNS. In osteoarthritis the tibia may have osteophytes anteriorly.

Indications for Injections

Aspiration of fluid can be useful in diagnosis of inflammatory arthritis or infection. Injection of corticosteroid may be useful for treating inflammatory arthritis or pain from various causes. Injection of hyaluronate has been shown in small studies to be helpful for osteoarthritis. Injection of anesthetic may also be useful diagnostically in determining the origin of pain.

Equipment

- Needle: 22-gauge, 1.5-inch needle and appropriate syringe
- Injectate
  - For anesthesia or diagnostics, 2–4 mL of local anesthet-ic is adequate.
  - For inflammatory conditions, 1 mL of an injectable cor-ticosteroid can be added.
- Use a high-frequency linear array transducer.

Author's Preferred Technique

a. Patient position
   i. The patient may sit or lie on the back end of a table with knee flexed about 90 degrees and the foot placed flat on the front end of the table (Figure 80-2).
   ii. The ankle should be in 30–45 degrees of plantarflex-ion, which opens up the anterior joint space and straightens the anterior surface of the skin, making probe placement easier.
b. Transducer position
   i. Oriented long axis to the axis of the foot.
   ii. Just medial to tibialis anterior tendon. There should be no tendons, nerves, or blood vessels overlying the view of the joint space.
   iii. The tibiotalar joint should be near the center of the field of view.
c. Needle orientation relative to the transducer
   i. In plane
d. Needle approach
   i. Distal to proximal, at a slight downward angle, just superficial to the talar dome
e. Target
   i. Anterior recess of the joint line, just deep to the joint capsule (Figure 80-3)

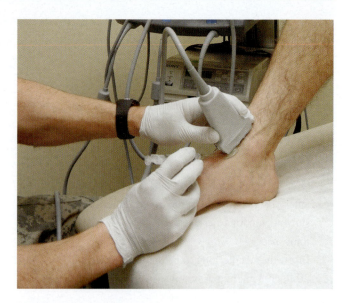

FIGURE 80-2 ■ Patient, transducer, and needle position for an in-plane, long-axis to the ankle tibiotalar joint injection.

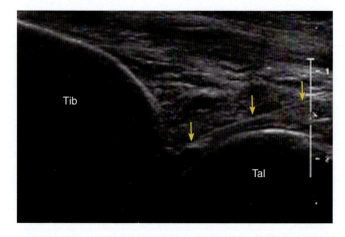

FIGURE 80-3 ■ Ultrasound image of in-plane long-axis to the an-terior tibiotalar joint injection (yellow arrows point to the needle). Tal, talus; Tib, tibia.

f. Pearls and Pitfalls
   i. There is a risk of perforation of a tendon or neuro-vascular structure because of improper lateral place-ment of the transducer.
   ii. The angle of needle entry can be too steep, which can impact the talar dome.

Alternate Technique 1

a. Transducer position
    i. Oriented long axis to the axis of the foot.
    ii. The tibiotalar joint should be near the center of the field of view.
b. Needle orientation relative to the transducer
    i. Out of plane
c. Needle approach
    i. Medial to lateral or lateral medial depending on patient position.
    ii. Judge entry depth based on the ultrasound image depth (Figure 80-4).
    iii. Use a walk-down technique.
d. Target
    i. Anterior recess of joint line, just deep to the joint capsule visualizing the needling tip in an out-of-plane view (Figure 80-5).

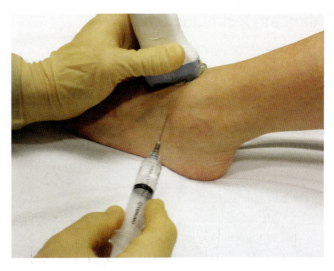

FIGURE 80-4 ■ Patient, transducer, and needle position for an out-of-plane, long-axis to the ankle tibiotalar joint injection.

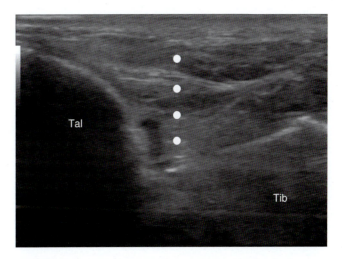

FIGURE 80-5 ■ Ultrasound image of anterior tibiotalar joint injection, out of plane and long axis to the tibiotalar joint using a walk-down technique (dots). Tal, talus; Tib, tibia.

Alternate Technique 2

a. Transducer position
   i. Oriented short axis to the distal tibia.
   ii. The transducer is moved distally until the hyper-echoic tibia disappears and the more hypoechoic joint is visualized above the level of the talar dome; the nerve artery and vein will be anterior to the joint.
b. Needle orientation relative to the transducer
   i. In plane (Figure 80-6)
c. Needle approach
   i. Medial to lateral or lateral medial depending on patient position
d. Target
   i. Midportion of the joint (Figure 80-7)
   ii. The appropriate depth can be verified by changing to a long-axis view of the ankle joint and visualizing the needle tip in an out-of-plane view.

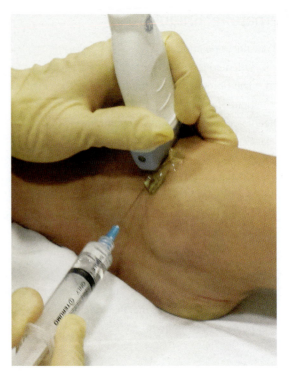

FIGURE 80-6 ■ Patient, transducer, and needle position for in-plane, short axis to ankle tibiotalar joint injection.

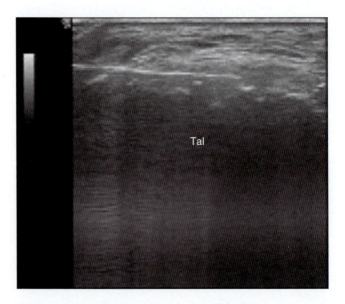

FIGURE 80-7 ■ Ultrasound image of needle in plane and short axis to the tibiotalar joint.

References

1. Nazarian LN, Rawool NM, Martin CE, Schweitzer ME. Synovial fluid in the hindfoot and ankle: detection of amount and distribution with US. *Radiology* 1995;197:275–278.

2. Wisniewski SJ, Smith J, Patterson DG, et al. Ultrasound-guided versus nonguided tibiotalar joint and sinus tarsi injections: a cadaveric study. *P M R* 2010 April;2:277–281.

Kevin deWeber, MD, FAAFP, FACSM

KEY POINTS

- Use a 22–25-gauge, 1.5-inch needle.
- Use a high-frequency linear array transducer.
- Orient the transducer parasagittally lateral to the Achilles tendon with beam directed slightly inferiorly.
- Image the talocalcaneal and tibiotalar joint spaces.
- Insert the needle long axis at steep angle, passing just over calcaneus.
- Alternate approaches can be used but are closer to tendons, nerves, and vessels.

Pertinent Anatomy

The subtalar (talocalcaneal) joint is comprised of three facets—posterior, middle, and anterior—between the calcaneus inferiorly and the talus superiorly. The posterior facet is the largest and most important. The subtalar joint confers most of the inversion and eversion motion of the hindfoot.

Common Pathology

Severe inversion ankle injuries that rupture the calcaneofibular ligament can lead to moderate instability of the subtalar joint. Injuries that rupture deeper ligaments in the sinus tarsi area, such as the cervical ligament and talocalcaneal ligament, can lead to marked instability during inversion. Such injuries may produce a subtalar joint effusion. Fractures and severe chondral contusions or the talus and/or calcaneus may lead to degenerative arthritis. The subtalar joint is a victim of inflammatory arthritides such as rheumatoid arthritis, reactive arthritis (Reiter syndrome), and gout.

Ultrasound Imaging Findings

Distension of the joint capsule from the joint space can be seen with effusion or infection.

Indications for Injections

Aspiration of fluid for diagnostic testing can lead to an accurate diagnosis of infection, gout, or other inflammatory arthritis. Injection of anesthetic may be useful diagnostically in determining the origin of vague hindfoot pain.

Injection Technique

Based on a cadaveric study, there are three possible injection approaches—anterolateral, posterolateral, and posteromedial.[1] All three are technically feasible and accurate, but the posterolateral approach is recommended because of its further distance from nerves, vessels, and tendons and its use of a long-axis needle approach.

Equipment

- Needle: 22- or 25-gauge, 1.5-inch needle
- Injectate: 3–5 mL of a local anesthetic with or without an injectable corticosteroid
- High frequency linear array transducer

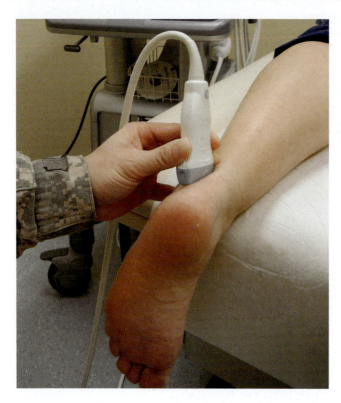

FIGURE 81-1 ■ Patient, transducer, and ultrasound positions for posterolateral approach to left subtalar joint.

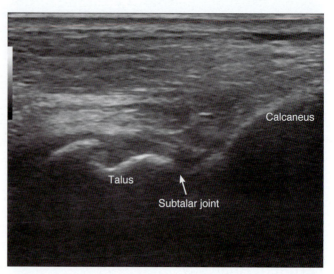

FIGURE 81-2 ■ Ultrasound view of normal anatomy of posterolateral ankle.

Author's Preferred Technique

a. Patient position
   i. Prone on table, with foot hanging over the edge and ankle in dorsiflexion (Figure 81-1)
b. Transducer Position
   i. Lateral to Achilles tendon in parasagittal plane, with beam angled slightly inferiorly toward calcaneus (Figure 81-2)
c. Needle orientation relative to the transducer
   i. Long axis, angling steeply over downsloping calcaneus (Figure 81-3)
d. Needle approach
   i. Enter at a steep downward angle, just superficial to the posterolateral calcaneus (see Figure 81-3)
e. Target
   i. With the tibia, talus, and calcaneus in view, the needle is directed to the talocalcaneal joint space, just deep to the capsule (Figure 81-4)

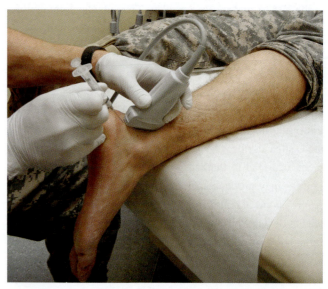

FIGURE 81-3 ■ Needle approach for posterolateral subtalar joint injection of a right ankle.

f. Pearls and Pitfalls

   i. This is a relatively difficult position to achieve with the probe and a steep angle to achieve with the needle, possibly making needle visualization difficult. Use of needle localization software is helpful.

   ii. When a subtalar joint effusion is present, an aspiration can be done as above, or at another location if capsular distension is more pronounced.

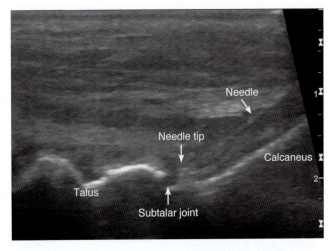

FIGURE 81-4 ▪ Ultrasound view of a posterolateral subtalar joint injection.

Reference

1. Henning T, Finoff JT, Smith J. Sonographically guided posterior subtalar joint injections: anatomic study and validation of 3 approaches. *PMR* 2009 Oct;1:925–931.

Keith Hardy, MD

KEY POINTS

- Use a 25-gauge, 1.5-needle directed posteromedial (out-of-plane approach).
- Use a high-frequency linear array transducer in a sagittal oblique orientation.
- Only the initial entry is easily visible with ultrasound.
- Final depth may be determined by feel.

Pertinent Anatomy

The sinus tarsi (also known as tarsal sinus) is a cone-shaped cavity located in the lateral aspect of the foot between the neck of the talus and the anterosuperior aspect of the calcaneus. It serves as a boundary between the posterior and anterior subtalar joints and contains fat, an arterial anastomosis, joint capsules, nerve endings, and five ligamentous structures—the medial, intermediate, and lateral roots of the inferior extensor retinaculum as well as the cervical ligament and the ligament of the tarsal canal. The sinus tarsi is not encapsulated[1] (Figure 82-1).

Common Pathology

The pathogenesis of sinus tarsi syndrome has remained poorly understood. Trauma is the most commonly described cause of sinus tarsi syndrome. The sinus tarsi can also be affected by inflammatory conditions such as ankylosing spondylitis, rheumatoid arthritis, and gout. Ganglion cysts may be present. Alignment abnormalities such as pes planus and cavus may also be implicated. Described hypotheses for pain have included interosseus ligament injury, synovial pinching, fibrotic vascular changes, and nociceptive abnormalities.[1]

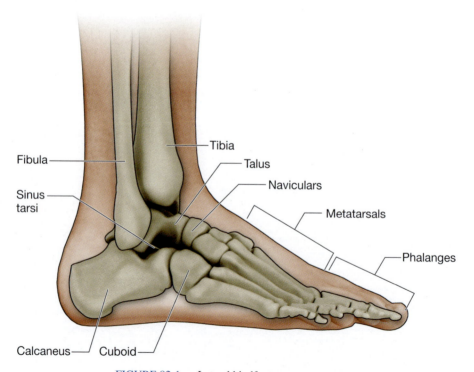

FIGURE 82-1 ■ Lateral hindfoot osseous anatomy.

Ultrasound Imaging Findings

The transducer is placed in a coronal oblique plane such that the transducer spans from the anterior process of the calcaneus to the talar neck. After identifying the osseous calcaneus and talar neck, the transducer is translated proximally and rotated and tilted to provide the best visualization of the sinus tarsi. In this view, the sinus tarsi appears as a soft tissue space extending posteriorly (deep on the ultrasound screen) between the calcaneus and talus (Figure 82-2).

Indications for Injections of the Sinus Tarsi

Injection of the sinus tarsi can be performed for patients with recalcitrant lateral foot pain that is refractory to conservative measures including antiinflammatory medication, splinting, and functional rehabilitation including exercises targeting the Achilles tendon, peroneal tendons, and proprioception. Wisniewski et al. were the first to examine sinus tarsi injection accuracy. Using palpation, they had a 35% accuracy rate in 20 injections in cadavers. Their ultrasound-guided injections were 90% accurate.[2] Clinical outcomes for guided versus unguided injections have not been studied.

Equipment

- ▪ Needle: 25-gauge, 1.5-inch needle
- ▪ Injectate
  - • 1 mL of a local anesthetic
  - • 1 mL of an injectable corticosteroid
- ▪ High-frequency linear array transducer

Author's Preferred Technique

a. Patient position (Figure 82-3)
   i. Supine
   ii. Ankle slightly inverted and plantar flexed
b. Transducer position
   i. Coronal oblique plane spanning the talar neck and the anterior process of the calcaneus, rotated and tilted to optimize the view of the sinus tarsi

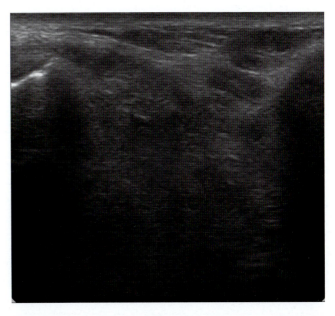

FIGURE 82-2 ▪ Ultrasound appearance of the sinus tarsi with the transducer positioned in a sagittal oblique orientation with the talus to the left and the calcaneus to the right in the image.

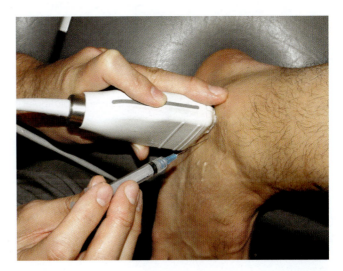

FIGURE 82-3 ▪ Out-of-plane needle approach from anterior to posteromedial with the transducer positioned in a sagittal oblique position.

c. Needle orientation relative to the transducer
   i. Out of plane
d. Needle approach (Figures 82-4 and 82-5)
   i. Posteromedial.
   ii. Use walk-down technique.
e. Target
   i. Sinus tarsi
f. Pearls and Pitfalls
   i. Ultrasound guidance allows visualization in the initial phase of the injection, but once beyond the margins of the talus and calcaneus, "feel" must be used to gauge the appropriateness of depth. The needle is generally brought to rest against an osseus structure.

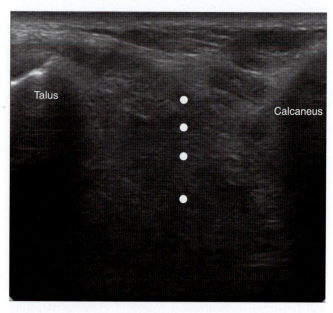

FIGURE 82-4 ■ Ultrasound appearance of the step-down needle insertion technique.

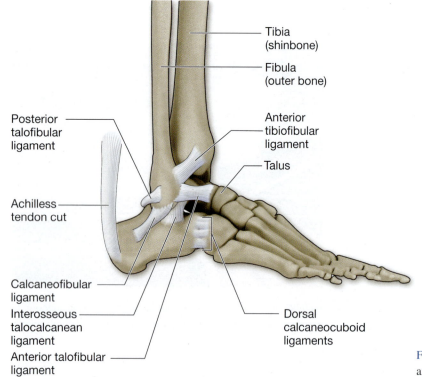

FIGURE 82-5 ■ Sinus tarsi and lateral hindfoot and lateral ankle anatomy.

References

1. Lektrakul N, Chung CB, Lai Ym, et al. Tarsal sinus: arthrographic, MR imaging, MR arthrographic, and pathologic findings in cadavers and retrospective study data in patients with sinus tarsi syndrome. *Radiology* 2001 Jun;219(3):802–810.

2. Wisniewski SJ, Smith J, Patterson DG, Carmichael SW, Pawlina W. Ultrasound-guided versus nonguided tibiotalar joint and sinus tarsi injections: a cadaveric study. *PMR* 2010 Apr;2(4):277–281.

Keith Hardy, MD

KEY POINTS

- Use a 25–27-gauge, 1.5-inch needle in plane or out of plane.
- Use a high-frequency linear array transducer in long-axis orientation to the joint for injection guidance.
- Avoid multiple tendons and neurovascular structures.

- Survey the area in a short-axis orientation to the neurovascular and ligament structures.
- Choose appropriate needle insertion based on the patient's tendon and neurovascular anatomy.

Pertinent Anatomy

The talonavicular joint is a ball and socket synovial joint. A fibrous capsule incompletely encloses the joint. The plantar calcaneonavicular (spring) ligament supports the head of the talus and spans the medial inferior portion of the joint. The tibionavicular portion of the deltoid ligament covers the medial joint line, and the dorsal talonavicular portion of the deltoid ligament is found over the dorsal joint line. Medially, the tibialis posterior, extensor hallucis longus tendon, the long saphenous vein, and the saphenous nerve and branches may traverse the joint. The tibialis anterior tendon, intermediate branch of the superficial fibular nerve, and the medial tarsal arteries are found over the dorsomedial joint. Dorsolaterally, the lateral branch of the deep peroneal nerve and lateral tarsal artery may be found superficial to the joint. The dorsalis pedis artery and the medial terminal branch of the deep fibular nerve are found deep to the inferior extensor retinaculum on the dorsum of the joint. The branches of the superficial fibular nerve (dorsal digital nerves) are found more superficially (Figure 83-1).

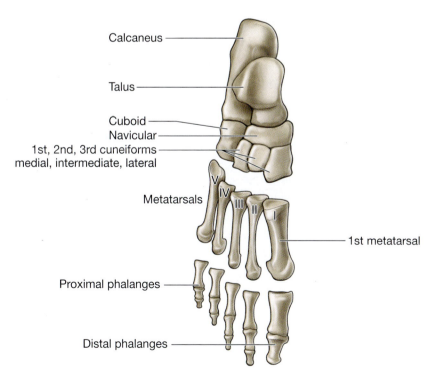

FIGURE 83-1 ■ Dorsal foot osseous anatomy. (Reproduced with permission from Morton DA, Foreman KB, Albertine KH, eds. *The Big Picture: Gross Anatomy*. New York: McGraw-Hill; 2011: figure 34-2C.)

Common Pathology

The talonavicular joint can be affected by osteoarthritis, inflammatory arthritis, posttraumatic arthritis, tarsal coalition, diabetic neuropathic arthropathy, and congenital abnormalities such as club foot. Pain can result from biomechanical inefficiencies that lead to abnormal stress across the joint. The talonavicular joint is a vital contributor to the stability of the medial arch, and a collapsed arch often involves significant derangement of the talonavicular joint. Pain with walking, tenderness over the hindfoot, swelling, stiffness, and deformity can result from talonavicular joint pathology.

Ultrasound Imaging Findings

A high-frequency linear array transducer at a frequency of 8–12Hz or higher and set to a depth less than 3 cm is used to identify the pertinent talonavicular joint anatomy. The transducer is placed in a sagittal plane to view the dorsal aspect of the joint. An axial transducer orientation across the dorsum of the joint aids in identifying the important traversing neurovascular and tendon structures as described above (Figure 83-2). Osteophytes, joint space narrowing, erosions, joint effusion, and increased Doppler signal with synovitis may be seen with ultrasound.

Indications for Injections of the Talonavicular

Injection of the talonavicular joint can be performed for patients with recalcitrant hindfoot pain that is refractory to conservative measures including antiinflammatory medication and functional rehabilitation including exercises targeting ankle proprioception, strengthening, and flexibility. The anatomy is complicated and, therefore, palpation-guided injections are difficult. Historically, these injections have often been injected using fluoroscopic guidance. This author is not aware of studies describing the success rate of unguided- or ultrasound-guided talonavicular joint injections. Computed tomography has been described as an alternative for guiding injection into challenging joints.[1] Outcome data for talonavicular injections guided or unguided are not available.[2]

Equipment

- ■ Needle: 25-gauge, 1.5-inch needle
- ■ Injectate
  - • 1 mL of a local anesthetic
  - • 1 mL of injectable corticosteroid
- ■ High-frequency linear array transducer

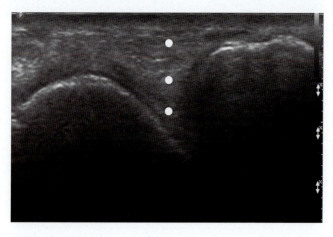

FIGURE 83-2 ■ Ultrasound appearance of the step-down needle insertion (see *white dots*) technique.

Author's Preferred Technique

a. Patient position
   i. Supine.
   ii. Ankle in a comfortable position slightly plantarflexed.
b. Transducer position
   i. Sagittal across the dorsal joint (Figure 83-3)
c. Needle orientation relative to the transducer
   i. Out of plane
d. Needle approach
   i. Medial to lateral.
   ii. Use step-down technique.
e. Target
   i. Talonavicular joint, subcapsular space
f. Pearls and Pitfalls
   i. Identify all relevant structures between the insertion point and target, including saphenous vein, branches of the saphenous nerve, medial tarsal arteries, and tibialis anterior tendon.
   ii. Prior to inserting the needle, use the ultrasound transducer to scan and mark the intended insertion point to avoid neurovascular and tendon structures.
   iii. A paper clip can be used to cast an acoustic shadow deep to the transducer to precisely identify the correct insertion point for the short-axis needle technique.

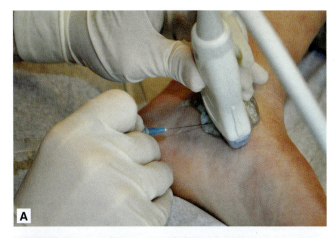

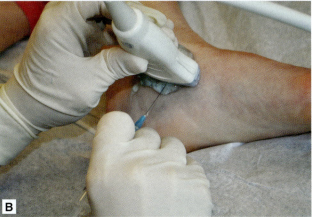

FIGURE 83-3 ■ Sagittal approach (out of plane) to the talonavicular joint.

Alternate Technique

Standoff Technique, Long-Axis Needle View

a. Patient position
   i. Supine
   ii. Ankle in slight plantarflexion
b. Transducer position
   i. Step off with sterile gel, long axis to the joint across the dorsal or medial joint (Figure 83-4).
   ii. The transducer can be angled (tilted off the skin proximally, with heaped up gel) to allow a fully visible proximal to distal needle insertion pathway.
c. Needle orientation relative to the transducer
   i. In plane
d. Needle approach
   i. Proximal to distal

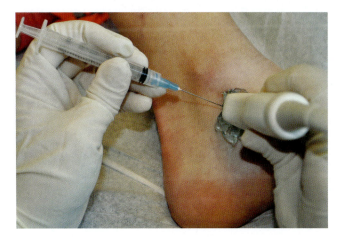

FIGURE 83-4 ■ In-plane needle approach from medial to lateral with the transducer positioned longitudinally across the joint.

e. Pearls and Pitfalls

   i. A proximal-to-distal needle approach allows for a needle trajectory that matches the contour of the head of the talus to achieve the appropriate depth of insertion into the joint.

   ii. Scan the region in axial orientation to appreciate the various traversing tendons and neurovascular structures.

   iii. The long-axis constant needle visualization technique is often preferred as it allows constant visualization of the needle to avoid the important surrounding structures. However, it can be more technically demanding for the novice injectionist. If a proper preinjection survey is performed, the short-axis, step-down technique is often more easily performed. Damage to sensory nerve branches has been associated with muscle atrophy and neuropathic pain.[3,4]

References

1. Saifuddin A, Abdus-Samee M, Mann C, Singh D, Angel JC. CT guided diagnostic foot injections. *Clin Radiol* 2005;60: 191–195.

2. Sofka CM, Adler RS. Ultrasound-guided interventions in the foot and ankle. *Semin Musculoskelet Radiol* 2002 Jun;6(2): 163–168.

3. Lui Th, Chan LK. Safety and efficacy of talonavicular arthroscopy in arthroscopic triple arthrodesis. A cadaveric study. *Knee Surg Sports Traumatol Arthrosc* 2010 May;18(5):607–611. Epub March 9, 2010.

4. Hammond AW, Phisitkul P, Femino J, Amendola A. Arthroscopic debridement of the talonavicular joint using dorsomedial and dorsolateral portals: a cadaveric study of safety and access. *Arthroscopy* 2011 Feb;27(2):228–234. Epub October 27, 2010.

Arthur Jason De Luigi, DO, FAAPMR, DAPM

KEY POINTS

- Use a 25-gauge, 1.5-inch needle.
- Use a high-frequency linear array transducer at a depth of less than 3 cm.
- The dorsalis pedis should be identified on sonographic evaluation prior to injection to avoid intraarterial needle placement.

- Using a medial-to-lateral approach allows the clinician direct access to the joint while avoiding the dorsalis pedis artery.

The tarsometatarsal (TMT) joint is an arthrodial joint also known as the *Lisfranc joint* named after Jacques Lisfranc de St. Martin, a French surgeon from around the eighteenth century.

Pertinent Anatomy (Figure 84-1)

The joint is comprised of articulations of the tarsal bones (first, second, and third cuneiforms and the cuboid) and the metatarsal bones. The first through third metatarsal bones articulate with their respective first through third cuneiform bones. However, the keystone of the joint is the second metatarsal, which is wedged in a tight recess between the first and third cuneiforms. The fourth metatarsal articulates with both the cuboid and the third cuneiform, and the fifth metatarsal with the cuboid.[1]

The bones of the TMT joint are connected by dorsal, plantar, and interosseous ligaments. The Lisfranc ligament is the main stabilizer of the first and second metatarsal joints. It is a strong oblique ligament that extends from the plantar-lateral aspect of the medical cuneiform. It passes in front of the interosseous ligament between the first and second cuneiforms and inserts onto the plantar-medial aspect of the second metatarsals.[1]

The dorsalis pedis artery crosses the TMT joint and typically dives between the bases of the first and second metatarsals to form the plantar arterial arch. The dorsalis pedis should be identified on sonographic evaluation prior to injection to avoid intraarterial needle placement.

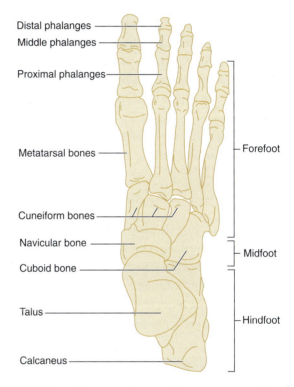

FIGURE 84-1 ■ Diagram of normal bony anatomy of the foot. (Reproduced with permission from Tintinalli JE, Stapczynski JS, Cline DM, et al., eds. *Tintinalli's Emergency Medicine: A Comprehensive Study Guide*. 7th ed. New York: McGraw-Hill; 2011: figure 274-1A.)

Common Pathology

Lisfranc (TMT) joint injuries are rare, and range from sprains to fracture-dislocations. The injuries are typically through direct or indirect trauma. Direct trauma is secondary to an external force striking the foot. However, indirect trauma would occur via a force being transmitted to a "stationary" foot so that the weight of the body becomes a deforming force by torque, rotation, or compression; such as a falling off a horse with one's foot in the stirrup. Fractures of the base of the second metatarsal should always raise suspicions of TMT injury.[2–9]

The TMT joint is the most common site (70%) for neuropathic arthropathy, also known as *Charcot joint*. The medial aspect is affected more commonly than the lateral TMT joint. There is progressive degeneration of joint marked by bony destruction, bone resorption, and eventual deformity. The onset is typically insidious, and can lead to deformity, ulceration, infection, and amputation. It can occur in conditions leading to a peripheral polyneuropathy, such as diabetes mellitus.[10] The TMT joint also infrequently develops osteoarthritis, typically posttraumatically, and is rarely involved in other arthritides.

Ultrasound Image Findings

The Lisfranc joint is best visualized in long axis using a high-frequency linear array transducer at depth of less than 3 cm. Common findings include fracture or dislocation, cortical irregularities, and joint effusions. Ligamentous injuries can also be identified with laxity or disruption noted on dynamic evaluation by applying a plantar flexion force to the distal aspect of the foot.

Indications for Injection

Injection of the TMT joint can be performed as a diagnostic procedure for patients suspected of TMT pain or as therapeutic injection for patients with recalcitrant pain that is unresponsive to rest, icing, antiinflammatories and physical therapy.

Injection of the TMT joint has been described based on palpation without additional guidance by Khosla et al. The success rate of palpation based unguided injections was 21% into the first TMT joint and 29% into the second TMT joint.[11] Both fluoroscopic and ultrasound-guided injections have been described.[11,12] Ultrasound-guided injection has been described by Khosla and colleagues with a success rate of 64% with ultrasound-guided injection versus 89% with fluoroscopic guidance versus 25% with unguided injections.[11] Clinical outcomes of guided versus nonguided injection has not been described.

Equipment

- Needle: 25-gauge, 1.5-inch needle
- Injectate
  - 1 mL of a local anesthetic agent
  - 1 mL an injectable corticosteroid
- High-frequency linear array or linear array "hockey stick" transducer

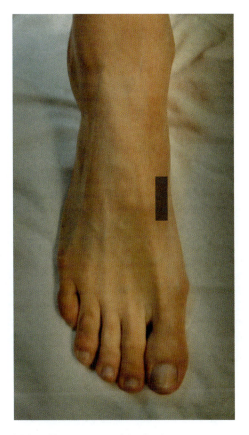

FIGURE 84-2 ■ Tarsometatarsal (patient).

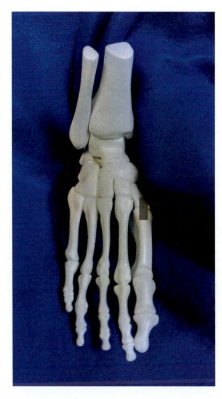

FIGURE 84-3 ■ Tarsometatarsal (anatomic).

Author's Preferred Technique

a. Patient position
   i. Supine position
   ii. Foot elevated versus foot flat with knee flexed
b. Transducer position
   i. If possible, orient the planes along conventional axes (transverse/longitudinal).
   ii. Identify the best view obtainable of the target site.
   iii. Anatomic sagittal (longitudinal) plane (Figures 84-2, 84-3, and 84-4).
c. Needle orientation relative to the transducer
   i. Out of plane
d. Needle approach
   i. Walk-down technique (Figure 84-5)
   ii. Medial to lateral
e. Target
   i. Mid portion of the TMT joint (see Figures 84-4 and 84-5)

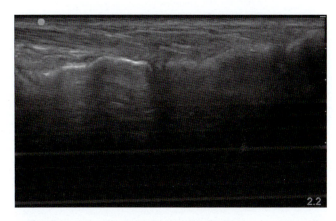

FIGURE 84-4 ■ Tarsometatarsal long-axis view.

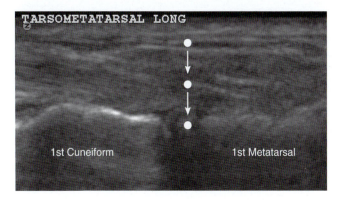

FIGURE 84-5 ■ Tarsometatarsal injection: Out of plane approach in long-axis view using a step down approach (dots).

f. Pearls and Pitfalls
    i. Identify the dorsalis pedis artery on the initial scan to ensure avoidance during needle placement.
    ii. The TMT joint can be accessed along any of the joint articulations, however, based on the author's clinical experience, it is recommended to access the joint between the first cuneiform and first metatarsal. Using a medial-to-lateral approach allows the clinician direct access to the joint, while avoiding the dorsalis pedis artery.

References

1. Gray H. Tarso-metatarsal articulations. In: Gray H, ed. *Gray's Anatomy*. 1st ed. Philadelphia, PA: Courage Books; 1901:290–291.
2. Arntz CT, Hansen ST Jr. Dislocations and fracture dislocations of the tarsometatarsal joints. *Orthop Clin North Am* 1987;18:105–114.
3. Brown DD, Gumbs RV. Lisfranc fracture-dislocations: report of two cases. *J Natl Med Assoc* 1991;83:366–369.
4. Curtis MJ, Myerson M, Szura B. Tarsometatarsal joint injuries in the athlete. *Am J Sports Med* 1993;21:497–502.
5. Heckman JD. Fractures and dislocations of the foot. In: Rockwood CA, Green DP, Bucholz RD, eds. *Rockwood and Green's Fractures in Adults*. vol 2. 3rd ed. Philadelphia, PA: Lippincott; 1991:2140–2151.
6. Mantas JP, Burks RT. Lisfranc injuries in the athlete. *Clin Sports Med* 1994;13:719–730.
7. Myerson M. The diagnosis and treatment of injuries to the Lisfranc joint complex. *Orthop Clin North Am* 1989;20:655–664.
8. Trevino SG, Kodros S. Controversies in tarsometatarsal injuries. *Orthop Clin North Am* 1995;26(2)229–238.
9. Wiley JJ. The mechanism of tarso-metatarsal joint injuries. *J Bone Joint Surg Br* 1971;53:474–482.
10. Sommer TC, Lee TH. Charcot foot: the diagnostic dilemma. *Am Fam Physician* 2001 Nov 1;64(9):1591–1598.
11. Khosla S, Thiele R, Baumhauer JF. Ultrasound guidance for intra-articular injections of the foot and ankle. *Foot Ankle Int* 2009 Sep;30(9):886–890.
12. Khoury NJ, El-Khoury GY, Saltzman CL, Brandser EA. Intraarticular foot and ankle injections to identify source of pain before arthrodesis. *Am J Roentgen* 1996 Sep;167(3):669–673.

Arthur Jason De Luigi, DO, FAAPMR, DAPM

KEY POINTS

- Use a high-frequency linear array transducer at a depth of less than 3 cm.
- Isolated pathology of the calcaneocuboid is rare and is typically secondary to trauma and osteoarthritis.
- *Cuboid syndrome* has been proposed to occur secondary to several causes such as excessive pronation, overuse, and due to inversion ankle sprain.

- Identify the peroneus longus tendon as it traverses the area along its course. Once the tendon is identified, the tendon can be avoided during the needle trajectory into the joint.

Pertinent Anatomy

The calcaneocuboid and talonavicular joints act as a functional unit known as the *transverse tarsal joint* (Figure 85-1).

Transverse tarsal joint motion ranges from 10 degrees of abduction and 15 degrees of adduction. Stability of the transverse tarsal joint is controlled by the position of the subtalar

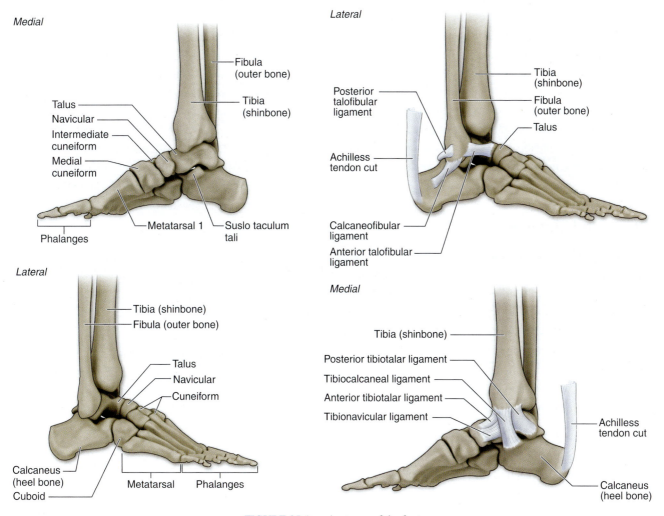

FIGURE 85-1 ■ Anatomy of the foot.

joint. Inversion of the subtalar joint places the axes of these joints in a nonparallel position leading to increased stability of the hindfoot. Whereas the flexibility of these joints is increased when the joints are in parallel, such as heel strike, when the calcaneus is everted (Figure 85-2).

The calcaneocuboid joint is between the calcaneus and the cuboid with connections by multiple ligaments (dorsal calcaneocuboid, plantar calcaneocuboid, long plantar, and the bifurcated ligament).[1] The calcaneocuboid joint is frequently described as among the least mobile joints of the foot. It is postulated that this is due to the relatively flat articular surfaces with some irregular undulations leading to motion being limited to a single rotation with some translation. The cuboid can rotate as much as 25 degrees about an oblique axis during inversion and eversion, also known as *obvolution-involuation*.[2]

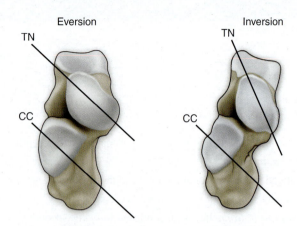

FIGURE 85-2 ■ The function of the transverse tarsal joint demonstrates that when the calcaneus is in eversion, the resultant axes of the talonavicular and calcaneocuboid joints are parallel or congruent. When the subtalar joint is in an inverted position, the axes are incongruent, giving increased stability to the midfoot.

Common Pathology

Isolated pathology of the calcaneocuboid is rare and is typically secondary to trauma and osteoarthritis. Rheumatoid arthritis frequently affects the foot in 90% of rheumatoid patients and almost always bilateral[3]; however, isolated calcaneocuboid involvement is uncommon. *Cuboid syndrome* has been described in the literature based on pain in the calcaneocuboid joint and has been proposed to occur secondary to several causes such as excessive pronation, overuse, and inversion ankle sprain.[4] Another cause of pain in the calcaneocuboid joint is cuboid subluxation or dislocation. Plantar flexion and abduction is the most common mechanism of injury of the calcaneocuboid joint.

Ultrasound Image Findings

The calcaneocuboid joint is best visualized in long axis using a high-frequency linear array transducer at a depth of less than 3 cm. Pathologic findings on sonographic evaluation include cuboid subluxation, cortical irregularities, calcifications, and joint effusions. Although not specific to the calcaneocuboid joint, pathology of the adjacent peroneus longus tendon may also be visualized.

Indications for Injection

Injection of the calcaneocuboid joint can be performed as a diagnostic procedure for patients suspected calcaneocuboid pain or as therapeutic injection for patients with recalcitrant

pain that is unresponsive to rest, icing, antiinflammatories and physical therapy.

Injection of the calcaneocuboid joint based on palpation (unguided) has been used anecdotally in clinical practice, although no literature exists to describe the technique. Therefore, no literature exists regarding the success rate of these unguided injections. Fluoroscopic-guided injections of calcaneocuboid joint were described by Khoury and colleagues,[5] and computerized tomography–guided injections have been described by Saifuddin and colleagues.[6] Ultrasound-guided injection has neither been described in the literature nor has success rates or clinical outcomes of guided injection versus unguided injections.

Equipment

■ Needle: 25-gauge, 1.5-inch needle
■ Injectate:
  • 1 mL of a local anesthetic
  • 1 mL of an injectable corticosteroid
■ High-frequency linear array or linear array "hockey stick" transducer

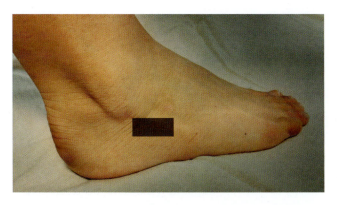

FIGURE 85-3 ■ Calcaneocuboid transducer placement lateral foot.

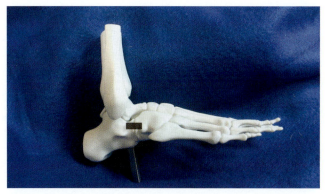

FIGURE 85-4 ■ Calcaneocuboid transducer placement anatomic.

Author's Preferred Technique

a. Patient position
    i. Supine position
    ii. Foot elevated and flat with knee flexed
b. Transducer position
    i. Image area of interest in two perpendicular planes.
    ii. If possible, orient the planes along conventional axes (transverse/longitudinal).
    iii. Identify the best view obtainable of the target site.
    iv. Anatomic sagittal (longitudinal) plane, out of plane, medial to lateral (Figures 85-3, 85-4, and 85-5).
c. Needle orientation relative to the transducer
    i. Out of plane
d. Needle approach
    i. Walk-down technique (Figure 85-6)
    ii. Lateral to medial
e. Target
    i. Calcaneocuboid joint (Figures 85-5 and 85-6)
f. Pearls and Pitfalls
    i. Identify the peroneus longus tendon, which passes adjacent to the joint.
    ii. Based on the author's clinical experience, it is best to identify the peroneus longus tendon as it traverses the area along its course. Once the tendon is identified, the tendon can be avoided during the needle trajectory into the joint.

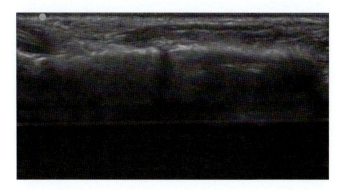

FIGURE 85-5 ■ Calcaneocuboid longitudinal.

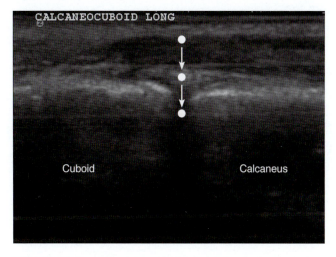

FIGURE 85-6 ■ Calcaneocuboid joint (longitudinal out of plane approach using step-down technique (dots)).

References

1. Gray H. Articulations of the tarsus. In: Gray H, ed. *Gray's Anatomy*. 1st ed. Philadelphia, PA: Courage Books; 1901:287–288.

2. Greiner TM, Ball KA. The calcaneocuboid joint moves with three degrees of freedom. *J Foot Ankle Res* 2008;1(Suppl 1):O39.

3. Mann JA, Chou LB, Ross SDK. Foot and ankle surgery. In: Skinner HB, ed. *Current Diagnosis and Treatment in Orthopedics*. New York: McGraw-Hill; 2006.

4. Durall CJ. Examination and treatment of cuboid syndrome: a literature review. *Sports Health* 2011 Nov-Dec;3(6):514–519.

5. Khoury NJ, El-Khoury GY, Saltzman CL, Brandser EA. intraarticular foot and ankle injections to identify source of pain before arthrodesis. *Am J Roentgenol* 1996 Sep;167(3):669–173.

6. Saifuddin A, Abdus-Samee M, Mann C, Singh D, Angel JC. CT guided diagnostic foot injections. *Clin Radiol* 2005 Feb;60(2): 191–195.

Eric Robert Helm, MD / Nicholas H. Weber, DO / Megan Helen Cortazzo, MD

KEY POINTS

- Use a 25-gauge, 1.5-inch needle in a short-axis approach.
- Use a high-frequency linear array transducer.
- The dorsomedial aspect of metatarsophalangeal (MTP) joint is ideal needle placement.
- Anatomic sagittal plane is the correct positioning.
- Use a walk-down technique.
- Stay dorsal to avoid medial hallucal nerve.

Pertinent Anatomy

The metatarsophalangeal (MTP) joint is a condyloid joint consisting of the articulation between the metatarsal bones of the foot and proximal phalanges of the toes. The joint capsule is stabilized by the extensor tendon dorsally, two lateral collateral ligaments, and heavy plantar ligaments. The plantar ligaments and metatarsal heads are connected to adjacent ligaments and heads by deep transverse metatarsal ligaments. At the first MTP joint, there are adjacent sesamoid bones within each of the heads of the flexor hallucis tendon. They act to reinforce the plantar plate of the joint capsule. The movements permitted in the MTP articulation are primarily flexion and extension, with limited abduction and adduction (Figure 86-1).

Common Pathology

The MTP joint can be injured by direct impact to the dorsal or plantar surface of the forefoot. Hyperextension of the MTP joint (specifically of the great toe) with an applied axial load can lead to a spectrum of injuries from plantar plate tear to phalangeal or metatarsal fracture or dislocation.

The MTP joint can become inflamed or irritated in rheumatologic conditions, such as gout, rheumatoid arthritis, psoriatic arthritis, and calcium pyrophosphate disease. Degenerative changes can also occur with aging, leading to clinically significant osteoarthritis. Hallux rigidus is a painful condition of the MTP joint of the great toe, characterized by restricted dorsiflexion.

Ultrasound Imaging Findings

The MTP joint is best visualized in long axis using a high-frequency linear array transducer and depth of less than 2 cm. Common findings include cortical irregularities, joint space narrowing, osteophytes and calcifications, synovial hypertrophy, and joint effusions.

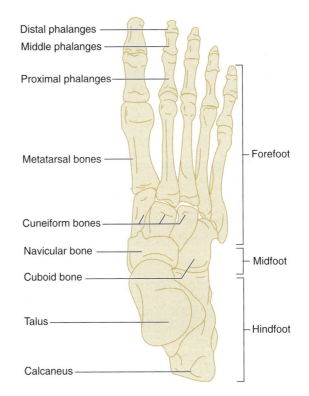

FIGURE 86-1 ■ Diagram of normal bony anatomy of the foot. (Reproduced with permission from Tintinalli JE, Stapczynski JS, Cline DM, et al., eds. *Tintinalli's Emergency Medicine: A Comprehensive Study Guide.* 7th ed. New York: McGraw-Hill; 2011: figure 274-1A.)

Indications for Injections of the Metatarsophalangeal Joint

Injection of the MTP joint can be performed for patients with recalcitrant pain that is unresponsive to rest, icing, antiinflammatories, orthotics, and physical therapy. Injection of the MTP joint has been described based on palpation by Boxer et al.[1] Ultrasound-guided injection has been described by Reach et al.,[2] with a success rate of 100% with guided injection of the first and second MTP joint. Clinical outcomes of guided versus nonguided joint procedures have been described by Balint et al.,[3] who showed successful intraarticular fluid aspiration in 97% of the ultrasound-guided group versus 32% in the unguided group. These findings were consistent with findings from Raza et al.,[4] who confirmed intraarticular needle placement in 96% of ultrasound-guided injections versus 59% of palpation-guided injections.

Equipment

- Needle: 25-gauge, 1.5-inch needle
- Injectate
  - 1 mL local anesthetic
  - 1 mL corticosteroid
- High-frequency linear array transducer

Author's Preferred Technique

a. Patient position
   i. Supine with knee flexed so foot is flat on examination table (Figure 86-2)
b. Transducer position
   i. Anatomic, sagittal plane over the dorsomedial aspect of the joint (Figure 86-3)
c. Needle orientation relative to the transducer
   i. Out of plane
d. Needle approach
   i. Medial to lateral (Figure 86-4) for first MTP
   ii. Medial to lateral or lateral to medial (Figure 86-5) for the second through fourth MTP
   iii. Walk-down technique
e. Target
   i. Dorsomedial aspect of the MTP joint (Figure 86-6)
f. Pearls and Pitfalls
   i. Stay dorsal to avoid the medial or lateral hallucal nerve.
   ii. The out-of-plane approach avoids extensor tendons.

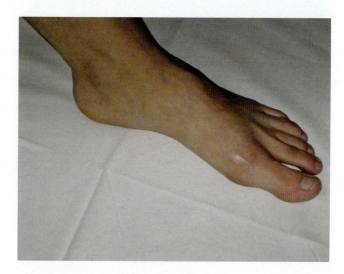

FIGURE 86-2 ■ Medial aspect of left foot.

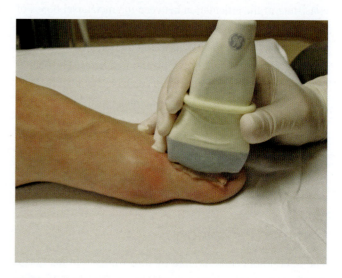

FIGURE 86-3 ■ Long-axis plane probe position over (MTP) metatarsophalangeal joint of great toe.

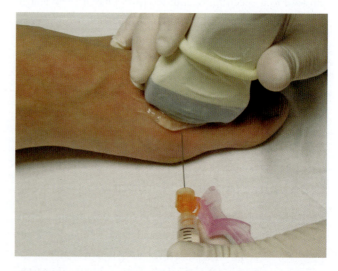

FIGURE 86-4 ■ Out-of-plane, medial-to-lateral needle approach to first (MTP) metatarsophalangeal joint.

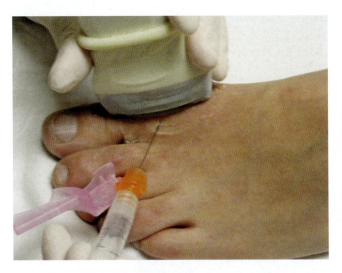

FIGURE 86-5 ▪ Out-of-plane, lateral-to-medial needle approach to first (MTP) metatarsophalangeal (MTP) joint.

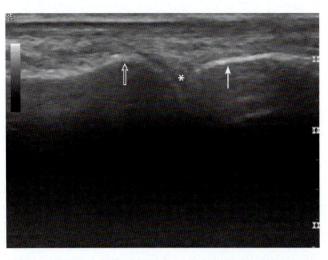

FIGURE 86-6 ▪ Long-axis imaging over the first metatarsophalangeal joint shows the metatarsal head (*open arrow*), metatarsophalangeal (MTP) joint space (*asterisk*), and proximal phalanx (*thin arrow*).

Alternate Technique

a. Patient position
   i. Supine with knee flexed so foot is flat on examination table (see Figure 86-2)
b. Transducer position
   i. Anatomic sagittal plane over the dorsomedial aspect of the joint just lateral or medial to extensor tendon (see Figure 86-3)
c. Needle orientation relative to the transducer
   i. In plane with standoff oblique technique
d. Needle approach
   i. Proximal to distal (Figure 86-7)
e. Target
   i. Proximal dorsal aspect of the MTP joint (see Figure 86-6)
f. Pearls and Pitfalls
   i. Stay dorsal to avoid the medial or lateral hallucal nerve.
   ii. The short-axis needle orientation is preferred to gain optimal access to the MTP joint and avoid surrounding neurovascular and tendinous structures.

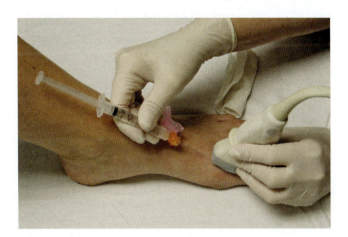

FIGURE 86-7 ▪ In-plane, proximal to distal needle approach to first metatarsophalangeal joint.

References

1. Boxer MC. Osteoarthritis involving the metatarsophalangeal joints and management of metatarsophalangeal joint pain via injection therapy. *Clin Podiatr Med Surg* 1994;11:125–132.
2. Reach JS, Easley ME, Chuckpaiwong B, Nunley JA. Accuracy of ultrasound guided injections in the foot and ankle. *Foot Ankle Int* 2009;30(3):239–242.
3. Balint PV, Kane D, Hunter J, et al. Ultrasound guided versus conventional joint and soft tissue fluid aspiration in rheumatology practice: a pilot study. *J Rheumatol* 2002;29(10):2209–2213.
4. Raza K, Lee CY, Pilling D, et al. Ultrasound guidance allows accurate needle placement and aspiration from small joints in patients with early inflammatory arthritis. *Rheumatology (Oxford)* 2003;42(8):976–979.

Eric Robert Helm, MD / Nicholas H. Weber, DO / Megan Helen Cortazzo, MD

KEY POINTS

- A 25-gauge, 1-inch needle is used in a short-axis approach.
- Use a high-frequency linear array transducer.

- Follow the anatomic sagittal plane.
- Use a walk-down technique.
- Stay dorsal to avoid interdigital nerves.

Pertinent Anatomy

The interphalangeal joint is a hinge joint consisting of the articulation between the phalanges of the toes. The joint capsule is stabilized by the extensor tendon dorsally, two collateral ligaments on each side, and plantar ligament on the flexor surface. The movements permitted in the interphalangeal joint articulation are primarily flexion and extension (Figure 87-1).

Common Pathology

The interphalangeal (IP) joint can be injured by direct impact to the dorsal or plantar surface of the forefoot. Common injuries of the IP joint range from collateral ligament tear to phalangeal fracture or dislocation. Common structural deformities include mallet, claw, and hammertoe.

The IP joint can also be inflamed or irritated in rheumatologic conditions, such as gout, rheumatoid arthritis, psoriatic arthritis, and calcium pyrophosphate disease. Degenerative changes can also occur with aging, leading to clinically significant osteoarthritis.

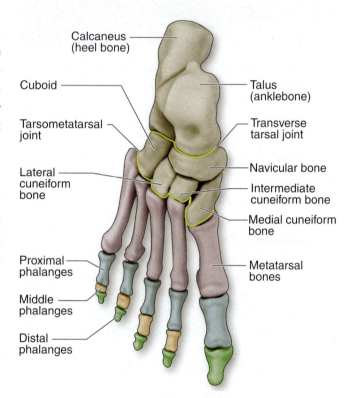

FIGURE 87-1 ■ Diagram of normal bony anatomy of the foot.

Ultrasound Imaging Findings

The IP joint is best visualized in long axis using a high-frequency linear array transducer at a depth of less than 2 cm. Common findings include cortical irregularities, joint space narrowing, calcifications, synovial hypertrophy, and joint effusions.

Indications for Injections of the Interphalangeal Joint

Injection of the IP joint can be performed for patients with recalcitrant pain that is unresponsive to rest, icing, antiinflammatories and physical therapy. Injection of the IP joint has been

described based on palpation by Boxer et al.[1] Ultrasound-guided injection has been described by Reach et al.,[2] with a success rate of 100% with guided injection in similar sized joints. Clinical outcomes of guided versus nonguided IP joint procedures have been described by Balint et al.,[3] who showed successful intraarticular fluid aspiration in 32% in the unguided group versus 97% success in the ultrasound-guided group. These findings were consistent with findings from Raza et al.,[4] who confirmed intraarticular needle placement in 59% of palpation-guided versus 96% of ultrasound-guided injections.

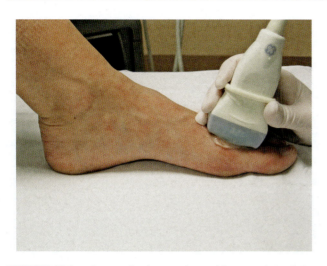

FIGURE 87-2 ■ Long-axis plane probe position over interphalangeal joints of great toe.

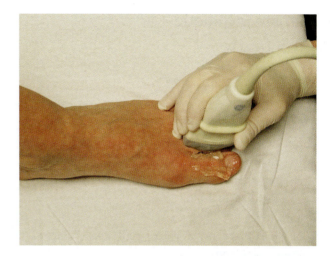

FIGURE 87-3 ■ Long-axis plane probe position over interphalangeal joints of second toe.

Equipment

■ Needle: 25-gauge, 1-inch needle
■ Injectate
   • 1 mL local anesthetic
   • 1 mL corticosteroid
■ High-frequency linear array transducer

Author's Preferred Technique

a. Patient position
    i. Supine
b. Transducer position
    i. Anatomic sagittal plane over the dorsal aspect of the joint (Figures 87-2 and 87-3)
c. Needle orientation relative to the transducer
    i. Out of plane
d. Needle approach
    i. Medial to lateral (Figure 87-4)
    ii. Lateral to medial (Figure 87-5)
e. Target
    i. Dorsomedial or dorsolateral aspect of the metatarsophalangeal joint (Figure 87-6)
f. Pearls and Pitfalls
    i. Stay dorsal to avoid the interdigital nerve.

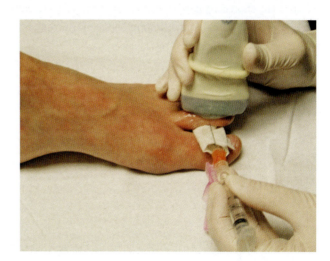

FIGURE 87-4 ■ Out-of-plane, medial-to-lateral needle approach to second distal interphalangeal joint.

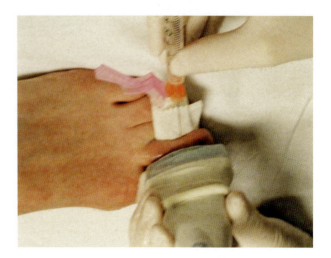

FIGURE 87-5 ■ Out-of-plane, lateral-to-medial needle approach to second distal interphalangeal joint.

Alternate Technique

a. Patient position
   i. Supine
b. Transducer position
   i. Anatomic sagittal plane over the dorsal aspect of the joint (see Figures 87-2 and 87-3)
c. Needle orientation relative to the transducer
   i. In plane
d. Needle approach
   i. Proximal to distal
e. Target
   i. Proximal dorsal aspect of the IP joint (Figure 87-7)
f. Pearls and Pitfalls
   i. Stay dorsal to avoid the interdigital nerve.
   ii. Avoid the extensor tendon.
   iii. The short-axis needle orientation is preferred to gain optimal access to the IP joint and avoid surrounding neurovascular structures.

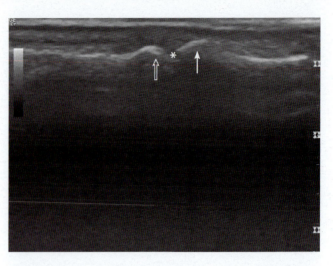

FIGURE 87-6 ■ Long-axis imaging over second interphalangeal joint shows the proximal phalanx (*open arrow*), proximal interphalangeal (PIP) joint space (*asterisk*), and distal phalanx (*thin arrow*).

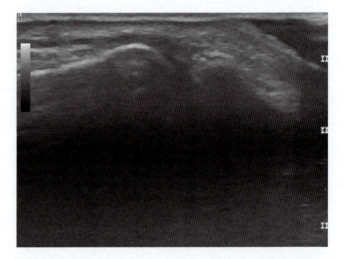

FIGURE 87-7 ■ Long-axis imaging over second interphalangeal joint demonstrates joint space opening with distal phalanx flexion.

References

1. Boxer MC. Osteoarthritis involving the metatarsophalangeal joints and management of metatarsophalangeal joint pain via injection therapy. *Clin Podiatr Med Surg*. 1994;11:125–132.
2. Reach JS, Easley ME, Chuckpaiwong B, Nunley JA. Accuracy of ultrasound guided injections in the foot and ankle. *Foot Ankle Int*. 2009;30(3):239–242.
3. Balint PV, Kane D, Hunter J, et al. Ultrasound guided versus conventional joint and soft tissue fluid aspiration in rheumatology practice: a pilot study. *Journal of Rheumatology*. 2002;29(10):2209–2213.
4. Raza K, Lee CY, Pilling D, et al. Ultrasound guidance allows accurate needle placement and aspiration from small joints in patients with early inflammatory arthritis. *Rheumatology (Oxford)*. 2003;42(8):976–979.

Nicholas H. Weber, DO / Eric Robert Helm, MD / Megan Helen Cortazzo, MD

KEY POINTS

- Use a 27-gauge, 1.25-inch needle with in-plane approach.
- Use a high-frequency linear array transducer.
- View the plantar aspect of the first metatarsal head.
- Follow the anatomic short-axis plane.
- Use a medial-to-lateral approach.
- A bursae injection with anesthetic is diagnostic.

Pertinent Anatomy

The sesamoid bones are located at the first metatarsal head, within the medial and lateral heads of the flexor hallucis brevis tendon. The abductor and adductor hallucis tendons have insertions onto the tibial (medial) and fibular (lateral) sesamoids, respectively. The deep transverse metatarsal ligament attaches to the fibular sesamoid. There is a small bursa located directly beneath each of the sesamoids. The sesamoid bones function to elevate the first metatarsal head to level with adjacent metatarsal heads and thus absorb and transmit weight through the forefoot, while also improving mechanical advantage in great toe flexion. The tibial sesamoid accepts the majority of weight bearing transmitted to the first metatarsal head (Figure 88-1).

Common Pathology

The sesamoid bones and metatarsosesamoid soft tissue area can be injured by direct impact to the plantar surface of the forefoot causing compression of the sesamoids against the metatarsal head.[1-7] Common injuries include fracture (typically caused by forced dorsiflexion of the metatarsophalangeal [MTP] joint seen in football and soccer players), subluxation, and osteonecrosis.[4] The sesamoid bones can also be inflamed or irritated in rheumatologic conditions, such as rheumatoid arthritis and osteoarthritis.[4] Sesamoiditis is pain mediated from the sesamoids of the great toe without known trauma. Inflammation of the bursa beneath the sesamoids results in swelling and pain with weight bearing or direct palpation, and is often misdiagnosed as sesamoiditis. The tibial sesamoid bone is more prone to injury, given its larger surface area, seen particularly in repetitive trauma such as that in jogging, long distance running and ballet. Patients with metatarsosesamoid pathology complain of point tenderness on the plantar aspect of the first metatarsal head that is worse with push off during activity and relieved with rest.

Ultrasound Imaging Findings

The metatarsosesamoid bones are best visualized in short axis using a high-frequency linear array transducer at a depth of less than 1 cm. Common findings include cortical irregularities, calcifications, and effusions. Bipartite or multipartite sesamoids are also important to identify, as 25% of the population will have a bipartite sesamoid and 85% are bilateral. A key difference is that bipartite sesamoids have smooth margins and fractures demonstrate irregular fracture lines.

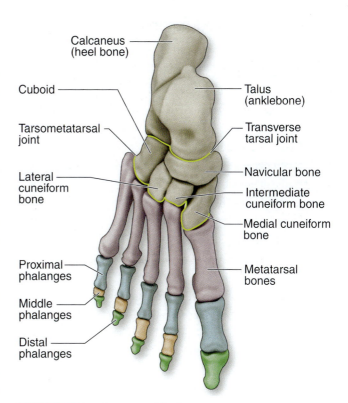

FIGURE 88-1 ■ Structure of the foot.

Indications for Metatarsosesamoid Injection

Injection of the metatarsosesamoid area can be performed for patients with recalcitrant pain that is unresponsive to rest, icing, antiinflammatories, orthotics, and physical therapy.[1-4] Injection of the metatarsosesamoid region based on palpation has not specifically been described. Ultrasound-guided injection has been described by Reach et al., with a success rate of 100%.[1] Clinical outcomes comparing guided versus non-guided joint procedures have been described by Balint et al. who showed successful intraarticular fluid aspiration in 32% unguided versus 97% success in the ultrasound-guided group.[2] These findings were consistent with findings from Raza et al., who confirmed intraarticular needle placement in 59% of palpation-guided versus 96% of ultrasound-guided injections.[3]

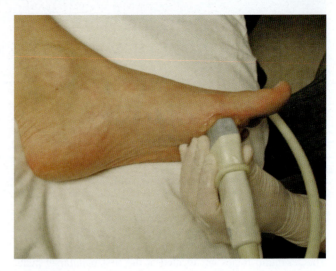

FIGURE 88-2 ■ Short-axis plane probe position over the metatarsosesamoid joint of great toe.

Equipment

■ Needle: 27-gauge, 1.25-inch needle
■ Injectate
  • 0.5 mL of a local anesthetic
  • 0.5 mL injectable corticosteroid
■ High-frequency linear array transducer

Author's Preferred Technique

a. Patient position
   i. Supine
b. Transducer position
   i. Anatomic short-axis plane over the first metatarsal head (Figure 88-2)
c. Needle orientation relative to the transducer
   i. In plane
d. Needle approach
   i. Medial to lateral (Figure 88-3)
e. Target
   i. Bursae (Figure 88-4)
   ii. Injection of metatarsosesamoid joint (Figure 88-5)
f. Pearls and Pitfalls
   i. Consider a first MTP joint injection unless a perisesamoid soft tissue injection is indicated.
   ii. Avoid the flexor hallucis brevis and abductor and adductor hallucis tendons.

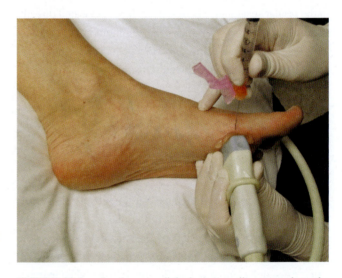

FIGURE 88-3 ■ In-plane, medial plantar needle approach to the first metatarsosesamoid joint.

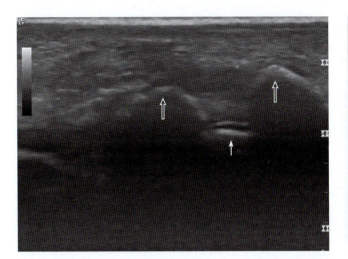

FIGURE 88-4 ■ Short-axis imaging over the metatarsosesamoid joint of great toe shows tibial sesamoid medially (*open arrow*), fibular sesamoid laterally (*open arrow*), and metatarsal head (*thin arrow*). Medial is to the right side of the image.

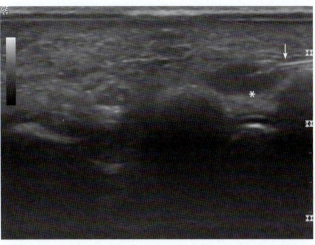

FIGURE 88-5 ■ Short-axis imaging over the metatarsosesamoid (MTS) joint of great toe shows the needle tip (*thin arrow*) clearing the tibial sesamoid and entering the MTS joint space (*asterisk*). Medial is to the right side of the image.

References

1. Reach JS, Easley ME, Chuckpaiwong B, Nunley JA. Accuracy of ultrasound guided injections in the foot and ankle. *Foot Ankle Int* 2009;30(3):239–242.
2. Balint PV, Kane D, Hunter J, et al. Ultrasound guided versus conventional joint and soft tissue fluid aspiration in rheumatology practice: a pilot study. *J Rheumatol* 2002;29(10):2209–2213.
3. Raza K, Lee CY, Pilling D, et al. Ultrasound guidance allows accurate needle placement and aspiration from small joints in patients with early inflammatory arthritis. *Rheumatology (Oxford)* 2003;42(8):976–979.
4. Boxer MC. Osteoarthritis involving the metatarsophalangeal joints and management of metatarsophalangeal joint pain via injection therapy. *Clin Podiatr Med Surg* 1994;11:125–132.
5. Madden CC, Netter, FH. *Netter's Sports Medicine*. Philadelphia, PA: Saunders/Elsevier; 2010:464–474.
6. Jenkins DB, Hollinshead WH. *Hollinshead's Functional Anatomy of the Limbs and Back*. Philadelphia, PA: Saunders; 1998:323–341.
7. Bracilovic A. *Essential Dance Medicine: Sesamoid Bones*. New York: Humana; 2009.

Nelson A. Hager, MS, MD / Alfred C. Gellhorn, MD

KEY POINTS

- Use a 25-gauge, 1.5-inch needle, short-axis view, in plane.
- A high-frequency, small footprint "hockey stick" transducer is ideal for the complex contours of the foot.
- In cross section, the tibialis anterior tendon is normally approximately twice as large as the other extensor tendons.
- The dorsal pedis artery and deep peroneal nerve may be identified in the interval between the tibialis anterior and extensor hallucis longus and should be avoided.

Pertinent Anatomy (Figure 89-1)

The tibialis anterior originates from the upper two-thirds of the lateral surface of the tibia, and after passing beneath the most medial compartments of the transverse and cruciate crural ligaments, it inserts onto the medial surface of the medial cuneiform and the plantar aspect of the base of first metatarsal bones of the foot.

The tendon is retained close to the talar head by the superomedial band and close to the medial cuneiform bone by the inferomedial band of the inferior extensor retinaculum, as well as by the transverse retinaculum band.[1]

Four extensor tendons lie alongside each other in the anterior ankle. The tibialis anterior is the largest and the most medial tendon. The tibialis anterior tendon appears to be approximately twice as large as the other extensor tendons in cross section. Each of the extensor tendons passes beneath the retinacula with tendon sheaths that protect them from mechanical friction (Figure 89-2).

The anterior tibial artery lies in a deeper position, just lateral to the extensor hallucis longus tendon. The deep peroneal nerve initially lies medial to the vessels and then crosses over them to descend lateral to the artery proceeding distally.[2]

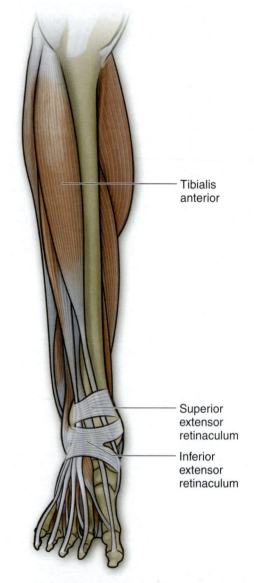

FIGURE 89-1 ■ Anterior view of the tibialis anterior muscle and tendon.

Tibialis anterior

Superior extensor retinaculum

Inferior extensor retinaculum

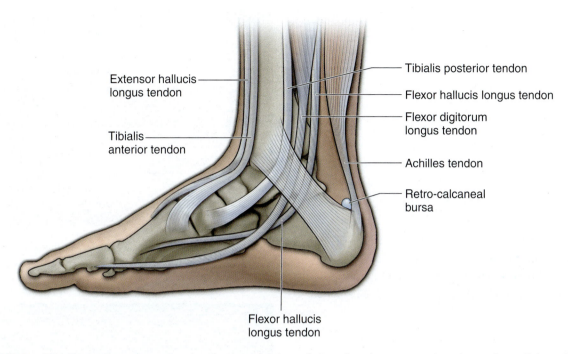

Extensor hallucis longus tendon

Tibialis anterior tendon

Tibialis posterior tendon

Flexor hallucis longus tendon

Flexor digitorum longus tendon

Achilles tendon

Retro-calcaneal bursa

Flexor hallucis longus tendon

FIGURE 89-2 ■ Tibialis anterior tendon and tendon sheath passing beneath the retinacula en route to insertion on the medial cuneiform.

Common Pathology

Abnormalities in the tibialis anterior tendon are generally less common than other tendons of the foot. One explanation provided is that the tendon is usually only exposed to minor mechanical stress owing to its straight course.[3]

Tibialis anterior tendon pathology typically presents as a rupture of the tendon or a distal insertional tendinopathy.[4] Rupture is rare and can be secondary to local trauma or spontaneous. Spontaneous rupture most frequently affects subjects older than 45 years of age.[5] Most tibialis anterior tendon tears occur within 3.5 cm of the insertion. This region on the distal tendon also corresponds to the primary region of tendon thickening associated with tendinosis.[4]

Tendinosis without rupture is often found in middle-aged patients and can be associated with other degenerative changes of the foot. It is characterized by a painful swelling over the distal tibialis anterior tendon and burning over the medial forefoot.[6] These patients can frequently have long-axis split tears in the tendons as well.[4]

The tibialis anterior tendon can also be injured in distance runners or football players who forcefully dorsiflex a plantar flexed foot against resistance, placing an eccentric stress on the tibialis anterior muscle.[7] In these patients, the tibialis anterior tendon can develop an inflammatory condition of the tendon sheaths from mechanical friction of the tendons beneath the retinacula.

Ultrasound Imaging Findings

Start with the transducer placed in the axial plane over the dorsal and medial aspect of the ankle from the musculotendinous junction proximally to the insertion distally on the first cuneiform. It can be evaluated on both the long and short axis from its myotendinous junction down to its boney insertion.

The ultrasound appearance of a distal tibialis anterior tendinopathy appears as the usual triad of a thickened, hypoechoic, and mildly hypervascular tendon. Ultrasound evaluation in the long axis usually demonstrates fusiform swelling of the tendon after it crosses the ankle joint and just before its insertion. These abnormalities are frequently accompanied by enthesopathic changes with hyperechoic calcifications at the tendon insertion. Fluid within the tibialis anterior tendon sheath was a common finding in patients with distal tendinosis.[4]

Tibialis anterior tendinitis is characterized by swelling of the synovium of the tendon sheath associated with hyperechoic thickening of the tendon sheath, hyperemia of the synovium (identified on Doppler imaging), and tendon sheath fluid collection.

Indications for Injections of the Tibialis Anterior Tendon Sheath

Therapeutic injections are indicated for patients with tenosynovitis or other painful tibialis anterior tendon injuries refractory to conservative therapy with relative rest, activity modification, ice, antiinflammatory medications, and physical therapy.

Relative contraindications to steroid injection include partial or complete tendon tear due to the potentially detrimental effect of steroids on tendon repair. Degenerative tear of the tibialis anterior tendon after corticosteroid injection has been described.[8]

To the authors' knowledge, there are no descriptions of image-guided injections of the tibialis anterior tendon. Outcomes for ultrasound-guided corticosteroid injections of the tibialis anterior tendon sheath have also not been reported.

Equipment

- Needle: 25-gauge, 1.5-inch needle
- Injectate
  - 0.5 mL of a local anesthetic
  - 0.5 mL of an injectable corticosteroid
- High-frequency hockey stick transducer

Author's Preferred Technique

a. Patient position
   i. Patient supine with the knee flexed to approximately 45 degrees with the ankle slightly plantar flexed and lying flat on the examination bed. Pillow bolsters can be used behind the knee and a rolled towel for optimal ankle positioning (Figure 89-3).
b. Transducer position
   i. Anatomic short-axis plane over the region of primary pathology (region of fusiform swelling, or tenosynovitis)
   ii. Short-axis view of the tibialis anterior tendon
c. Needle orientation relative to the transducer
   i. In plane, long axis
d. Needle approach
   i. Medial to lateral, which is the preferred given location of the dorsal pedis artery and deep peroneal nerve
e. Target
   i. Tibialis anterior tendon synovial sheath (Figure 89-4)

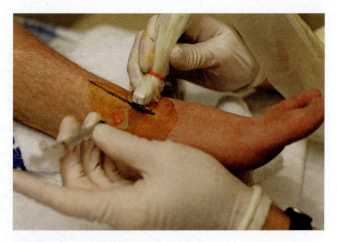

FIGURE 89-3 ▪ Tibialis anterior tendon sheath injection setup.

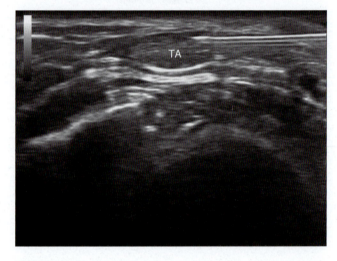

FIGURE 89-4 ▪ Ultrasound image of 25-gauge needle approaching the tibialis anterior tendon sheath from medial to lateral with the bevel within the tendon sheath. TA, tibialis anterior tendon sheath.

f. Pearls and Pitfalls
   i. The distal tibialis anterior tendon is tapered over the surface of the medial cuneiform and shows a hypoechoic pattern in its preinsertional portion as a result of anisotropy. The distal portion of this tendon is medial and not dorsal as might be expected. It may show a division prior to insertion that represents a normal variant and not a long-axis split of the distal tendon. It is important to identify a partial or complete tendon tear because of the potentially detrimental effect of steroids on tendon repair.

Alternate Technique

There are three bursae in association with the terminal portion of the tibialis anterior tendon. The first between the tendon and the cuneometatarsal joint. The second bursa lies between the tendon and the first cuneiform bone, and a third is superficial, located between the tendon and the overlying extensor retinaculum.[1]

Each of these can be targeted for intervention if characteristic findings of bursitis are noted on ultrasound, such as anechoic fluid collection, peribursal hyperemia on Doppler, and increased conspicuity of hyperechoic peribursal fat layers.

a. Patient position
    i. Patient position same as for the distal tendon sheath injection

b. Transducer position
    i. Anatomic short-axis plane over the region of primary pathology (region of noted bursa)
    ii. Short-axis view of the distal tibialis anterior tendon

c. Needle orientation relative to the transducer
    i. In plane, long axis

d. Needle approach
    i. Medial to lateral is preferred given the location of the dorsal pedis artery and deep peroneal nerve.

e. Target
    i. Interspace between the distal tibialis anterior tendon synovial sheath and the cuneometatarsal joint, the first cuneiform bone, and superficially between the tendon and the overlying extensor retinaculum.

References

1. Kelikian AS, ed. *Sarrafian's Anatomy of the Foot and Ankle: Descriptive, Topographic, Functional.* Philadelphia, PA: Lippincott Williams & Williams; 2011.
2. Bianchi S, Martinoli C. *Ultrasound of the Musculoskeletal System.* Berlin Heidelberg: Springer-Verlag; 2007: 785.
3. Scheller AD, Kasser JR, Quigley TB. Tendon injuries about the ankle. *Orthop Clin North Am* 1980;11:801–811.
4. Mengiardi B, Pfirrmann CW, Vienne P, et al. Anterior tibial tendon abnormalities: MR imaging findings. *Radiology* 2005 Jun; 235(3):977–984.
5. Dooley BJ, Kudelka P, Menelaus MB. Subcutaneous rupture of the tendon of tibialis anterior. *J Bone Joint Surg Br* 1980;62:471–472.
6. Beischer AD, Beamond BM, Jowett AJ, O'Sullivan R. Distal tendinosis of the tibialis anterior tendon. *Foot Ankle Int* 2009 Nov;30(11):1053–1059.
7. Simpson MR, Howard TM. Tendinopathies of the foot and ankle. *Am Fam Physician* 2009 Nov;80(10):1107–1114.
8. Velan, GJ, Hendel. Degenerative tear of the tibialis anterior tendon after corticosteroid injection—augmentation with the extensor hallucis longus tendon, case report. *Acta Orthop Scan* 1997;68(3):302–309.

Nelson A. Hager, MS, MD

Pertinent Anatomy

The peroneal tendon complex is composed of the peroneus brevis and longus muscles, the peroneus brevis and longus tendons, the common synovial sheath, the superior and inferior retinaculum, and the os peroneum. In the supramalleolar region, the peroneus longus tendon lies lateral to the peroneus brevis muscle and tendon. Distally, the peroneus brevis muscle decreases in size as it continues to its tendinous portion, and is tendinous by the time it reaches the retromalleolar region; at this point the peroneus longus tendon runs posterior and lateral to the peroneus brevis tendon. The osteofibrous tunnel, which houses the peroneal tendons and their synovial sheath, is formed by the bony retrofibular groove and the fibrous superior retinaculum. In some subjects, a small sesamoid bone, the os peroneum, is found inside the peroneus longus tendon at the level of the cuboid sulcus. The common synovial sheath surrounding the peroneus longus and brevis tendon divides into two distinct parts distally just posterior to the peroneal tubercle.[1]

Common Pathology

Traumatic injury may occur from a forceful contraction of the peroneal muscles usually with the ankle in plantarflexion and inversion. Classically, this occurs in skiing, football, ice skating, soccer, basketball, rugby, or gymnastics. Nontraumatic subluxation is associated with an anatomically shallow, flat, or absent retrofibular groove; chronic lateral ankle instability; severe pes planus; generalized ligamentous laxity; and neuromuscular diseases.[2] Intermittent instability may be either a subluxation or dislocation over the proximal malleolus or an intrasheath subluxation, where the tendons temporarily reverse their anteroposterior relationship. Tenosynovitis may be secondary to trauma, repetitive microtrauma, systemic joint disorders, or infection.

Indications for Injections of the Peroneal Tendon Sheath

Diagnostic injections with local anesthetic may be helpful in localizing pain and in surgical decision making. Therapeutic injections are indicated for patients with tenosynovitis or other painful peroneal tendon injuries refractory to conservative therapy with relative rest, activity modification, ice, antiinflammatory medications, and physical therapy. Relative contraindications to steroid injection include partial or complete tendon tear due to the potentially detrimental effect of steroids on tendon repair. Injections of the tendon sheath are described using fluoroscopy[3], palpation guidance, and ultrasound guidance.[4] Ultrasound-guided injections were found to be 100% accurate versus palpation-guided injections, which were 60% accurate.[4] Outcomes for ultrasound-guided corticosteroid injections of the peroneal tendon sheath have not been reported; using fluoroscopic tenography, 46% of patients with refractory peroneal tenosynovitis reported complete or near complete relief.[3]

Tendon Sheath Injection

Equipment

▪ Needle: 25-gauge, 1.5-inch needle
▪ Injectate
  • 0.5 mL of a local anesthetic
  • 0.5 mL of an injectable corticosteroid
▪ High-frequency, "hockey stick" transducer

Author's Preferred Technique

a. Patient position
   i. Patient supine
   ii. Lateral ankle facing superiorly, with towel roll placed under the medial ankle
   iii. Ankle positioned in inversion and plantarflexion
b. Transducer position (Figure 90-1A, B)
   i. Anatomic short-axis plane posterior to fibula in the retromalleolar groove
   ii. Short-axis view of peroneus longus and brevis tendons
c. Needle orientation relative to the transducer
   i. In plane
d. Needle approach
   i. Posterior to anterior
e. Target
   i. Common peroneal tendon synovial sheath
f. Pearls and Pitfalls
   i. Take care to distinguish fluid within the common peroneal sheath (tenosynovitis) from fluid related to a tear of the calcaneofibular ligament.
   ii. The peroneus quartus is a frequent anatomic variant present in up to 22% of subjects, and may be confused with a split of the peroneus brevis.

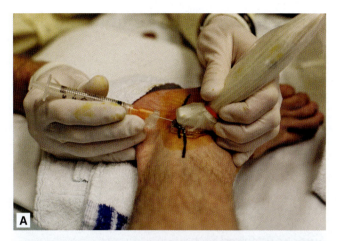

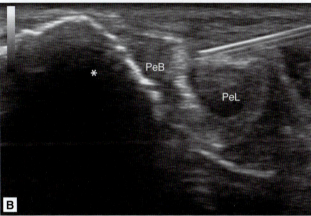

FIGURE 90-1 ▪ **A.** Peroneal tendon sheath injection: Posterior-to-anterior approach, using a small footprint transducer. The course of the peroneal tendons are indicated in black marker. **B.** Peroneal tendon sheath injection: At the level of the lateral malleolus, the peroneal tendons share a common synovial sheath. The lateral malleolus is seen to the left of the image (*asterisk*). Peroneus longus and brevis tendons are both visualized. PeB, peroneus brevis tendon; PeL, peroneus longus tendon.

Intratendinous Percutaneous Tenotomy of Peroneus Brevis

Equipment

▪ Needle
- 25-gauge, 1.5-inch needle for local anesthesia
- 18-gauge, 1.5-inch needle for tenotomy

▪ Injectate: Limited amount of local anesthetic to allow for adequate pain control during needle fenestration of the tendon

▪ High-frequency, "hockey stick" transducer

Author's Preferred Technique

a. Patient position
    i.   Patient supine
    ii. Lateral ankle facing superiorly, with towel roll placed under the medial ankle
    iii. Ankle positioned in inversion and plantarflexion
b. Transducer position (Figure 90-2A)
    i.   Long-axis view of peroneus brevis tendon at its insertion on fifth metatarsal
c. Needle orientation relative to the transducer (Figure 90-2B)
    i.   In plane
d. Needle approach
    i.   Proximal to distal
e. Target
    i.   Peroneus brevis insertion

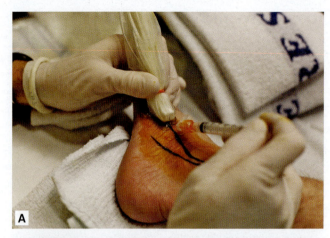

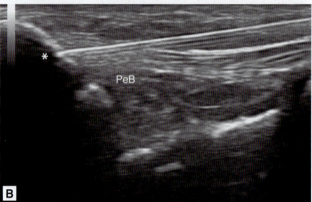

FIGURE 90-2 ▪ **A.** Peroneus brevis percutaneous tenotomy: Long-axis approach at the distal peroneus brevis at its insertion on the base of the fifth metatarsal. Course of the peroneal tendons are indicated in black marker. Patient is in the lateral decubitus position, with the foot supported on padding. **B.** Peroneus brevis percutaneous tenotomy: Peroneus brevis attachment to base of the fifth metatarsal. The needle (*asterisk*) should be well visualized given the superficial location of the injection. PeB, peroneus brevis tendon.

References

1. Bianchi S, Delmi M, Molini L. Ultrasound of peroneal tendons. *Semin Musculoskelet Radiol* 2010;14(03):292–306.
2. Bracker MD. *The 5-Minute Sports Medicine Consult (The 5-Minute Consult Series).* 2nd ed. Philadelphia, PA: Lippincott Williams & Wilkins; 2011:768.
3. Jaffee N, Gilula L. Diagnostic and therapeutic ankle tenography. *AJR Am J Roentgenol* 2001 Feb;176(2):365–371.
4. Muir JJ, Curtiss HM, Hollman J, Smith J, Finnoff JT. The accuracy of ultrasound-guided and palpation-guided peroneal tendon sheath injections. *Am J Phys Med Rehabil* 2011;90(7):564–571.

Luis Baerga-Varela, MD

KEY POINTS

- Use a 27-gauge, 1.25-inch or 25-gauge, 1.5-inch needle.
- Use a high-frequency linear array transducer.
- Either a short-axis or long-axis probe position may be used with an in-plane approach.
- Avoid injecting directly into the tendon.
- Avoid the sural nerve and saphenous vein laterally and the tibial nerve, artery, and veins medially.

Pertinent Anatomy

The Achilles tendon is the longest and strongest tendon in the body. It measures 12–15 cm in length and approximately 6 mm in cross-section. The tendon of the soleus muscle fuses with the aponeurosis of the two heads of the gastrocnemius, thus forming the Achilles tendon proximally. It travels distally, in the midline, posterior to the ankle inserting into the posterior surface of the calcaneus. The tendon rotates 90° with the medial fibers rotating posteriorly and the posterior fibers rotating laterally. In cross section, the Achilles tendon has a flat appearance proximally and a crescent shape distally, with a convex posterior aspect and a flat or concave anterior

aspect. Approximately 2–6 cm proximal to the insertion is an area of relative hypovascularity.[1]

The Achilles tendon is covered by a double-layered connective tissue membrane or paratenon. It is not a true sheath, since it has no synovium. The paratenon is very vascular and provides blood supply to the tendon.[2] Anterior to the tendon, Kager's fat pad separates the Achilles tendon from the flexor hallucis longus. Just proximal to the Achilles insertion in the posterior calcaneus, the retrocalcaneal bursa lies anterior to the tendon. Along the medial border of the Achilles, the long thin plantaris tendon is found in 90% of individuals. The sural nerve and saphenous vein are located on the lateral aspect of the Achilles tendon[1] (Figure 91-1).

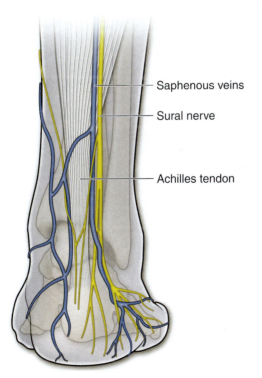
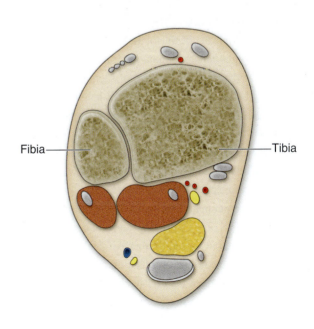

Saphenous veins

Sural nerve

Achilles tendon

Fibia

Tibia

FIGURE 91-1 ■ Posterior ankle anatomy: Achilles tendon (Ach), paratenon (P), Kager's fat pad (KF), plantaris tendon (Pl), sural nerve (Sn), saphenous vein (Sv), flexor hallucis longus muscle and tendon (FHL), tibial nerve (Tn), tibial artery and nerves (Ta), flexor digitorum longus tendon (FDL), posterior tibialis tendon (PT), peroneus longus tendon (PL), peroneus brevis muscle and tendon (PB), Tibia (Tib), and fibula (Fib).

Common Pathology

The Achilles tendon is susceptible to injury from overuse. These overuse injuries are very common in runners. Chronic tendinopathies can affect the tendon by itself, or in combination with adjacent tissues; for example, tendinopathy with paratenonitis or insertional tendinopathy and retrocalcaneal bursitis. Paratenonitis can be caused by overuse and biomechanical factors and is often seen in conjunction with tendinopathies. It may also be caused by seronegative arthritis and infections.[2]

Chronic tendinopathy of the Achilles tendon usually occurs in the proximal two-thirds. Occasionally, it occurs at the tendon insertion into the calcaneus.[3] Clinically, the patient reports pain and reduced performance. On examination, tendon thickening can be observed. Tendon gaps or defects must be evaluated, which would suggest a tendon tear.

Histological findings of chronic tendinopathy can include disorganized collagen fibers, increase in ground substance, and neovascularity.[4] Although there is no evidence of cellular inflammation in chronic tendinopathy, inflammation may play a role in early phases of tendinopathy.[5] The histologic changes in peritendinosis consist of fibrinous exudate, fibroblastic proliferation, and inflammatory cell infiltrate.[2]

Ultrasound Imaging Findings

The Achilles tendon and paratenon are best visualized in both long and short axis using a high-frequency linear array transducer and a depth of 1–2 cm. The depth may need to be adjusted if there is pathologic thickening of the tendon. The ankle should be placed in slight dorsiflexion, to place tension on the tendon fibers and avoid anisotropy because of sagging of the tendon. Care should be taken to evaluate the full length and width of the tendon, from the myotendinous junction to its insertion on the posterior calcaneus, in both long-axis and cross-sectional views. This will ensure that no focal zones of pathology will be missed. Contralateral side comparison should always be done.

Normal findings show the normal fibrillar pattern of the tendon with the paratenon seen as a slightly more echogenic rim. The thickness of the tendon varies with body habitus and individual height, but should be approximately 5–6 mm.[6] The fibers at the calcaneal insertion take on an oblique angle, so the probe angle needs to be adjusted to eliminate anisotropy. A common pitfall is to mistake this anisotropy with insertional tendinopathy (Figure 91-2).

Common pathologic findings of tendinopathy include increased interfibrillar distance (hypoechoic tendon appearance) and tendon thickening (Figure 91-3). Complete, partial

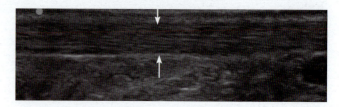

FIGURE 91-2 ■ Normal Achilles tendon (between *white arrows*).

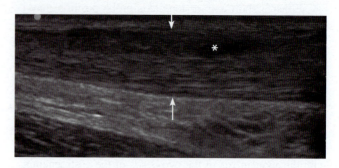

FIGURE 91-3 ■ Achilles tendinopathy: Achilles tendon (*white arrows*); area of tendinopathy (*asterisk*).

tears and full-thickness partial tears can be identified by gaps or fibrillar pattern interruption (Figure 91-4). Findings consistent with paratenonitis include irregular tendon margins, peritendinous effusion, and edema of the pre-Achilles tendon fat pad adjacent to the tendon (Figure 91-5).

Indications for Injections of the Achilles Paratenon

Injections of the Achilles paratenon can be performed in patients with inflammatory paratenonitis (seronegative arthritis) or patients with chronic Achilles tendinopathy not responsive to relative rest and physical therapy including modalities, stretching, and eccentric strengthening of the gastrocnemius-soleus complex. Whether corticosteroids should be injected into the Achilles paratenon is controversial.[7] Some authors argue that paratenon injections ultrasonography ensures that the corticosteroid is not injected intratendon, thus reducing risk of tendon rupture.[8] Other injectates described in the literature for treatment of Achilles tendinopathy and paratenonitis include: platelet-rich plasma and prolotherapy.

In a cadaveric study by Reach and Easley, 10 paratenons were injected with Indian-blue dye under sonography and later dissected, showing 100% injection accuracy with ultrasound.[9] To this author's knowledge, there are no studies on the accuracy of unguided paratenon injections.

Equipment

- Needle: 27-gauge, 1.25-inch needle or 25-gauge, 1.5-inch needle
- Injectate
  - 2–3.5 mL of a local anesthetic
  - 0.5–2 mL of an injectable corticosteroid
- High-frequency linear array transducer

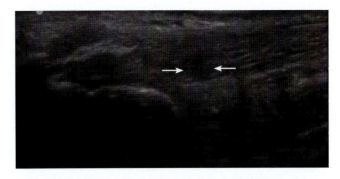

FIGURE 91-4 ■ Achilles tendon tear (between *white arrows*).

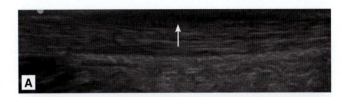

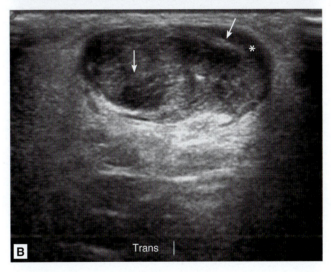

FIGURE 91-5 ■ Paratenonitis: **A.** Sagittal view of Achilles tendon with paratenonitis (*white arrow*). **B.** Short-axis view of Achilles tendinopathy with paratenonitis (*white asterisk*).

Author's Preferred Technique

a. Patient position (Figure 91-6)
   i. Prone
   ii. Foot hanging over edge of table
b. Transducer position 1
   i. Anatomic short-axis plane over Achilles tendon (cross-sectional view of tendon)
c. Needle orientation relative to transducer
   i. In plane
d. Needle approach
   i. Lateral to medial
e. Target (Figure 91-7)
   i. Anterior to paratenon (between paratenon and posterior Achilles tendon)
f. Pearls and Pitfalls
   i. Avoid the sural nerve and saphenous vein, which lie lateral to the Achilles tendon. Identify these prior to injection and maintain the needle posterior to the Achilles tendon. Alternatively, approach from medial to lateral, but be careful of the tibial nerve and artery posterior to the medial malleolus.
   ii. This is the author's preferred technique, because the needle is perfectly parallel to transducer and to the paratenon plane. This allows excellent visualization of the needle and reduces the risk of injecting the tendon itself.

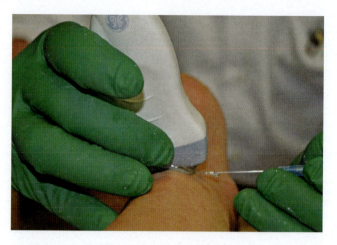

FIGURE 91-6 ■ Patient position, transducer position, and needle orientation: patient prone with foot slightly dorsiflexed over edge of examination table, transducer in anatomic short-axis plane and needle in plane with transducer from lateral to medial.

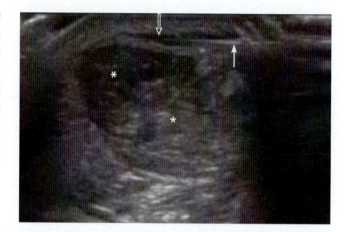

FIGURE 91-7 ■ Achilles paratenon injection short-axis approach: needle (*arrow*), paratenon (*open arrow*), short-axis view of Achilles tendon (*asterisk*), area of tendinopathy (*asterisk*).

Alternate Technique

a. Patient position
    i. Prone
    ii. Foot hanging over edge of table
b. Transducer position 2 (Figure 91-8)
    i. Anatomic sagittal plane over Achilles tendon (long axis over tendon)
c. Needle orientation relative to transducer
    i. In plane
d. Needle approach
    i. Proximal to distal
e. Target (Figure 91-9)
    i. Anterior to paratenon (between paratenon and posterior Achilles tendon)
f. Pearls and Pitfalls
    i. Because of the needle and syringe being in plane with the leg, there will be difficulties with the entry angle between needle and plane of paratenon. The needle can be bent at the hub to assist with this. Care must be taken to avoid going too deep and injecting within the tendon.

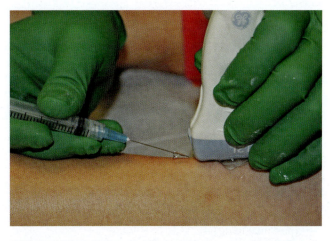

FIGURE 91-8 ▪ Patient position and transducer position and needle orientation: patient prone with foot slightly dorsiflexed over edge of examination table, transducer in anatomic sagittal plane and needle in plane with transducer.

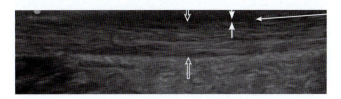

FIGURE 91-9 ▪ Achilles paratenon injection sagittal approach: Needle representation (*long arrow*), paratenon (*small arrows*), Achilles tendon (*open arrows*).

References

1. Martinolli C, Bianchi S. Ankle. In: Bianchi S, Martinolli C. *Ultrasound of the Musculoskeletal System.* 1st ed. Berlin: Springer; 2007:771–834.
2. Pierre-Jerome C, Moncayo V, Terk MR. MRI of the Achilles tendon: a comprehensive review of the anatomy, biomechanics, and imaging of overuse tendinopathies. *Acta Radiol* 2010 May;51(4):438–454.
3. Gibbon WW, Cooper JR, Radcliffe GS. Distribution of sonographically detected tendon abnormalities in patients with a clinical diagnosis of chronic Achilles tendinosis. *J Clin Ultrasound* 2000 Feb;28(2):61–66.
4. Maffulli N, Barrass V, Ewen SW. Light microscopic histology of Achilles tendon ruptures. A comparison with unruptured tendons. *Am J Sports Med* 2000;28:857–863.
5. Maffulli N, Sharma P, Luscombe LJ. Achilles tendinopathy: aetiology and management. *J R Soc Med* 2004;97:472–476.
6. Van Holsbeeck MT, Introcaso JH, *Musculoskeletal ultrasound.* St. Louis: Mosby-Year Book; 1991:1–327.
7. Speed CA. Corticosteroid injections in tendon lesions. *BMJ* 2001;323:382–386.
8. Wijesekera NT, Chew NS, Lee JC, et al. Ultrasound-guided treatments for chronic Achilles tendinopathy: an update and current status [Review]. *Skeletal Radiol* 2010 May;39(5):425–434. Epub February 1, 2010.
9. Reach JS, Easley ME, Chuckpaiwong B, Nunley JA 2nd. Accuracy of ultrasound guided injections in the foot and ankle. *Foot Ankle Int* 2009 Mar;30(3):239–242.

Bradley D. Fullerton, MD

KEY POINTS

- Use a high-frequency linear array transducer.
- Use a 21–27-gauge, 1.25–2-inch needle.
- The needle approach is at proximal two-thirds, short axis, and in plane (medial to lateral).
- The needle approach at insertion is long axis and in plane (proximal to distal).

- More than 80% of abnormal findings (ie, degeneration) are seen in the proximal two-thirds of the tendon.
- Major pitfall: The sural nerve lies lateral to the tendon may limit treatment effectiveness.

Pertinent Anatomy

The Achilles tendon is the longest (10–12 cm), thickest (5–6 mm), and strongest tendon in the body. The tendon is enveloped by paratenon (not a synovial sheath) medially, laterally, and dorsally. The sural nerve borders the lateral, proximal portion of the Achilles tendon (Figure 92-1).

Common Pathology

The Achilles tendon is relatively hypovascular 2–6 cm proximal to its insertion at the calcaneus; this is the most common location of tendinopathy and rupture related to tendon degeneration. Although tears are uncommon at the calcaneal insertion, tendinopathy can be seen in association with retrocalcaneal

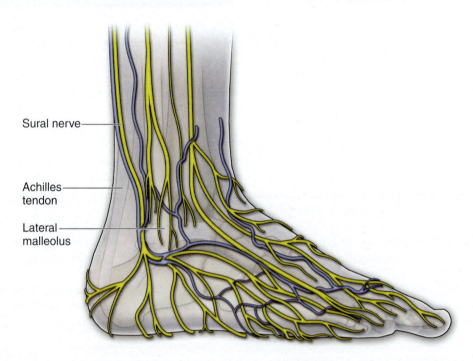

Sural nerve

Achilles tendon

Lateral malleolus

FIGURE 92-1 ■ Lateral view of the relationship between the sural nerve and Achilles tendon. The nerve courses from posterior to anterior near the soleus musculotendinous junction.

bursitis (ie, Haglund's deformity). The Achilles tendon is the most frequently involved tendon in metabolic disorders such as gout and hypercholesterolemia. Metabolic causes should be considered before injection, especially in bilateral disease.

Ultrasound Imaging Findings

The Achilles tendon should be visualized in long and short axis using a high-frequency linear array transducer at a frequency of 8–18 MHz and depth of 2–3 cm. Tendon fibers curve as they approach the calcaneal insertion resulting in anisotropy. Common pathologic findings include hypoechogenicity, thickening, heterogenous echotexture, loss of fibrillar pattern, neovascularization entering the tendon from the ventral surface, and tears within the proximal two-thirds of the tendon (Figure 92-2). Disruption of the dorsal surface of the tendon with high-power color Doppler flow near the disruption has been associated with partial ruptures.[6] Complete ruptures appear as focal defects in the tendon with intact paratenon. Acoustic shadowing at the torn ends of the tendon, increased through transmission at the defect and fat herniation into the defect can also be seen in complete rupture. At the distal tendon, tendinopathy involves the deep portion and is usually associated with retrocalcaneal bursitis.[1] Enthesophytes, seen as hyperechoic foci or linear array signal with posterior acoustic shadowing, are common at the calcaneal insertion.

Indications for Percutaneous Tenotomy, Fenestration, and Injection of the Achilles Tendon

Percutaneous treatment with tenotomy, intratendinous injection, extratendinous injection, or a combination of these can be performed for patients with recalcitrant pain that is unresponsive to activity modification, nonsteroidal antiinflammatory drugs (NSAIDs), orthotic treatment, stretching, and physical therapy.[6] A systematic review of randomized controlled trials (RCTs) found no benefit of corticosteroid injection for Achilles tendinopathy.[2] An RCT showed no additional benefit of one platelet-rich plasma (PRP) injection versus saline injection in a population that had not failed eccentric training prior to injection.[3] A 6–12-week eccentric training program should be tried for noninsertional Achilles tendinopathy prior to injection therapy.[4] Yelland et al. found that palpation-guided extratendinous injection of dextrose combined with eccentric exercise provided more rapid recovery of function than exercise or injection alone.[5]

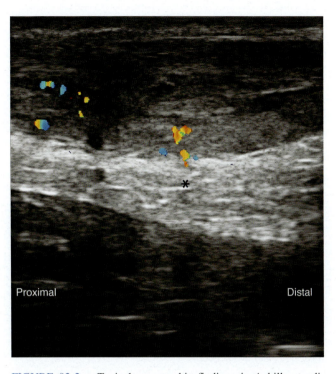

Proximal   Distal

FIGURE 92-2 ■ Typical sonographic findings in Achilles tendinosis. The tendon is thickened with loss of normal fibrillar pattern, diffuse hypoechoic signal, and neovascularization. The *asterisk* is located in Kager's fat pad deep to a neovessel entering the ventral surface of the tendon.

Multiple ultrasound-guided injection techniques for chronic Achilles tendinopathy have been reported in case series and small randomized trials. For noninsertional disease, a series of sonography-guided sclerosing injections of abnormal neovessels at the ventral tendon using polidocanol were effective in 19 of 20 consecutive patients in a RCT crossover design study.[6] A series of sonography-guided, intratendinous injections of 25% dextrose (ie, prolotherapy) in 108 consecutive tendons (with midbody and/or insertional disease) resulted in significant improvements in pain as measured by a visual analog scale at rest, with activities of daily living, and with sport.[7] Clinical improvement was sustained for a year or more in both the polidocanol and dextrose studies. Finnoff et al. reported success with percutaneous needle tenotomy using 18–19-gauge needles followed by PRP.[8] Neither dextrose nor PRP injections for Achilles tendinopathy unresponsive to eccentric exercise have been studied in and RCT. Clinical outcomes of nonguided versus guided injection have not been described.

Midbody Achilles Tendinopathy

Equipment

■ Needle
- 27-gauge, 1.25-inch needle (for dextrose)
- 25-gauge, 1.5-inch needle (for PRP)

■ Injectate
- 2–4 mL 25% dextrose and 0.5% local anesthetic OR
- 2–4 mL autologous PRP (delivered in multiple locations; approximately 0.5 mL per location)

■ High-frequency linear array transducer

Author's Preferred Technique

a. Patient position (Figure 92-3)
   i. Prone
   ii. Foot hanging off table
b. Transducer position
   i. Anatomic axial plane, short axis to tendon
c. Needle orientation relative to the transducer
   i. In plane
d. Needle approach (Figures 92-3 and 92-4)
   i. Medial to lateral
   ii. Skin entry parallel to probe
e. Target
   i. Region of hypoechoic-heterogenous echotexture, thickening, neovessels, and/or anechoic tears within midbody Achilles tendon

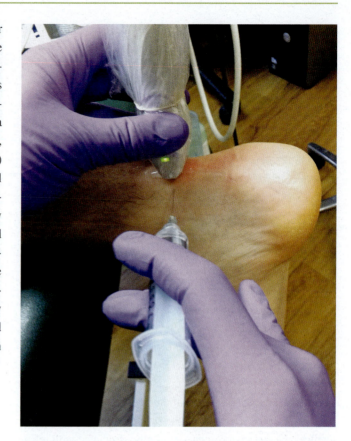

FIGURE 92-3 ■ Medial view of right ankle. Patient, transducer, and needle position for proximal Achilles tendinopathy fenestration and injection.

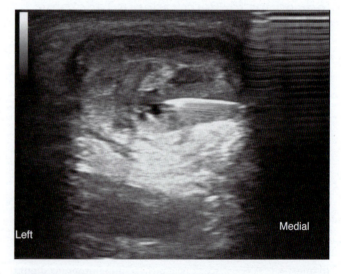

FIGURE 92-4 ■ Short-axis view of Achilles tendinopathy. The needle approaches in plane with the probe from medial to lateral. The needle bevel is seen approaching a round anechoic structure, likely a neovessel.

f. Pearls and Pitfalls
  i. The preinjection of 1–2 mL 1% lidocaine via a 30-gauge, 1-inch needle improves tolerance for anxious patients.

Alternate Technique

a. Patient position (see Figure 92-3)
  i. Prone
  ii. Foot hanging off table
b. Transducer position
  i. Anatomic axial plane, short axis to tendon
c. Needle orientation relative to the transducer
  i. Out of plane
d. Needle approach (Figures 92-5 and 92-6)
  i. Distal to proximal or proximal to distal
  ii. Use walk-down technique
e. Target
  i. Region of hypoechoic-heterogenous echotexture, thickening and/or anechoic tears within midbody Achilles tendon

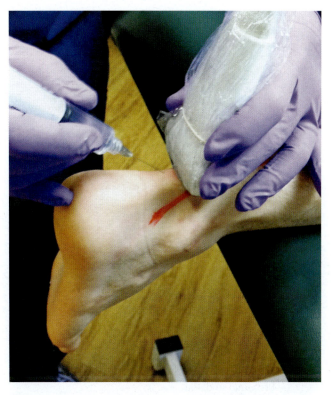

FIGURE 92-5 ▪ Lateral view of right ankle. Alternate technique for Achilles fenestration and injection with out-of-plane needle approach. The *red line* indicates the actual course of the sural nerve seen on sonography in this patient.

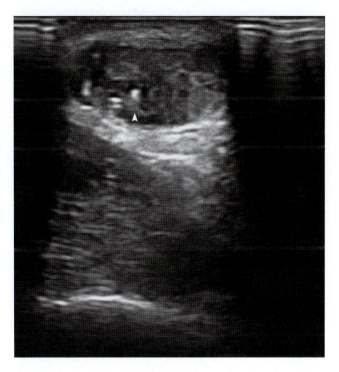

FIGURE 92-6 ▪ Short-axis view of Achilles tendinopathy with out-of-plane needle approach. The needle tip is seen as hyperechoic dot just superior to the *arrowhead*. Kager's fat pad is hyperechoic layer deep to the *arrowhead* and flexor hallucis longus muscle is deep to Kager's fat pad.

Insertional Achilles Tendinopathy

Equipment

- Needle
  - 25-gauge, 2-inch needle (for dextrose or PRP)
  - 18–21-gauge, 2–3-inch needle (for needle tenotomy)
- Injectate
  - 2-4 mL 25% dextrose and 0.5 % lidocaine OR
  - 2-4 mL autologous PRP (delivered in multiple locations; 0.5–1 mL per location)

Author's Preferred Technique

a. Patient position
  i. Prone
  ii. Foot hanging off table
b. Transducer position
  i. Anatomic sagittal plane, long axis to tendon
c. Needle orientation relative to the transducer
  i. In plane
d. Needle approach (Figures 92-7 and 92-8)
  i. Proximal to distal
  ii. Skin entry 20–30 degrees from parallel to probe
e. Target
  i. Region of calcification, hypoechoic-heterogenous echotexture, thickening, and/or anechoic tears at the Achilles tendon insertion into the calcaneus
f. Pearls and Pitfalls
  i. The preinjection of 1–2 mL 1% lidocaine via 30-gauge, 1-inch needle is mandatory before tenotomy.
  ii. Calcification and enthesophytes require more fenestration using larger gauge needles (18–19 gauge).

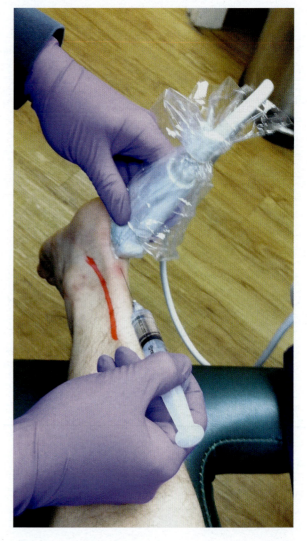

FIGURE 92-7 ■ Patient, transducer, and needle position for treatment of insertional Achilles tendinopathy. Dorsal view of the lateral, right ankle with course of the sural nerve in *red*.

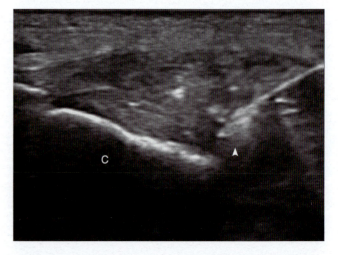

FIGURE 92-8 ■ Long-axis view of insertional Achilles tendinopathy tenotomy. The *arrowhead* points to the bevel of an 18-gauge needle. C, calcaneal enthesis of the Achilles tendon.

Alternate Technique

a. Patient position
   i. Prone
   ii. Foot hanging off table
b. Transducer position
   i. Anatomic axial plane, short axis to tendon
c. Needle orientation relative to the transducer
   i. Out of plane
d. Needle approach (Figure 92-9)
   i. Proximal to distal
   ii. Use walk-down technique
e. Target
   i. Region of calcification, hypoechoic-heterogenous echotexture, thickening, and/or anechoic tears at the Achilles tendon insertion into the calcaneus
f. Pearls and Pitfalls
   i. The preinjection of 1–2 mL 1% lidocaine via 30-gauge, 1-inch needle is mandatory before tenotomy.
   ii. Calcification and enthesophytes require more fenestration using larger gauge needles (18–19 gauge).

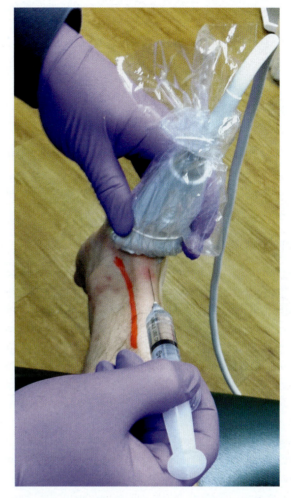

FIGURE 92-9 ■ Alternate technique for treatment of insertional Achilles tendinopathy. Transducer is short axis to the tendon insertion with out-of-plane needle approach.

References

1. Gibbon WW, Cooper JR, Radcliffe GS. Distribution of sonographically detected tendon abnormalities in patients with a clinical diagnosis of chronic Achilles tendinosis. *J Clin Ultrasound* 2000;28(2):61–66.
2. Coombes BK, Bisset L, Vicenzino B. Efficacy and safety of corticosteroid injections and other injections for management of tendinopathy: a systematic review of randomised controlled trials. *Lancet* 2010;376(9754):1751–1767.
3. de Vos RJ, Weir A, van Schie HTM, et al. Platelet-rich plasma injection for chronic Achilles tendinopathy: a randomized controlled trial. *JAMA* 2010;303(2):144–149.
4. Shalabi A, Kristoffersen-Wilberg M, Svensson L, et al. Eccentric training of the gastrocnemius-soleus complex in chronic Achilles tendinopathy results in decreased tendon volume and intratendinous signal as evaluated by MRI. *Am J Sports Med* 2004;32(5):1286–1296.
5. Yelland MJ, Sweeting KR, Lyftogt JA, et al. Prolotherapy injections and eccentric loading exercises for painful Achilles tendinosis: a randomised trial. *Br J Sports Med* 2011;45(5):421–428.
6. Alfredson H, Ohberg L. Sclerosing injections to areas of neovascularisation reduce pain in chronic Achilles tendinopathy: a double-blind randomised controlled trial. *Knee Surg Sports Traumatol Arthrosc* 2005;13(4):338–344.
7. Ryan M, Wong A, Taunton J. Favorable outcomes after sonographically guided intratendinous injection of hyperosmolar dextrose for chronic insertional and midportion Achilles tendinosis. *AJR Am J Roentgenol* 2010;194(4):1047–1053.
8. Alfredson H, Masci L, Ohberg L. Partial mid-portion Achilles tendon ruptures: new sonographic findings helpful for diagnosis. *Br J Sports Med* 2011;45(5):429–432.
9. Finnoff JT, Fowler SP, Lai JK, et al. Treatment of chronic tendinopathy with ultrasound-guided needle tenotomy and platelet-rich plasma injection. *PM R* 2011;3(10):900–911.
10. Alfredson H, Cook J. A treatment algorithm for managing Achilles tendinopathy: new treatment options. *Br J Sports Med* 2007;41(4):211–216.

Mandy Huggins, MD / Gerard A. Malanga, MD

Pertinent Anatomy

The retrocalcaneal bursa lies in the posterior ankle between the posterior calcaneus and distal Achilles tendon. Anatomically speaking, the calcaneus, the Achilles tendon insertion on the calcaneus, and the retrocalcaneal bursa are very intimately related (Figure 93-1). Kager's fat pad lies superior to the posterior calcaneus and anterior to the Achilles tendon. The sural nerve is also located in the posterior ankle, between the Achilles tendon and the lateral malleolus. It is a cutaneous sensory nerve that supplies the skin of the posterolateral aspect of the distal third of the leg and the lateral aspect of the dorsal foot and fifth digit. The sural nerve is accompanied by the small saphenous vein.

The retrocalcaneal bursa can occasionally be seen on ultrasound in asymptomatic individuals and is considered to be normal if its anteroposterior diameter measures less than 2.5–3 mm.[1,2] It may change shape with plantarflexion and dorsiflexion of the ankle.[2]

Common Pathology

Retrocalcaneal bursitis can be isolated, but can also be associated with inflammatory disorders or chronic trauma. A prominence on the posterolateral calcaneus (often referred to a Haglund's deformity) can lead to mechanical irritation of the tendon insertion and the bursa. One must distinguish between a Haglund's deformity and Haglund's disease, which is a clinical picture of a painful retrocalcaneal bursa, insertional Achilles tendinopathy, a Haglund's deformity, and sometimes retro-Achilles bursitis.[3] When inflamed, the bursa will appear as an enlarged, comma-shaped hypoechoic structure between the Achilles tendon and the calcaneus. Hypervascularity and thickening of the distal Achilles tendon may be seen.[1,2]

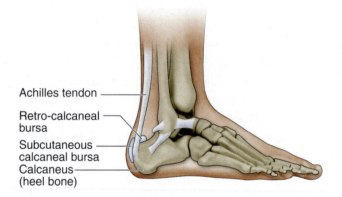

Achilles tendon
Retro-calcaneal bursa
Subcutaneous calcaneal bursa
Calcaneus (heel bone)

FIGURE 93-1 ■ Retrocalcaneal anatomy.

Indications for Injection

Pain can persist despite other conservative treatment (ice, nonsteroidal antiinflammatory drugs, orthotics, heel pads, physical therapy modalities) for this condition. A retrocalcaneal bursa injection with local anesthetic and steroid should be considered before surgical excision of the bursa. Ultrasound guidance for this procedure has been described and may improve clinical outcome versus palpation-guided injections,[4–6] although exact accuracy of guided and unguided injections has not been studied. Steroid injection is contraindicated if septic bursitis is suspected. The Achilles tendon should be avoided.

Equipment

- Needle: 25-gauge, 1.5-inch needle
- Injectate
  - 0.5 mL local anesthetic
  - 0.5 mL injectable corticosteroid
- High-frequency linear array transducer

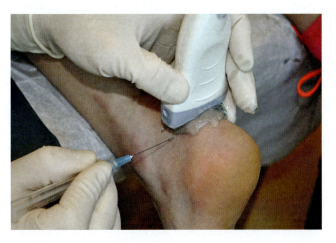

FIGURE 93-2 ■ Transducer position and needle approach to retrocalcaneal bursa.

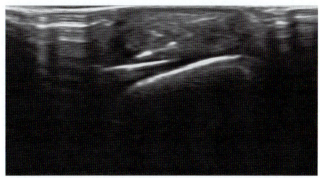

FIGURE 93-3 ■ Ultrasound image of needle approach to retrocalcaneal bursa.

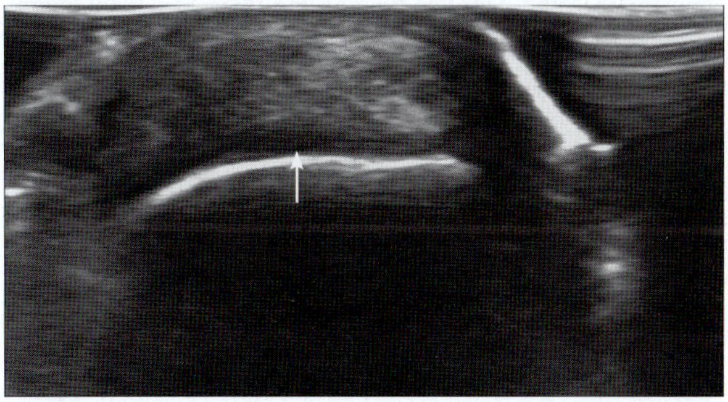

FIGURE 93-4 ■ Ultrasound image of the retrocalcaneal bursa on short axis deep to Achilles tendon (*arrow*).

Author's Preferred Technique

a. Patient position
    i.   Prone
    ii. Foot off edge of table to allow neutral flexion
b. Transducer position
    i.   Transducer in short-axis plane (Figure 93-2)
c. Needle orientation relative to the transducer
    i.   In plane
d. Needle approach
    i.   Lateral to medial (Figure 93-3)
e. Target
    i.   Hypoechoic structure between the Achilles tendon and the calcaneus (Figure 93-4)
f. Pearls and Pitfalls
    i.   Avoid injecting the Achilles tendon
    ii. Avoid the sural nerve

References

1. Jacobson, JA. In: *Fundamentals of Musculoskeletal Ultrasound*. Philadelphia, PA: Saunders; 2007:282–294.
2. Bianchi S, Martinoli C. In: *Ultrasound of the Musculoskeletal System*. Berlin Heidelberg: Springer; 2007:774–834.
3. Alfredson H, Cook J. In: Brukner P, Khan K. *Clinical Sports Medicine*. 3rd rev. ed. Spring Hill, Australia: McGraw-Hill; 2009: 605–606.
4. Sofka CM, Adler, RS, Positano R, et al. Haglund's syndrome: diagnosis and treatment using sonography. *HSS J* 2006 Feb;2(1):27–29.
5. Brophy DP, Cunnane F, Fitzgerald O, Gibney RG. Technical report: ultrasound guidance for injection of soft tissue lesions around the heel in chronic inflammatory arthritis. *Clin Radiol* 1995;50: 120–122.
6. Checa A, Chun W, Pappu R. Ultrasound-guided diagnostic and therapeutic approach to retrocalcaneal bursitis. *J Rheumatol* 2011; 38:391–392.

Mandy Huggins, MD / Gerard A. Malanga, MD

KEY POINTS

- Use a 25-gauge, 1.5-inch needle.
- Use a high-frequency linear array transducer in short-axis plane.
- The retro-Achilles bursa is not visualized in normal states.
- Use a long-axis, in-plane, medial-to-lateral approach.

Pertinent Anatomy

The retro-Achilles bursa is located in the posterior ankle, superficial to the Achilles tendon and deep to subcutaneous tissue (Figure 94-1) and is not visualized on ultrasound in normal states.[1,2] The sural nerve and saphenous vein are also located in the posterior ankle, between the Achilles tendon and the lateral malleolus. This cutaneous, sensory nerve supplies the skin of the posterolateral aspect of the distal third of the leg and the lateral aspect of the dorsal foot and fifth digit.

Common Pathology

Retro-Achilles bursitis is usually a result of local mechanical irritation, usually from footwear, or Haglund's disease. This bursitis is seen on ultrasound as a localized fluid collection

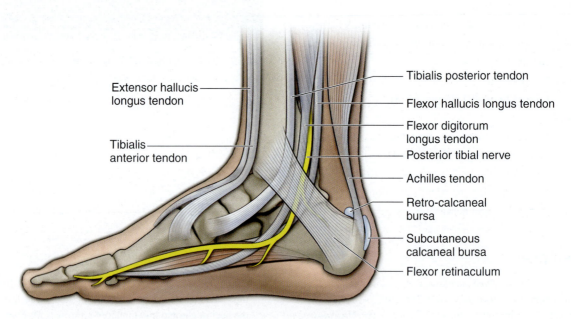

Extensor hallucis longus tendon

Tibialis anterior tendon

Tibialis posterior tendon

Flexor hallucis longus tendon

Flexor digitorum longus tendon

Posterior tibial nerve

Achilles tendon

Retro-calcaneal bursa

Subcutaneous calcaneal bursa

Flexor retinaculum

FIGURE 94-1 ■ Anatomy of retro-Achilles bursa.

within the subcutaneous tissue superficial to the Achilles tendon (Figure 94-2). Hypervascularity may also be seen. Care should be taken not use excessive pressure with the transducer, as the bursa can easily be compressed.[2]

Indications for Injection

Injection of the retro-Achilles bursa can be performed for patients with pain that is recalcitrant to shoe modification, ice, and nonsteroidal antiinflammatory drugs. It is reasonable to consider this therapeutic option before surgery.[3,4] The accuracy of palpation-guided and ultrasound-guided injections of the retro-Achilles bursa has not been studied. Steroid injection is contraindicated if septic bursitis is suspected. The Achilles tendon should be avoided.

Equipment

- Needle: 25-gauge, 1.5-inch needle
- Injectate
  - 0.5 mL injectable corticosteroid
  - 0.5 mL local anesthetic
- High-frequency linear array transducer

Author's Preferred Technique

a. Patient position
   i. Prone
   ii. Foot off edge of table to allow neutral flexion
b. Transducer position
   i. Transducer in short-axis plane (Figure 94-3)
c. Needle orientation relative to the transducer
   i. In plane
d. Needle approach
   i. Lateral to medial (Figure 94-4)
e. Target
   i. Superficial to the Achilles tendon
f. Pearls and Pitfalls
   i. Avoid injecting the Achilles tendon.
   ii. Avoid the sural nerve.

References

1. Jacobson, JA. In: *Fundamentals of Musculoskeletal Ultrasound*. Philadelphia, PA: Saunders; 2007:282–294.
2. Bianchi S, Martinoli C. In: *Ultrasound of the Musculoskeletal System*. Berlin Heidelberg: Springer; 2007:774–834.
3. Alfredson H, Cook J. In: Brukner P, Khan K. *Clinical Sports Medicine*. 3rd rev. ed. Spring Hill, Australia: McGraw-Hill; 2009:605–606.
4. Fessell DP, Jacobson JA. Ultrasound of the hindfoot and midfoot. *Radiol Clin North Am* 2008 Nov;46(6):1027–1043.

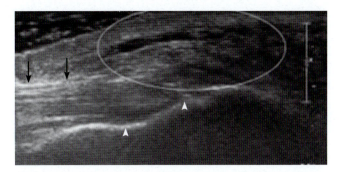

FIGURE 94-2 ■ Ultrasound image of long axis of retro-Achilles bursa. Superficial portion of Achilles tendon (*black arrows*) and deep portion of the tendon (*white arrow heads*) with retro-Achilles region circled.

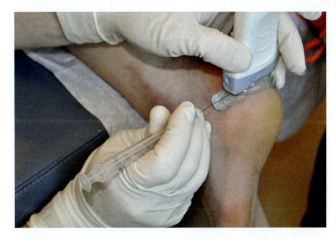

FIGURE 94-3 ■ Approach to ultrasound-guided injection of retro-Achilles bursa.

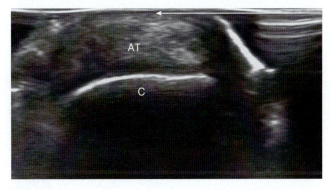

FIGURE 94-4 ■ Ultrasound view short axis to the Achilles tendon, demonstrating in-plane needle approach (*white arrow*) to the retro-Achilles region, superficial to the Achilles tendon. AT, achilles tendon; C, calcaneus.

Christopher J. Visco, MD

KEY POINTS

- Use a high-frequency linear array transducer.
- Use a 25- or 27-gauge, 1.5-inch needle, in plane for tendon sheath injection.
- Use a 19- or 20-gauge, 2-inch needle, in plane for tendon fenestration.

- Identify associated structures including flexor retinaculum and accessory navicular.
- Pitfalls include not adequately pre-scanning for the neurovascular structures.
- Use a standoff approach from anterior to posterior for tendon sheath injection.

Pertinent Anatomy

The tibialis posterior tendon is an extension of its associated muscle in the deep compartment, which originates from the interosseus membrane, posterior tibia, and fibula. The long myotendinous junction of the bipennate muscle extends to a few centimeters above the medial malleolus. The flexor retinaculum helps to constrain the tendon against the shallow retromalleolar groove as it becomes the most medial and superficial structure travelling with the flexor digitorum longus, flexor hallucis longus, and neurovascular bundle (Figure 95-1). The tibialis posterior muscle and tendon are most elongated during the terminal stance phase of gate when the foot is in full pronation (plantarflexion, adduction, and inversion). As the muscle contracts, the medial longitudinal arch forms, and subsequent rigidity is conferred to the foot. The distal tendon courses anterior to the sustentaculum tali and subsequently has a broad and complex attachment, which dynamically supports the medial longitudinal arch. The tendon divides less than 2 cm proximal to the navicular, and then further distally, with insertions on the navicular, cuboid, cuneiforms, and metatarsals 2, 3, and 4.[1] A portion of the flexor hallucis brevis attaches to the plantar cuneometarsal extension of the tibialis posterior tendon. The tendon sheath, which may contain a small amount of physiologic fluid extends distally to the first tendon division. An accessory navicular may be seen in approximately 5%, located at just proximal to the navicular, and can be confused with an avulsion fracture or calcific tendinopathy.

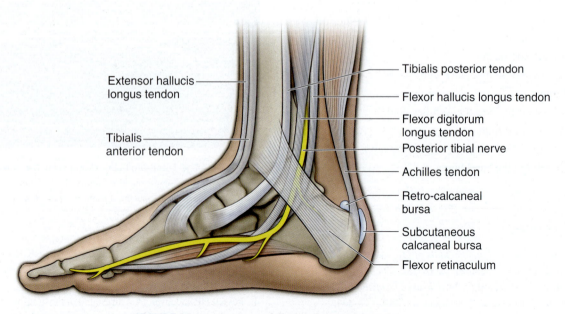

Extensor hallucis longus tendon

Tibialis anterior tendon

Tibialis posterior tendon

Flexor hallucis longus tendon

Flexor digitorum longus tendon

Posterior tibial nerve

Achilles tendon

Retro-calcaneal bursa

Subcutaneous calcaneal bursa

Flexor retinaculum

FIGURE 95-1 ■ Anatomy of the tibialis posterior tendon.

Common Pathology

The tibialis posterior tendon is prone to developing tendon injury owing to its retromalleolar position, distal angulation, and high force transfer. Most commonly degenerative changes will occur either in the retromalleolar tendon or at the distal insertion on the navicular. Tendinopathic changes of the tibialis posterior tendon often occurs insidiously without direct trauma or injury. Focal degeneration or a longitudinal split-thickness tear can occur. An accessory navicular may be associated with aberrant anatomy of the distal portion of the tibialis posterior tendon and local degenerative changes. Repeated loading across the tendon may lead to inflammation, relative ischemia, tendinopathic changes, or subluxation. Tendinitis or tenosynovitis may occur acutely, particularly in association with lateral ankle injury, but this is less common than degenerative disease of the tibialis posterior tendon. Associated predisposing pathology may include systemic rheumatic disease or local factors such as subtalar joint osteoarthritis, flexor retinaculum thickening, or rupture. In patients with tibialis posterior dysfunction, the foot often remains flexible in a relatively pronated position and may present with a valgus hind foot and swelling over the medial ankle.

Ultrasound Imaging Findings

The tibialis posterior is best visualized in short axis using a high-frequency linear array transducer at a depth of 2–3 cm (the most superficial scanning occurs at the medial malleolus). Common findings include abnormal thickening of the tendon; irregularity of normal fibrillar architecture in short axis; relative hypoechoic appearance; increased diameter in short axis; fluid in or thickening of the tendon sheath (Figure 95-2). Fluid can best be appreciated just proximal or distal to the retromalleolar groove. Associated findings may include a thickened or ruptured flexor retinaculum or an accessory navicular that appears intratendinous and occur concomitantly with local tendon degenerative changes (not to be confused with a calcific tendinopathy). Tendon subluxation anteriorly over the medial malleolus may be tested dynamically with light pressure in short axis, the foot in a dorsiflexed position while resisting supination.

Indications

Injection of the tibialis posterior tendon sheath can be considered for patients with recalcitrant pain tendonitis or tenosynovitis that is unresponsive to rest, icing, nonsteroidal antiinflammatory drugs, bracing, orthotics, and adequate physical therapy. It may also be indicated in earlier intervention for acute inflammatory states, particularly when rapid return to activity is needed. Injection of the tibialis posterior tendon sheath has been described based on palpation (ie, unguided). The success rate of these unguided injections has been found to be 100% in one small study.[2] Ultrasound-guided injection has been described without discussion of success rates and no comparison to unguided injections.[3,4] Clinical outcomes of guided versus guided injection *has not* been described. There is no description of contraindications based on ultrasound findings, although injection of corticosteroid directly into a tendinopathy or a partial-thickness tear could predispose to tendon rupture.

Needle fenestration of the posterior tibialis tendon may be considered for those patients with a focus of tendinopathy that is recalcitrant to conservative care. Ultrasound findings that may help determine indications include thickening, hypoechoic tissue, irregularity, and tenderness to sonopalpation in a focal area of the tibialis posterior tendon. An intrasubstance calcification may also be observed and targeted for needle fenestration. There is no literature regarding the success rate of performing these procedures.

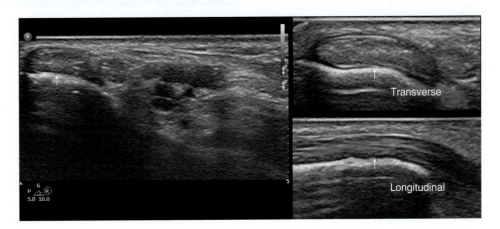

FIGURE 95-2 ▪ Ultrasound image of the tibialis posterior tendon: short- and long-axis views. Normal fluid around the tendon (*arrow*).

Tibialis Posterior Tendon Sheath Injection

Equipment

■ Needle: 25- or 27-gauge, 1.5-inch needle
■ Injectate
  • 2 mL of local anesthetic
  • 1 mL of injectable corticosteroid
■ High-frequency linear array transducer

Author's Preferred Technique

a. Patient position
   i. Anterior approach: Seated or supine with hip in external rotation and a small pillow or bolster under the lateral malleolus (Figure 95-3A)
   ii. Posterior approach: Same as anterior, or alternatively prone with foot off the end of plinth and slight hip internal rotation
b. Transducer position
   i. Short axis to the tendon in the anatomic axial position, posterior to the medial malleolus
c. Needle orientation relative to the transducer
   i. In plane
d. Needle approach
   i. Anterior to posterior (Figures 95-4A, B and 95-5A)
   ii. Posterior to anterior
e. Target
   i. Tendon sheath (not intratendinous)
f. Pearls and Pitfalls
   i. Identify and avoid the neurovascular bundle.
   ii. Identify an accessory navicular if present; do not confuse with intrasubstance calcification.
   iii. The anterior approach (anterior to posterior) is preferred and advantageous to avoid the neurovascular structures and allows for the shortest distance to the tendon. When using the anterior approach, it can help to use the standoff technique.
   iv. The posterior approach is helpful in certain situations, such as a deep retromalleolar groove or skin or positioning issues.

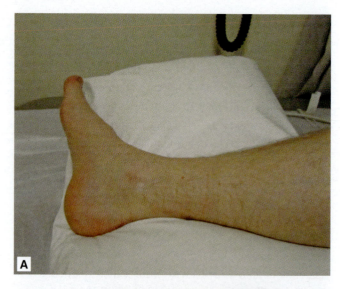

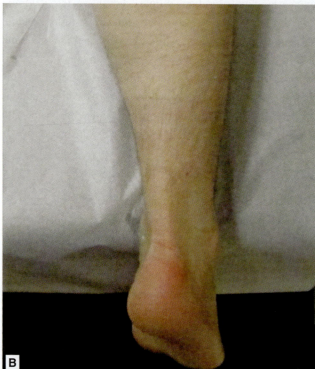

FIGURE 95-3 ■ Patient positioning for ultrasound-guided injection (**A**) and fenestration (**B**) of the tibialis posterior tendon.

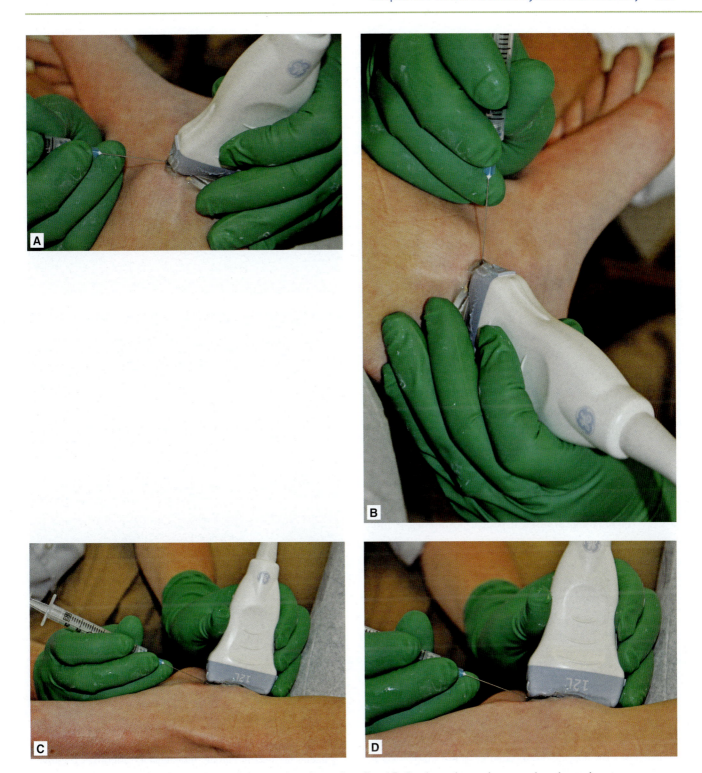

FIGURE 95-4 ■ **A** and **B**. In-plane, long-axis approach to the tendon. **C** and **D**. In-plane, short-axis approach to the tendon.

Tibialis Posterior Tendon Fenestration

Equipment

▪ Needle: 19- or 20-gauge, 2-inch needle
▪ Injectate
  • 2 mL of local anesthetic
  • 2 mL long-acting anesthetic
▪ High-frequency linear array transducer

Author's Preferred Technique

a. Patient position
   i. Prone with foot off the end of plinth and slight hip internal rotation; this position may be preferred for approaching distal pathology (Figure 95-3B).
   ii. Alternatively, seated or supine with hip in external rotation and a small pillow or bolster under the lateral malleolus, similar to the tendon sheath injection position.
b. Transducer position
   i. Long axis to the tendon in the anatomic coronal position, posterior to the medial malleolus, or distally at the navicular insertion
c. Needle orientation relative to the transducer
   i. In plane
d. Needle approach
   i. Distal to proximal (Figures 95-4C, D and 95-5B), or proximal to distal if patient positioning is more conducive
e. Target
   i. Intratendinous
f. Pearls and Pitfalls
   i. Identify and avoid neurovascular structures.
   ii. Identify an accessory navicular if present; do not confuse with intrasubstance calcification.

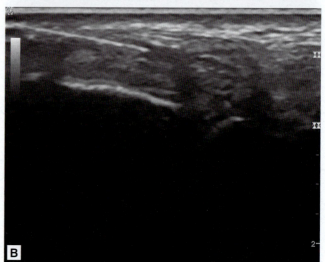

FIGURE 95-5 ▪ Ultrasound image of needle within tibialis posterior tendon sheath.

References

1. Pastore D, Dirim B, Wangwinyuvirat M, et al. Complex distal insertions of the tibialis posterior tendon: detailed anatomic and MR imaging investigation in cadavers. *Skelet Radiol* 2008;37(9):849–855.
2. Cooper AJ, Mizel MS, Patel PD, Steinmetz ND, Clifford PD. Comparison of MRI and local anesthetic tendon sheath injection in the diagnosis of posterior tibial tendon tenosynovitis. *Foot Ankle Int* 2007;28(11):1124–1127.
3. Brophy DP, Cunnane G, Fitzgerald O, Gibney RG. Technical report: ultrasound guidance for injection of soft tissue lesions around the heel in chronic inflammatory arthritis. *Clin Radiol* 1995;50(2):120–122.
4. Sofka CM, Adler RS. Ultrasound-guided interventions in the foot and ankle. *Semin Musculoskelet Radiol* 2002;06(2):163–168.

Johan Michaud, MD, FRCPC

KEY POINTS

- Use a 25-gauge, 1.5-inch needle.
- Use a high-frequency linear array transducer with a depth around 2 cm.
- Most pathologic cases are at the level of the ankle where the flexor hallucis longus (FHL) tendon can be identified between the posterior tubercles of the talus.

- Careful identification of the tibial posterior neurovascular bundle, located close to the FHL, is mandatory to avoid complication during this injection.
- At the ankle level, the in-plane approach with the entry point lateral to the Achilles tendon provides a safer approach with better needle visualization.

Pertinent Anatomy

The flexor hallucis longus (FHL) muscle is located deep in the posterior leg, anterior to the Achilles tendon. The strong FHL tendon reflects over the posterior aspect of the talus between its lateral and medial posterior tubercles and then it continues its course distally under the sustentaculum tali. At the ankle level, the FHL tendon is located in the tarsal tunnel, along with flexor digitorum longus (FDL) tendon, the tibialis posterior (TP) tendon, the posterior tibial artery and veins, and the tibial nerve. Distal to the sustentaculum tali, the FDL tendon crosses over the FHL tendon, at the so-called knot of Henry. In the distal sole, the FHL tendon passes between the hallux sesamoid bones to insert into the plantar aspect of the distal phalanx[1] (Figure 96-1).

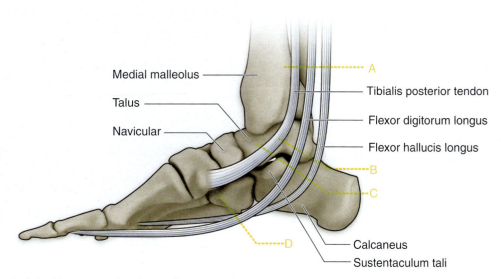

FIGURE 96-1 ■ Medial ankle anatomy showing the flexor hallucis longus tendon in relation to the retro malleolar area. *Yellow dotted lines* (A–D), probe positions for the ultrasound images of Figure 96-2A–D.

Common Pathology

Pathology can be located at three levels along the course of the FHL, but the most common is at the ankle level, being part of the posterior ankle syndrome.[2,3] FHL tenosynovitis at the ankle can also be the cause of a tarsal tunnel syndrome. It is well described in ballet dancers, runners, and those participating in jumping activities.[4,5] The pathology is usually a tenosynovitis of the FHL at the posterior talus level,[2,6] but partial or complete FHL rupture has also been also described.[7] Patients usually complain of a dull pain in the posteromedial ankle and arch of the foot that can mimic plantar fasciitis. It is usually secondary to mechanical overuse, but it can also be a sequela of a malleolus or calcaneus fracture[8] or secondary to an anatomical variant such as low inserted muscle fibbers on the FHL tendon. Rarely the pathology can be located more distally in the foot, either at the knot of Henry, creating an intersection syndrome with the FDL tendon[9] or at the level of the metatarsophalangeal (MTP) joint with a stenosing tenosynovitis of the FHL tendon at the sesamoid area.[10]

Ultrasound Imaging Finding

The FHL tendon is easily located on ultrasound using a short-axis scan in the medial retromalleolar area; it is located posterior to the TP and FDL tendons and deep to the tibial neurovascular bundle (Figure 96-2A). A good landmark is the cortical groove between the two tubercles of the posterior talus where the FHL is located (Figure 96-2B). Starting from the retromalleolar area, the FHL can be scanned distally, in short axis, passing below the sustentaculum tali (Figure 96-2C) and then crossing the FDL at the knot of Henry (Figure 96-2D) and, finally, in the sole of the foot until passing between the sesamoid bones of the hallux (see Figure 96-6B). The most common ultrasound pathologic finding will be tenosynovitis with fluid accumulation in the tendon sheath (Figure 96-3A).

Indications for FHL injection

FHL injection can be performed in nonresponders to conservative therapy. It can also be used as diagnostic test in unclear cases of posterior ankle pain. Unguided FHL tendon injection has been described but the success rate is unknown, and it is considered difficult because of the proximity of the tibial neurovascular bundle.[4,5,8] Ultrasound-guided FHL injection has been described with 100% accuracy.[8,11] Clinical outcomes of guided versus unguided technique are not known.

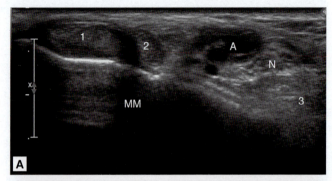

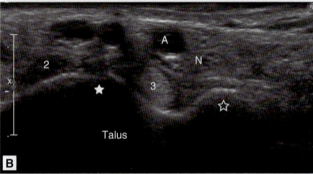

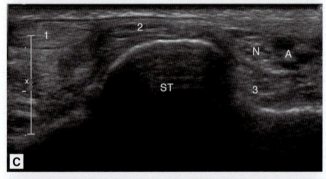

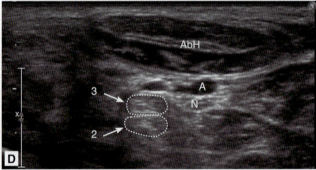

FIGURE 96-2 ■ **A–D.** Ultrasound images of normal flexor hallucis longus (FHL) tendon in short axis. See the *yellow lines* A–D in Figure 96-1 for the corresponding probe positions. 1, tibial posterior tendon; 2, flexor digitorum longus tendon; 3, flexor hallucis longs tendon; A, tibial posterior artery and veins; AbH, abductor hallucis muscle; Cal, calcaneus; MM, medial malleolus; N, tibial nerve; ST, sustentaculum tali; *void star*, posterolateral process of talus; *white star*, posteromedial process of talus.

Equipment

■ Needle: 25-gauge, 1.5-inch needle
■ Injectate
  • 1 mL of local anesthetic
  • 1 mL of injectable corticosteroid
■ High-frequency linear array transducer

Author's Preferred Technique

a. Patient position
   i. Prone position with ankle supported on a towel
b. Transducer position
   i. Anatomical axial plane in medial retromalleolar area. Identification in short axis of the TP, FDL, and neurovascular bundle (see Figure 96-2A). Slightly distal, locate the FHL tendon in short axis between the tubercles of posterior talus (see Figure 96-2B).
c. Needle orientation relative to the transducer
   i. In plane
d. Needle approach
   i. Lateral to medial: entry point lateral to Achilles tendon (Figure 96-3A, B)
   ii. Lateral to medial: entry point medial to Achilles tendon (Figure 96-4A, B)
   iii. Continuous needle progression under ultrasound monitoring until target reached
e. Target
   i. The FHL tendon sheath
f. Pearls and Pitfalls
   i. Be sure to identify and avoid tibial nerve and vessels.
   ii. A smaller "hockey stick" probe and an oblique standoff of gel can help when the entry point is medial to the Achilles tendon.
   iii. The author's preference for the needle approach is lateral to the Achilles tendon (see Figure 96-3A, B).

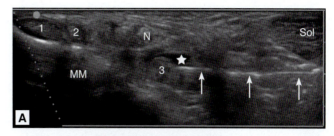
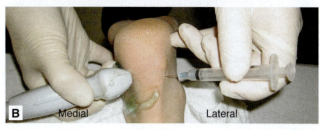

FIGURE 96-3 ■ In-plane ultrasound-guided injection of the flexor hallucis longus (FHL) tendon using an entry point for the needle lateral to the Achilles tendon. **A.** Ultrasound short-axis image of a tenosynovitis of the FHL and needle. **B.** Clinical corresponding image. 1, tibial posterior tendon; 2, flexor digitorum longus tendon; 3, FHL tendon; MM, medial malleolus; N, tibial nerve; Sol, soleus muscle; *white arrows*, needle; *white star*, fluid in FHL tendon sheath.

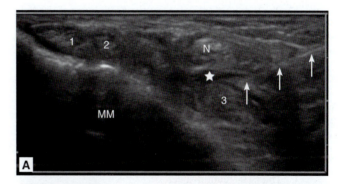
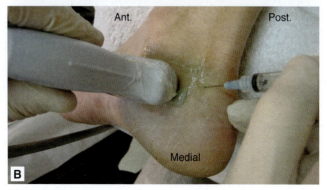

FIGURE 96-4 ■ In-plane ultrasound-guided injection of the flexor hallucis longus (FHL) using an entry point for the needle medial to the Achilles tendon. **A.** Ultrasound short-axis image of a tenosynovitis of the FHL and needle. **B.** Clinical corresponding image. 1, tibial posterior tendon; 2, flexor digitorum longus tendon; 3, FHL tendon; MM, medial malleolus; N, tibial nerve; *white arrows*, needle; *white star*, fluid in FHL tendon sheath.

Alternate Technique 1

a. Patient position
    i. Prone position with ankle supported on a towel
b. Transducer position
    i. Oblique axial plane in the medial arch of the foot. Identification of the FHL in short axis at the level of the sustentaculum tali and follow in the short axis distally until crossing with FDL tendon (Figures 96-2D and 96-5A, B).
c. Needle orientation relative to the transducer
    i. In plane
d. Needle approach
    i. Medial to lateral (see Figure 96-5A, B)
e. Target
    i. The crossing point between FHL and FDL tendons

Alternate Technique 2

a. Patient position
    i. Prone position with ankle supported on a towel
b. Transducer position
    i. Plantar short-axis plane at the MTP level of the hallux. Identification of the FHL in short axis at the level, or just proximal, to the sesamoid bones area (Figure 96-6A–C).
c. Needle orientation relative to the transducer
    i. In plane
d. Needle approach
    i. Medial to lateral (see Figure 96-6A)
e. Target
    i. The FHL tendon sheath

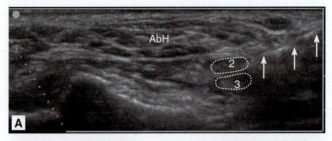

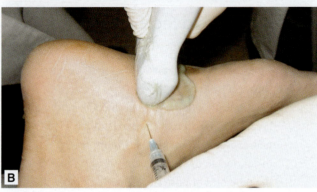

FIGURE 96-5 ▪ In-plane ultrasound-guided injection of the flexor digitorum longus (FDL) tendon crossing over the flexor hallucis longus (FHL) tendon (notch of Henry). **A.** Ultrasound short-axis image of the FDL and FHL crossing over and the needle. **B.** Clinical corresponding image. 1, tibial posterior tendon; 2, FDL tendon; 3, FHL tendon; AbH, abductor hallucis; *white arrows*, needle.

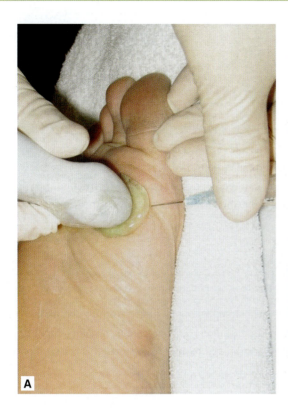
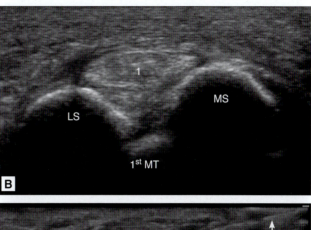
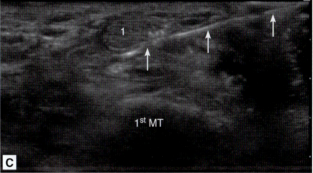

FIGURE 96-6 ■ In-plane ultrasound-guided injection of the flexor hallucis longus (FHL) at the metatarsophalangeal (MTP) joint level. **A.** Clinical corresponding image with needle direction from medial to lateral. **B.** Ultrasound short-axis image of the FHL tendon between the medial and lateral hallucis sesamoid bones. **C.** Ultrasound short-axis image of FHL tendon sheath injection proximal to the sesamoid bones, with needle. 1, FHL tendon; 1st MT, first metatarsal; LS, lateral sesamoid bone; MS, medial sesamoid bone; *white arrows,* needle.

References

1. Schuenke M, Schulte E, Schumacher U. *Thieme Atlas of Anatomy: General Anatomy and Musculoskeletal System.* New York: Georg Thieme Verlag; 2006.
2. Michelson J, Dunn L. Tenosynovitis of the flexor hallucis longus: a clinical study of the spectrum of presentation and treatment. *Foot Ankle Int* 2005 Apr;26(4):291–303.
3. Schulhofer SD, Oloff LM. Flexor hallucis longus dysfunction: an overview. *Clin Podiatr Med Surg* 2002 Jul;19(3):411–418, vi.
4. Sammarco GJ, Cooper PS. Flexor hallucis longus tendon injury in dancers and nondancers. *Foot Ankle Int* 1998 Jun;19(6):356–362.
5. Theodore GH, Kolettis GJ, Micheli LJ. Tenosynovitis of the flexor hallucis longus in a long-distance runner. *Med Sci Sports Exerc* 1996 Mar;28(3):277–279.
6. Lynch T, Pupp GR. Stenosing tenosynovitis of the flexor hallucis longus at the ankle joint. *J Foot Surg* 1990 Jul-Aug;29(4):345–348.
7. Wei SY, Kneeland JB, Okereke E. Complete atraumatic rupture of the flexor hallucis longus tendon: a case report and review of the literature. *Foot Ankle Int* 1998 Jul;19(7):472–474.
8. Mehdizade A, Adler RS. Sonographically guided flexor hallucis longus tendon sheath injection. *J Ultrasound Med* 2007 Feb;26(2):233–237.
9. Boruta PM, Beauperthuy GD. Partial tear of the flexor hallucis longus at the knot of Henry: presentation of three cases. *Foot Ankle Int* 1997 Apr;18(4):243–246.
10. Sanhudo JA. Stenosing tenosynovitis of the flexor hallucis longus tendon at the sesamoid area. *Foot Ankle Int* 2002 Sep;23(9):801–803.
11. Reach JS, Easley ME, Chuckpaiwong B, Nunley JA 2nd. Accuracy of ultrasound guided injections in the foot and ankle. *Foot Ankle Int* 2009 Mar;30(3):239–342.

John C. Hill, DO, FACSM, FAAFP / Matthew Leiszler, MD

KEY POINTS

- Use a 22–27-gauge, 1.5-inch needle.
- Use a high-frequency linear array transducer with lateral decubitus or prone position.
- Use a medial-to-lateral approach.
- The most common location of pathology is near the origin of the plantar fascia at the medial tuberosity of the calcaneus.

- The needle is placed next to the aponeurosis in the perifascial region.
- Pain can be reduced significantly by first placing a posterior tibial nerve block.

Pertinent Anatomy

The plantar fascia (aponeurosis) is a strong multilayered band of fibrous tissue with origin at the medial and lateral calcaneal tubercles. Distally, it attaches to the plantar plates of the metatarsophalangeal joints, forming the medial longitudinal arch of the foot.[1] The plantar fascia is thickest in the central portion and thinner in the medial and lateral portions (Figure 97-1).

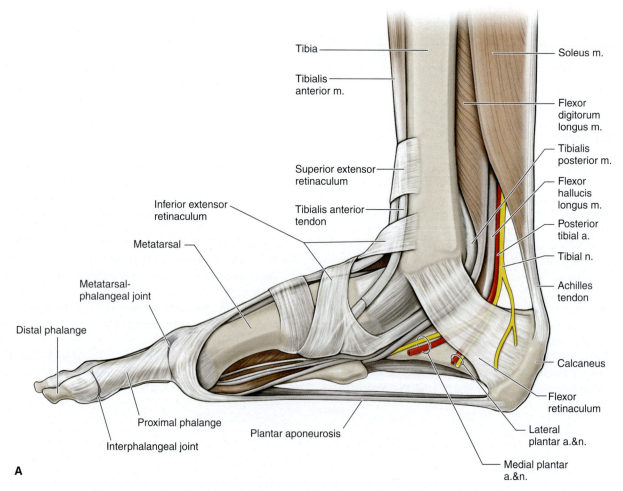

A

FIGURE 97-1 ■ **A.** Planter fascia viewed from medial side of foot. (Reproduced with permission from Morton DA, Foreman KB, Albertine KH, eds. *The Big Picture: Gross Anatomy*. New York: McGraw-Hill; 2011: figure 38-1.)

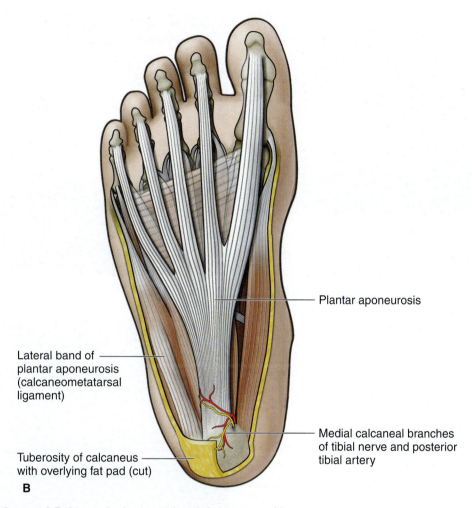

Plantar aponeurosis

Lateral band of plantar aponeurosis (calcaneometatarsal ligament)

Medial calcaneal branches of tibial nerve and posterior tibial artery

Tuberosity of calcaneus with overlying fat pad (cut)

B

FIGURE 97-1 ■ (*Continued*) **B.** Planter fascia viewed from inferior aspect of foot.

Common Pathology

The etiology of plantar fasciitis is likely multifactorial, including biomechanical and gait abnormalities. Reduced ankle dorsiflexion, increased body mass index, and work-related weight-bearing activities have been reported as independent risk factors.[2] The plantar fascia can be injured by overuse, leading to repeated micro tears near the origin of the fascia. Fasciitis may be a misnomer, as histologic findings are more consistent with a degenerative fasciosis without acute inflammation than a true inflammatory process. The area of irritation is found at the medial tuberosity of the calcaneus near the origin of the fascia and can be easily palpated when the fascia is placed on tension.[3]

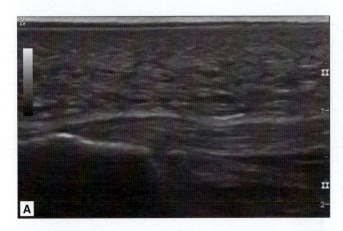

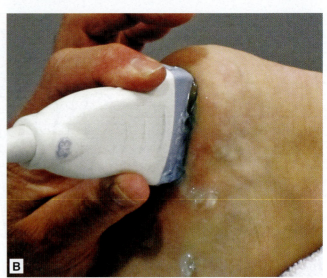

FIGURE 97-2 ■ **A.** Normal plantar fascia, long-axis view. **B.** Transducer location for long-axis image of plantar fascia.

Ultrasound Imaging Findings

The plantar fascia is best visualized in long axis and short axis using a high-frequency linear array transducer at a depth of less than 3 cm. Normal findings include a well-organized, uniform, hyperechoic pattern of collagen. Common pathological findings include thickening of the plantar fascia, as well as disorganized or hypoechoic appearance of the fascia. Often lateral bands of fascia are normal in appearance, and the hypoechoic medial bands are obvious in contrast (Figures 97-2 and 97-3).

Indications for Injections of the Plantar Fascia

Injection of the plantar fascia is reserved for patients with persistent pain that is unresponsive to rest, activity modification, ice massage, orthotics, stretching, heel cups, and night splints. Injection of the plantar fascia has been described based on palpation (ie, unguided).[4] Ultrasound-guided injection has been described by Kane et al.[5] Kane also reported clinical success rates of ultrasound-guided to palpation-guided corticosteroid injection, and found an overall response rate of 93% in ultrasound-guided injection and 80% in palpation-guided injections.[6]

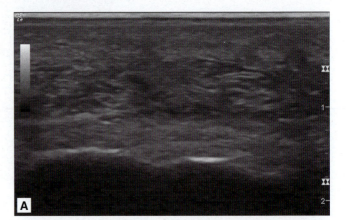

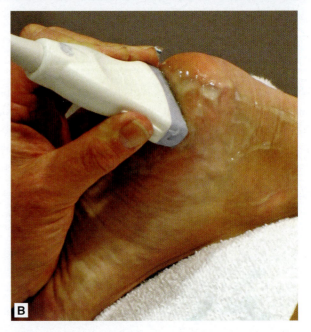

FIGURE 97-3 ■ **A.** Normal plantar fascia, short-axis view. **B.** Transducer location for short-axis image of plantar fascia.

Equipment

■ Needle and injectate
  • Use a 27-gauge, 1.5-inch needle for injection of 2.5 mL of a local anesthetic in the medial subcutaneous tissue along the approach to the location of pathology to ensure complete anesthesia (Figure 97-4).
  • Transition to a 22-gauge, 1.5-inch needle for injection of solution of a local anesthetic and 1 mL of injectable corticosteroid at the proximal perifascial location of pathology.
■ High-frequency linear array transducer

Author's Preferred Technique

a. Patient position
   i. Prone or lateral decubitus position
   ii. Lateral side of affected foot should be toward the table
b. Transducer position
   i. Short axis on plantar aspect of foot with plantar fascia in short axis overlying area of pathology
c. Needle orientation relative to the transducer
   i. Long axis
d. Needle approach (Figure 97-5)
   i. In plane
   ii. Visualize needle approaching from lateral aspect of field of view along same plane as pathology, sliding the needle under the plantar fascia in the perifascial space.
e. Target
   i. Location between calcaneus and hypoechoic and mixed echogenicity near origin of medial to central portion of plantar fascia
f. Pearls and Pitfalls
   i. Plantar fascia is thin in this location, leading to difficulty when injecting without ultrasound guidance.
   ii. The area of pathology is nearly always medial; therefore lateral approach should be avoided.
   iii. Peppering or a single injection of corticosteroid on the proximal side of the plantar fascia reduces risk of steroid causing atrophy of the fat pad.
   iv. Use color flow Doppler prior to injection to identify vessels adjacent to the medial calcaneal nerve to avoid nerve injury.
   v. Calcaneal stress fracture should be considered and ruled out prior to plantar fascia corticosteroid injection.

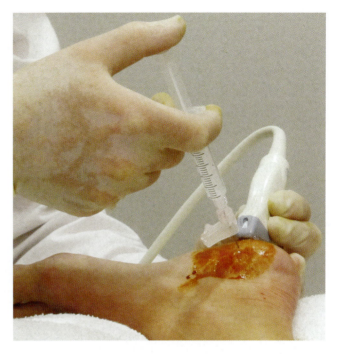

FIGURE 97-4 ■ Transducer and needle placement for ultrasound-guided plantar perifascial injection.

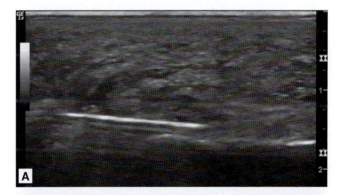

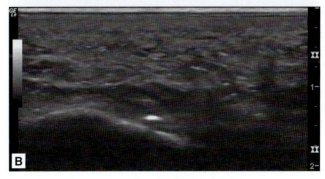

FIGURE 97-5 ■ **A.** Needle approaching from lateral side of image injecting under plantar fascia, in perifascial space. **B.** White dot represents out of plane view of needle under the plantar fascia, in perifascial space.

vi. Although corticosteroids have historically been injected, the rationale for this has been questioned given the lack of inflammatory cells on histologic studies.

vii. A medial-to-lateral approach is preferred because of increased accuracy in directing the needle into the exact location of the pathology, which typically involves the medial one-third of the plantar fascia.

viii. There is decreased pain with this approach, as well as decreased risk of injection into the fat pad and therefore, it possibly could be done without a posterior tibial nerve block. However, this block is often performed prior to this injection for patient comfort.

Alternate Technique

a. Patient position
    i. Prone on table with foot at edge of table
b. Transducer position
    i. On medial aspect of foot, perpendicular to heel pad
c. Needle orientation relative to transducer
    i. In plane
d. Needle approach
    i. Through the plantar aspect of heel, direct needle at a 45-degree angle under the location of pathology
    ii. Visualize needle approaching from the lateral field of view parallel to the plane of pathology
e. Target
    i. Location between calcaneus and hypoechoic and mixed echogenicity near origin of the medial to central portion of plantar fascia

f. Pearls and Pitfalls
    i. Consider using a posterior tibial nerve block because the approach through plantar aspect of heel pad will cause increased pain due to innervation of sole of foot; with nonguided injection, there is also an increased risk of unintentionally injecting fat pad leading to fat pad atrophy.
    ii. The exact location of the needle is not as clear in the medial aspect of the plantar fascia.

References

1. Karabay N, Toros T, Hurel C. Ultrasonographic evaluation in plantar fasciitis. *J Foot Ankle Surg* 2007;46(6):442–446.
2. Riddle DL, Pulisic M, Pidcoe P, et al. Risk factors for plantar fasciitis: a matched case-control study. *J Bone Joint Surg Am* 2003;85-A(7):1338.
3. Saunders S, Longworth S. *Injection Techniques in Orthopaedics and Sports Medicine: A Practical Manual for Doctors and Physiotherapists.* 3rd ed. St. Louis: Elsevier; 2006: section 3, 140.
4. Ball EM, McKeeman HM, Patterson C, et al. Steroid injection for inferior heel pain: a randomized controlled trial. *Ann Rheum Dis.* 2013;72:996–1002.
5. Kane D, Greaney T, Bresnihan B, et al. Ultrasound guided injection of recalcitrant plantar fasciitis. *Ann Rheum Dis* 1998;57:383–384.
6. Kane D, Greaney T, Shanahan M, et al. The role of ultrasonography in the diagnosis and management of idiopathic plantar fasciitis. *Rheumatology (Oxford)* 2001;40(9):1002–1008.

John C. Hill, DO, FACSM, FAAFP / Matthew Leiszler, MD

KEY POINTS

- Use a high-frequency linear array transducer.
- The most common location of pathology is near the origin of the plantar fascia at the medial tuberosity of the calcaneus.
- First placing a posterior tibial nerve block reduces pain significantly.

- Use a high frequency linear array transducer.
- Medial to lateral approach preferred.
- The plantar approach is more painful.

Pertinent Anatomy

The plantar fascia (aponeurosis) is a strong multilayered band of fibrous tissue with origin at the medial and lateral calcaneal tubercles. Distally, it attaches to the plantar plates of the metatarsophalangeal joints, forming the medial longitudinal arch of the foot.[1] The plantar fascia is thickest in the central portion and thinner in the medial and lateral portions (Figure 98-1).

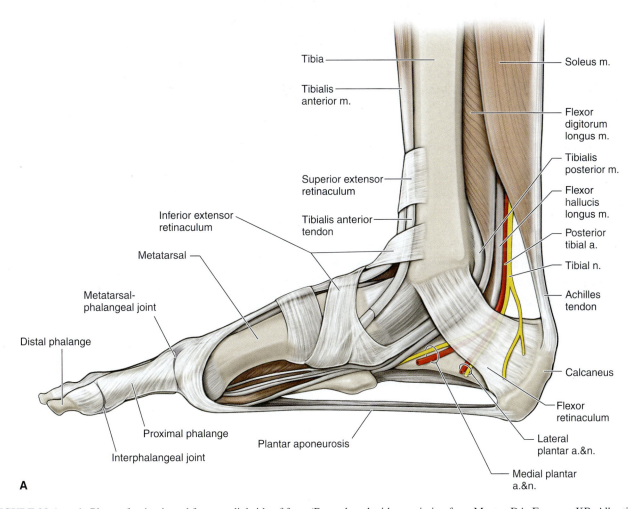

A

FIGURE 98-1 ■ **A.** Planter fascia viewed from medial side of foot. (Reproduced with permission from Morton DA, Foreman KB, Albertine KH, eds. *The Big Picture: Gross Anatomy*. New York: McGraw-Hill; 2011: figure 38-2.)

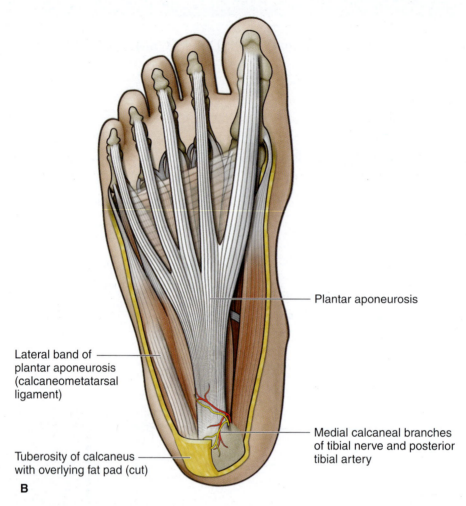

Plantar aponeurosis

Lateral band of plantar aponeurosis (calcaneometatarsal ligament)

Medial calcaneal branches of tibial nerve and posterior tibial artery

Tuberosity of calcaneus with overlying fat pad (cut)

B

FIGURE 98-1 ■ (*Continued*) **B.** Plantar fascia viewed from inferior aspect of foot.

Common Pathology

The etiology of plantar fasciitis is likely multifactorial, including biomechanical and gait abnormalities. Reduced ankle dorsiflexion, increased body mass index, and work-related weight-bearing activities have been reported as independent risk factors.[2] The plantar fascia can be injured by overuse, leading to repeated micro tears near the origin of the fascia. Fasciitis may be a misnomer, as histologic findings are more consistent with a degenerative fasciosis without acute inflammation than a true inflammatory process. Most often, the location of pathology is near the origin of the fascia at the medial tuberosity of the calcaneus.

Ultrasound Imaging Findings

The plantar fascia is best visualized in long axis (Figure 98-2) and short axis using a high-frequency linear array transducer at a depth of less than 3 cm. Normal findings include a well-organized, uniform, hyperechoic pattern of collagen. Common pathological findings include thickening of the plantar fascia, as well as disorganized or hypoechoic appearance of the fascia. Often lateral bands of fascia are normal in appearance, and the hypoechoic medial bands are obvious in contrast.

Indications for Injections of the Plantar Fascia

Injection of the plantar fascia is reserved for patients with persistent pain that is unresponsive to rest, activity modification, ice massage, orthotics, stretching, heel cups, and night splints. Injection of the plantar fascia has been described based on palpation (ie, unguided).[3] Ultrasound-guided injection has been described by Kane et al.[4] Kane also reported clinical success rates of ultrasound-guided to palpation-guided corticosteroid injection, and found overall response rate of 93% in ultrasound-guided injection and 80% in palpation-guided injections.[5] Accuracy of injection with palpation and ultrasound-guided injections has not been described.

Equipment

- ▦ Needle and injectate
  - Begin with a 27-gauge, 1.5-inch needle for injection of 2.5 mL of a local anesthetic in subcutaneous tissue along the approach to the location of pathology to ensure complete anesthesia.
  - Transition to an 18-gauge, 1.5-inch needle for injection of solution of both a short- and long-acting anesthetic 1–2 mL of each, and 1 mL of an injectable corticosteroid at location of pathology.
- ▦ High-frequency linear array transducer

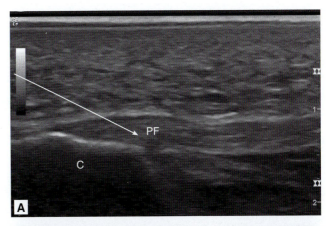

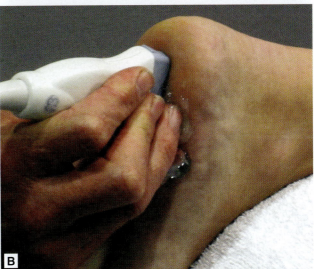

FIGURE 98-2 ■ **A.** Long-axis view of the normal plantar fascia with in-plane injection from posterior to anterior. **B.** Transducer placement for long-axis image of the plantar fascia. C, calcaneus; PF, plantar fascia.

Author's Preferred Technique

■ Place a posterior tibial nerve block (see Chapter 99)

a. Patient position (Figure 98-3)

   i. Prone or lateral decubitus position

   ii. Lateral side of affected foot should be toward the table

b. Transducer position (see Figure 98-3)

   i. Short axis on plantar aspect of foot with plantar fascia in short axis overlying area of pathology

c. Needle orientation relative to the transducer (Figure 98-4)

   i. In plane

d. Needle approach (Figures 98-4 and 98-5)

   i. Medial to lateral.

   ii. Visualize needle approaching from lateral aspect of field of view along same plane as pathology.

e. Target

   i. Location of hypoechoic and mixed echogenicity near origin of medial to central portion of plantar fascia

f. Pearls and Pitfalls

   i. The plantar fascia is thin in this location, leading to difficulty when injecting without ultrasound guidance.

   ii. The area of pathology is nearly always medial; therefore a lateral approach should be avoided.

   iii. Corticosteroids are not warranted because of the lack of any true inflammatory response. Peppering, percutaneous tenotomy technique is preferred and shown to have superior results over single corticosteroid injection.[3]

   iv. Use color flow Doppler prior to injection to identify vessels adjacent to the medial calcaneal nerve to avoid nerve injury.

   v. Calcaneal stress fracture should be considered and ruled out prior to plantar fascia corticosteroid injection.

   vi. Less pain is usually experienced with this injection technique.

Alternate Technique

a. Patient position (Figure 98-2B)

   i. Prone on table with foot at edge of table

b. Transducer position (see Figure 98-2B)

   i. On medial aspect of foot, perpendicular to heel pad

c. Needle orientation relative to transducer (Figure 98-2A)

   i. In plane

d. Needle approach (see Figure 98-2A)

   i. Posterior to anterior or anterior to posterior

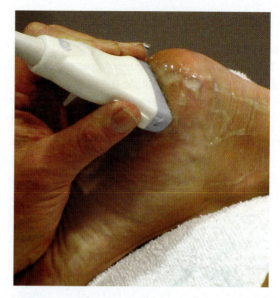

FIGURE 98-3 ■ Transducer placement for short-axis image of the plantar fascia.

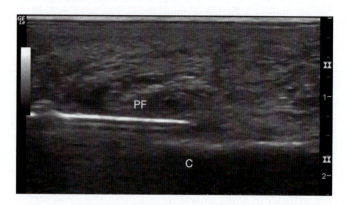

FIGURE 98-4 ■ Short-axis view of the abnormal plantar fascia with in-plane, medial-to-lateral approach to the area of pathology. C, calcaneus; PF, plantar fascia.

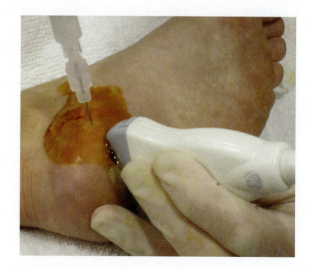

FIGURE 98-5 ■ Short-axis, in-plane approach to the plantar fascia from medial to lateral.

navasdf......

e. Target
   i. Location of hypoechoic and mixed echogenicity near origin of the medial to central portion of plantar fascia
f. Pearls and Pitfalls
   i. This approach should be done with a posterior tibial nerve block because the approach through the plantar aspect of the heel pad is not the first option because of increased pain with the plantar approach caused by innervation of the sole of the foot; with nonguided injection, there is also the increased risk of unintentionally injecting the fat pad leading to fat pad atrophy.
   ii. This technique is preferred for needle tenotomy or biologic injection into the fascia.

References

1. Karabay N, Toros T, Hurel C. Ultrasonographic evaluation in plantar fasciitis. *J Foot Ankle Surg* 2007;46(6):442–446.
2. Riddle DL, Pulisic M, Pidcoe P, et al. Risk factors for plantar fasciitis: a matched case-control study. *J Bone Joint Surg Am* 2003;85-A(7):1338.
3. Kalaci A, Cakici H, Hapa O, et al. Treatment of plantar fasciitis using four different local injection modalities: a randomized prospective clinical trial. *J Am Podiatr Med Assoc* 2009;99(2):108–113.
4. Kane D, Greaney T, Bresnihan B, et al. Ultrasound guided injection of recalcitrant plantar fasciitis. *Ann Rheum Dis* 1998;57:383–384.
5. Kane D, Greaney T, Shanahan M, et al. The role of ultrasonography in the diagnosis and management of idiopathic plantar fasciitis. *Rheumatology (Oxford)* 2001;40(9):1002–1008.

John C. Hill, DO, FACSM, FAAFP / Matthew Leiszler, MD / Jay E. Bowen, DO

KEY POINTS

- Use a 22-gauge, 1.5–2-inch needle.
- Use a high frequency linear array transducer with lateral decubitus or prone position.
- The tibial nerve is accessible near the medial malleolus next to posterior tibial artery.
- Visualizing the nerve in short axis is quite simple.
- The needle approach is in plane to the transducer, which is short axis to the nerve.

Pertinent Anatomy

Tibial Nerve

The sciatic nerve originates from the fourth and fifth lumbar and first and second sacral roots. The sciatic nerve is compromised of the peroneal and tibial nerves. If extrapelvic, they divide variably from the gluteal region, classically taught middle distal third of the thigh, or popliteal fossa. The tibial component is generally from the L5–S2 root levels, but can have contributions from L4–S3. The tibial nerve travels from the popliteal fossa into the posterior compartment of the lower leg moving medial as it travels distally at the ankle.

Tarsal Tunnel

The tarsal tunnel is on the medial aspect of the ankle and is divided into an upper (tibiotalar) compartment and a lower (talocalcaneal), "classic" compartment (Figure 99-1). This is bounded superficially by the deep aponeurosis in the upper and flexor retinaculum in the lower tunnel and has an osseous floor (medial surface of the talus, the inferomedial navicular, the sustentaculum tali, and the curved medial surface of the calcaneus). The flexor retinaculum, also called the *laciniate ligament*, attaches to the medial malleolus (tibia) and then angles obliquely inferior and posterior attaching to the posterior superior calcaneus and blending with the fascia over the dorsum of the heel.

The tibial nerve bifurcates from 1.3 cm proximal to the medial malleolus tip[1] to 14.3 cm proximal (Bareither).[2] However, Bilge used the inferior border of the flexor retinaculum as a reference point and found splitting of the nerve at the reference point 12% and distal 4% of the time without bifurcation

significantly proximal to the tunnel.[3] This dissection study noted the diameter was 5.8 ± 0.8 mm at the right ankle and 6.03 ± 0.91 mm on the left. An ultrasound study (Jain S)[4] noted 6.3 ± 3.2 mm^2 with a range from 2–15.7. Alshami et al.[5] noted excellent reliability in measuring the tibial nerve ultrasonographically 1 cm proximal to the tarsal tunnel and found that ≥1.8 mm^2 side-to-side difference could be clinically significant.

The contents of the tarsal tunnel from anterior to posterior consist of the posterior tibial tendon, flexor digitorum longus tendon, posterior tibial neurovascular bundle, and flexor hallucis longus muscle or at times its tendon.

If the tibial nerve does not bifurcate, it will trifurcate into the medial and lateral plantar nerves and the medial calcaneal nerve distal to the tarsal tunnel (Figures 99-2 and 99-3). Ninety-three percent of the time, the tibial bifurcation occurs within 2 cm of an imaginary line drawn between the middle of the medial malleolus and the midcalcaneus.[6] Calcaneal branches can have highly variable anatomy. Most individuals (79%) have a single calcaneal nerve, usually arising from the posterior tibial nerve, but sometimes arising from the lateral plantar nerve. About 21% of individuals have multiple calcaneal branches originating from the posterior tibial nerve, lateral plantar nerve, medial plantar nerve, or from a combination of these. Others have noted greater variability with one to three branches of the medial calcaneal nerve.[7] This can make isolated block of the nerve complicated. The calcaneal branches travel over the abductor hallucis muscle and supply sensation to the medial heel. The medial calcaneal nerve(s) penetrate the flexor retinaculum and innervate the skin over the medial and posterior heel (Didia).[8]

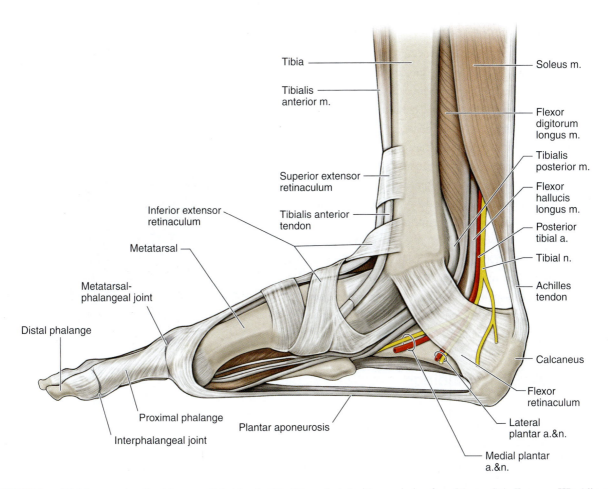

FIGURE 99-1 ■ Tibial nerve visualized from medial side of ankle. (Reproduced with permission from Morton DA, Foreman KB, Albertine KH, eds. *The Big Picture: Gross Anatomy*. New York: McGraw-Hill; 2011: figure 38-1.)

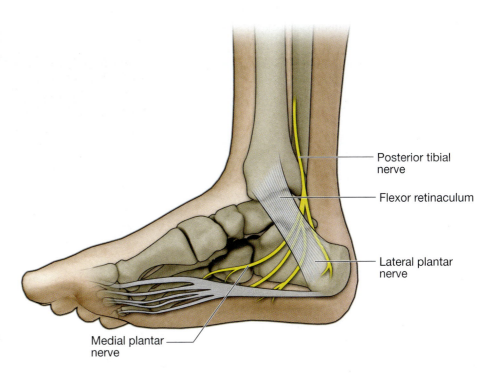

FIGURE 99-2 ■ Bifurcation of the medial and lateral plantar nerves.

Common Pathology

Tarsal tunnel syndrome typically involves entrapment of the tibial nerve or its branches causing medial foot and digits 1–3 pain and/or altered sensations.[9] Typically, there is a Tinel sign at the tunnel and at times altered sensation on examination most commonly in the medial plantar nerve distribution. There are many proposed etiologies, but increased pressure within the tunnel is the commonality if a history of direct trauma is not present.

Chronic heel pain can be from entrapment of the first branch of the lateral plantar nerve beneath the deep fascia of the abductor hallucis muscle and/or beneath the medial edge of the quadratus plantae fascia. This condition is called *Baxter's neuritis*.

Jogger's foot is a term to signify medial plantar nerve compression usually in the region of the navicula and abductor hallucis. The patient usually complains of medial arch pain when running and should be considered in the differential diagnosis and treatment of plantar fasciosis.

Ultrasound Imaging Findings

The tibial nerve is best visualized in short axis using a high-frequency linear array transducer at a depth of less than 2 cm. The nerve can be located one-third of the way from the apex of the heel to a point midway between the navicular tuberosity and the prominence of the medial malleolus (Figure 99-4). Normal findings include well-organized, uniform, mixed echogenicity of the nerve bundles on end, similar to the end of a broom. With the transducer placed transversely on the ankle just behind the medial malleolus, short-axis images of the posterior tibia, flexor digitorum, and flexor hallucis longus tendons are visualized. The posterior tibial artery can be seen pulsating, and next to this is the tibial nerve (see Figure 99-7).

Indications

Tibial nerve injections can be performed to block pain from a plantar foot procedure for patient comfort, greater ease for the physician, and potentially a reduced risk.[10] Prior to performing plantar fascia procedures, a tibial nerve effective anesthesia can be provided on the plantar aspect of the foot. The otherwise painful plantar fascia injection can now be done painlessly. If curetting and cautery are required for plantar warts, this block may also provide effective anesthesia, especially if the warts are located near the heel. It can be part of an anesthetic ankle block (including the peroneal [deep and superficial], sural and, at times, the saphenous) for surgery. Another reason is a new concept with promise—ultrasound-guided

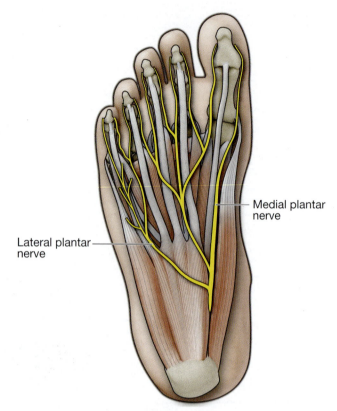

FIGURE 99-3 ■ Medial and plantar nerves at the plantar foot.

Medial plantar nerve

Lateral plantar nerve

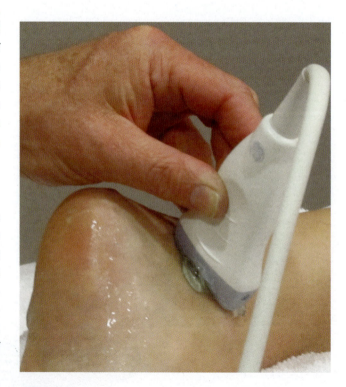

FIGURE 99-4 ■ Transducer placement over short axis of tibial nerve.

percutaneous hydroneuroplasty (UPHN). This is based in the theory that a portion of a nerve becomes adherent to the surrounding fascial tissue, as nerves are designed to glide through with some normal amount of movement. However, symptoms develop from fascial "gluing," some type of entrapment most commonly at a tunnel or scar tissue. Using ultrasound to visualize the nerve at a pathological site, determined by clinical examination without or without nerve swelling, the needle can be directed to the nerve and fluid, usually dilute anesthesia, injected to mechanically free the nerve from the surrounding tissue. If the nerve is swollen at the "tarsal tunnel," ultrasound can guide a corticosteroid injection or UPHN can be performed. A lateral plantar nerve block can be helpful in differentiating the cause of foot pain that may atypical for tarsal tunnel symptoms or plantar fasciosis (which can also include some traction on Baxter's nerve).

Equipment

- ■ Needle: 22-gauge 1.5–2-inch needle
- ■ Injectate
  - • Nerve block: 2 mLs local anesthetic ± injectable corticosteroids
  - • Nerve hydrodissection and decompression: 5–10 mL total solution (combination of normal saline, local anesthetic, ± dextrose solution)
- ■ High-frequency linear array transducer

Author's Preferred Technique

a. Patient position (see Figure 99-4)
  i. Prone or lateral decubitus position
  ii. Lateral side of affected foot should be toward the table
b. Transducer position (see Figure 99-4)
  i. Transverse on medial ankle posterior to medial malleolus viewing nerve in short axis
c. Needle orientation relative to the transducer (Figure 99-5)
  i. In plane
d. Needle approach (Figures 99-5 and 99-6)
  i. Posterior to anterior
e. Target (see Figure 99-6)
  i. Location of speculated bundles of mixed echogenicity characteristic of the nerve next to the pulsating posterior tibial artery, easily seen with Doppler imaging (Figure 99-7)

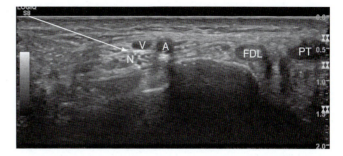

FIGURE 99-5 ■ Ultrasound image of tibial nerve next to posterior tibial artery and veins, both in short axis, just inferior to medial malleolus. *Arrow* demonstrates in-plane needle approach from posterior to anterior, avoiding the adjacent vessels. A, artery; FDL, flexor digitorum longus; N, nerve; PT, posterior tibial tendon; V, vein.

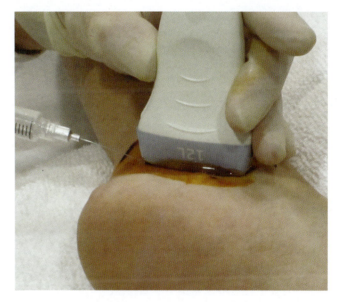

FIGURE 99-6 ■ Transducer and needle placement for tibial nerve block at the medial malleolus.

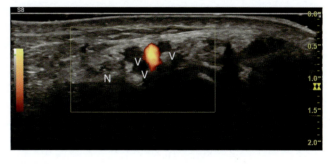

FIGURE 99-7 ■ Ultrasound image of tibial nerve (N) and veins (V) demonstrating Doppler flow in nearby artery.

f. Pearls and Pitfalls

   i. Care should be taken to place the needle next to artery and nerve, and not in these structures.

   ii. Following the injection, massaging the area for 30 seconds may increase the effectiveness of the block.

   iii. Use color flow Doppler prior to injection to identify posterior tibial vessels adjacent to tibial nerve to further help avoid nerve injury.

   iv. Wait approximately 5 minutes for the block to fully set up before beginning other procedures (ie, percutaneous needle tenotomy of plantar fascia).

References

1. Horwitz MT. Normal anatomy and variations of the peripheral nerves of the leg and foot. *Arch Surg* 1938;36:626.

2. Bareither, DJ, Genau JM, Massaro JC. Variation in the division of the tibial nerve: application to nerve blocks. *J Foot Surg* 1990;(29):581–583.

3. Bilge O, Ozer MA, Govsa F. Neurovascular branching in the tarsal tunnel. *Neuroanatomy* 2003;2:39–41.

4. Jain S, Visser LH, Praveen TLN, Rao PN, Surekha T, et al. High-resolution sonography: a new technique to detect nerve damage in leprosy. *PLoS Negl Trop Dis* 2009;3(8):e498. doi 10.1371/journal.pntd.0000498.

5. Alshami AM, Cairns CW, Wylie BK, Souvlis T, Coppieters MW. Reliability and size of the measurement error when determining the cross-sectional area of the tibial nerve at the tarsal tunnel with Ultrasonography. *Ultrasound Medicine Biol* 2009;35(7):1098–1102.

6. Havel PE, Ebraheim NA, Clark SE, et al. Tibial nerve branching in the tarsal tunnel. *Foot Ankle* Dec 1988;9(3):117–119.

7. Dellon AL, Kim J, Spaulding SM. Variations in the origin of the medial calcaneal nerve. *J Am Podiatr Med Assoc* 2002;92(2):97–101.

8. Didia BC, Horsefall AU. Medial calcaneal nerve. An anatomical study. *J Am Podiatr Med Assoc* 1990;80(3):115–119.

9. Pecina MM, Krmpotic-Nemanic J, Markiewitz AD. *Tunnel Syndromes*. 3rd ed. Boca Raton, FL: CRC Press; 2001.

10. Soares LG, Brull R, Chan VW. Teaching an old block a new trick: ultrasound-guided posterior tibial nerve block. *Acta Anaesthesiol Scan* 2008;52(3):446–447.

Amy X. Yin, MD / Joanne Borg Stein, MD

KEY POINTS

- A 25-gauge, 2-inch nerve block needle is recommended.
- A high-frequency linear array transducer may be used.
- Saphenous nerve block at the ankle may be used for local anesthetic for foot pain.
- It is also used for regional ankle anesthesia for foot and ankle procedures.

- Place the patient in the supine position with foot in plantarflexion.
- Use and anterior-to-posterior approach.

Pertinent Anatomy

The saphenous nerve is the sensory terminal branch of the femoral nerve. The saphenous nerve branches off the femoral nerve in the femoral triangle and travels with the superficial femoral vein and artery within the adductor (Hunter's) canal. It lies deep to the sartorius muscle until it reaches the distal thigh, where it becomes subcutaneous by piercing the fascia lata between the tendons of the gracilis and sartorius muscles. At the knee, the infrapatellar nerve branches off.

The saphenous nerve then runs distally behind the medial border of the tibia with the great saphenous vein. At the distal third of the lower leg, it divides into two branches. One branch continues along the margin of the tibia and ends at the ankle, and the other branch travels with the great saphenous vein down the anteromedial aspect of the ankle into the foot (Figure 100-1).

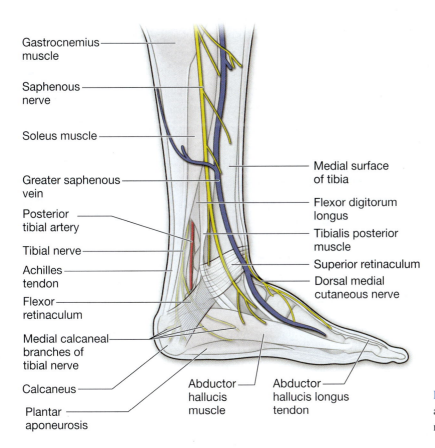

Gastrocnemius muscle
Saphenous nerve
Soleus muscle
Greater saphenous vein
Posterior tibial artery
Tibial nerve
Achilles tendon
Flexor retinaculum
Medial calcaneal branches of tibial nerve
Calcaneus
Plantar aponeurosis
Abductor hallucis muscle
Abductor hallucis longus tendon

Medial surface of tibia
Flexor digitorum longus
Tibialis posterior muscle
Superior retinaculum
Dorsal medial cutaneous nerve

FIGURE 100-1 ■ Anatomy of the anteromedial ankle showing the saphenous vein and saphenous nerve running anterior to the medial malleolus.

The branch of the saphenous nerve at the ankle provides sensory innervations to the medial side of the foot. This occasionally includes the metatarsophalangeal joints of the big toe.

Common Pathology

The saphenous nerve is the longest terminal branch of the femoral nerve and is susceptible to a variety of injury along its pathway. Injury from direct trauma, stretching, compression, or regional muscle and tendon pathology may occur, such as with contact and ball sports. The saphenous nerve is especially vulnerable to injury within the adductor (Hunter's) canal or after it becomes subcutaneous at the medial knee. Iatrogenic causes of saphenous neuralgia may include saphenous vein harvest for coronary artery bypass graft procedures, arthroscopic knee surgeries, medial knee joint injections, varicose vein surgeries, and high ankle surgeries or injuries.

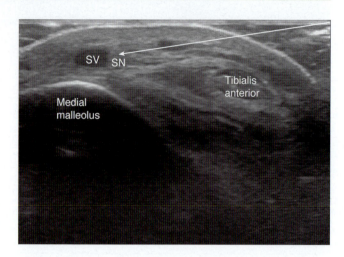

FIGURE 100-2 ▪ Ultrasound of the saphenous nerve (SN) at the medial ankle. Also visualized are the greater saphenous vein (SV), tibialis anterior tendon, and the medial malleolus. *Arrow* indicates needle angle of entry for in-plane approach from anterior to posterior.

Ultrasound Imaging Findings (Figure 100-2)

The ultrasound-guided saphenous nerve block at the ankle may be performed with a high-frequency linear array transducer.[1] For localization, the greater saphenous vein of the leg should first be identified at the anterior ankle between the tibialis anterior tendon and the medial malleolus. The saphenous vein is usually no more than 1–2 cm deep to the skin.[2] The saphenous nerve should then be visualized running next to the greater saphenous nerve. At the ankle, the saphenous nerve lies subcutaneously about 1 cm (11.5 mm for males and 10 mm for females) anterior to the medial malleolus.[3] It often is inferolateral to the vein.[1]

Of note, the patient may experience neuropathic pain with sonopalpation over the nerve. Adjacent muscle or tendon injury pattern or edema may also be visualized.

Indications for Saphenous Nerve Block at the Ankle

Saphenous nerve blocks at the ankle may be considered for patients with recalcitrant neuropathic pain of the foot from saphenous neuralgia. Conservative treatment should first be attempted. Associated pathology such as adjacent tendon or muscle injury or scar tissue should also be addressed.

Ankle blockade targets the saphenous nerve along with the tibial, sural, deep fibular (peroneal), and superficial fibular (peroneal) nerves. Ankle block can be used for analgesia of the foot for diagnostic and therapeutic purposes, such as for

patients with spastic talipes equinovarus and sympathetically mediated pain.[4]

In addition, foot and ankle surgeries are increasingly performed in an outpatient ambulatory setting. Regional ankle nerve block anesthesia is well suited for these procedures and for postprocedural pain. Foot and ankle procedures that may be performed with regional ankle anesthesia include incision and drainage of abscesses, foreign body removal, bunionectomies, radical toenail or ganglion excisions, Morton's or plantar neuromectomies, plantar fasciotomies, or even partial amputations.[3] Ankle blockade has the advantage of decreased morbidity and mortality, and more rapid recovery compared with spinal or general anesthesia.

Perineural injection of the saphenous nerve by landmark palpation can be and has been performed. However, ultrasound guidance will allow greater accuracy of injection by direct visualization of the saphenous nerve, greater saphenous vein, and associated structures.

Equipment

- Needle: 22-gauge 1.5–2-inch needle
- Injectate
  - Nerve block: 2 mL local anesthetic ± injectable corticosteroids
  - Nerve hydrodissection and decompression: 5–10 mL total solution (combination of normal saline, local anesthetic, ± dextrose solution)
- High-frequency linear array transducer

Author's Preferred Technique

a. Patient position (Figures 100-3 and 100-4)

    i. Supine with the foot in plantarflexion and the anteromedial ankle exposed.

    ii. The foot can be propped up or elevated with a pillow.[3,4]

    iii. Alternative position: supine with the knee flexed and foot on the bed.[3]

b. Transducer position

    i. Anatomic axial plane: anterior to the medial malleolus

c. Needle orientation relative to the transducer

    i. In plane

d. Needle approach (see Figures 100-3 and 100-4)

    i. Anterior to posterior preferred (see Figures 100-2 and 100-3).

    ii. Alternative: Posterior to anterior approach may also be performed (see Figure 100-4).[1]

e. Target (see Figure 100-2)

    i. Perineural circumferential spread of injectate spread around the saphenous nerve at the ankle

f. Pearls and Pitfalls

    i. The saphenous nerve may not be well distinguished. Thus, perivenous spread around the greater saphenous vein may be alternatively targeted because the saphenous nerve lies next to the vein.[2]

    ii. There is great anatomic variation and branching of the distal saphenous nerve and branching may occur above the level of an ankle block.[2] Nerve block at a higher level or nerve block of additional nerves may be required for analgesia or anesthesia.

    iii. Although of low likelihood, intraneural or intravascular injection is still a possible risk.

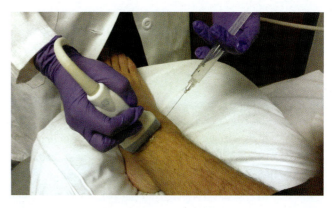

FIGURE 100-3 ■ Supine position: Anterior to posterior, in-plane needle approach is illustrated.

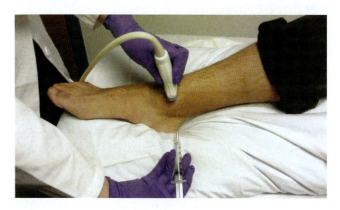

FIGURE 100-4 ■ Supine position: Posterior to anterior, in-plane needle approach is illustrated.

References

1. Breneman S. Ultrasound-guided ankle block. In: Bigeleisen PE, et al., eds. *Ultrasound-Guided Regional Anesthesia and Pain Medicine.* Philadelphia, PA: Lippincott Williams & Wilkins; 2010: 140–144.

2. Orebaugh SL, Moreno M, Breneman SM, Bigeleisen PE. Ultrasound-guided saphenous nerve block. In: Bigeleisen PE, et al., eds. *Ultrasound-Guided Regional Anesthesia and Pain Medicine.* Philadelphia, PA: Lippincott Williams & Wilkins; 2010: 108–113.

3. Schabort D, Boon JM, Becker PJ, Meiring JH. Easily identifiable bony landmarks as an aid in targeted regional ankle blockade. *Clin Anat* 2005 Oct;18(7):518–526.

4. Mulchandani H, Awad IT, McCartney CJ. Ultrasound-guided nerve blocks of the lower limb. In: Narouze SN, ed. *Atlas of Ultrasound-Guided Procedures in Interventional Pain Management.* 1st ed. New York: Springer; 2010:255–258.

5. Bodner G. Nerve Compression Syndromes. In: Peer S, Bodner G, et al., eds. *High-Resolution Sonography of the Peripheral Nervous System.* 2nd ed. Springer; 2008:106–108.

Rahul Naren Desai, MD / Jevon Simerly

KEY POINTS

- Use a high-frequency linear array transducer in the short-axis plane, relative to the course of the nerve and adjacent long bones.
- The sural nerve is formed from sensory branches of tibial and common fibular nerve. It is in the posterior-lateral lower leg, deep to peroneal tendons, and then courses to the lateral foot and little toe.
- Inject along the course (from the fibrous arch, to the lateral foot), depending on the craniocaudal level of pain and symptoms.

Pertinent Anatomy

The sural nerve (SN) provides sensory innervation to the posterior and lateral lower leg, lateral malleolus, lateral heel, lateral foot up to the base of the fifth toe. The nerve is formed from contributing branches of the tibial nerve (medial sural cutaneous nerve), and common fibular nerve (lateral sural cutaneous nerve). In the calf, the nerve is superficially located in the subcutaneous tissues, travelling with the small saphenous vein (SSV), along the lateral border of the Achilles tendon (AT). It then courses toward the lateral malleolus and runs deep to the peroneal tendon sheath. It extends to the fifth metatarsal base, branching into lateral and medial terminal branches (Figure 101-1).

Common Pathology

The SN is susceptible to neural lesions, without perineural connective tissue involvement. Compression neuropathy occurs secondary to trauma, such as chronic ankle sprains and fractures of the fifth metatarsal and os peroneum.

Lesions in the fibro-osseous tunnels cause nerve compression, most prominently in the lateral aspect of the heel or foot. These include ganglion cysts, varicosities, bone and joint abnormalities, tumors, tenosynovitis, and supernumerary or hypertrophic muscles.

Compromise of the SN at the superficial sural aponeurosis is rare and usually seen in athletes older than 30 years of age.

Ultrasound Imaging Findings

The best position to observe the SN is along its short axis, as it travels with the lesser saphenous vein(s). The ultrasound transducer is placed in the short-axis position, relative to the limb,

and is placed at the middle to lower third of the calf. When the short-axis image of the SSV is seen, the SN usually appears as an ovoid structure that is moderately echogenic and lays posterior and lateral to the SSV. It is ovoid, echogenic, and demonstrates a characteristic fascicular, honeycomb pattern of peripheral nerves. These structures (nerve, and vein) lie between the AT posteriorly, and the peroneal myotendinous units laterally. The transducer can then be slowly moved to track the course of the nerve, as it travels distally, and finally dives deep to the peroneal tendons (Figure 101-2).

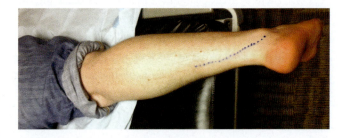

FIGURE 101-1 ■ Surface mapping of the sural nerve.

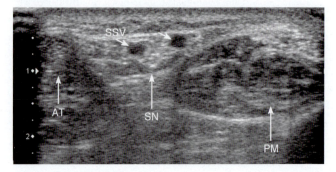

FIGURE 101-2 ■ Ultrasound of sural nerve (SN) travelling with small saphenous vein (SSV), between Achilles tendon (AT), and peroneal muscle (PM) bellies.

Indications for Injections of the Sural Nerve

Injection of the SN can be performed for patients with pain syndromes that are along the SN distribution of the lower leg and foot, which are unresponsive to conservative therapies. It may also be used as a diagnostic procedure to secure or rule out diagnosis.

Equipment

■ Needle
  • Use a 25-gauge, 1.5-inch needle.
  • A 25-gauge or 23-gauge 5/8-inch butterfly needle with short tubing can be helpful in very thin patients.
■ Injectate
  • 3-4 mLs local anesthetic (combination of both short and long acting)
  • 1 mL injectable corticosteroid
■ High-frequency linear array transducer

Author's Preferred Technique

a. Patient position
  i. Prone with affected lower leg externally rotated (see Figure 101-1)
  ii. Contralateral decubitus with effected leg on top
b. Transducer position (Figure 101-3)
  i. Short axis with respect to nerve course (along long axis of limb, then tracking deep to and along course of peroneal tendons)
c. Needle orientation relative to the transducer
  i. In plane (Figure 101-4).
  ii. Out of plane may be needed at ankle level.
d. Needle approach
  i. Author's preference is to start from posterior medial approach (lateral to the AT), and direct needle laterally toward the nerve. The injectionist is standing on the contralateral side of the bed (Figure 101-5).
  ii. Alternatively, use a lateral-to-medial approach from the ipsilateral side the bed, with the screen positioned on the opposite side.

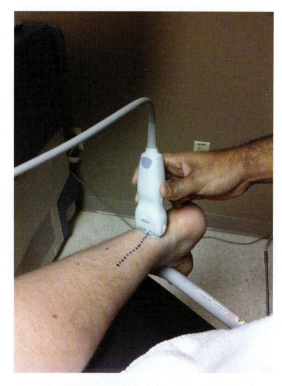

FIGURE 101-3 ■ Transducer position.

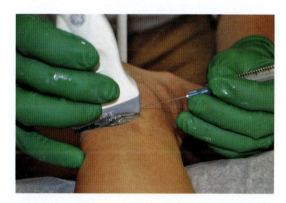

FIGURE 101-4 ■ Sural nerve injection approach: In plane short axis to the nerve.

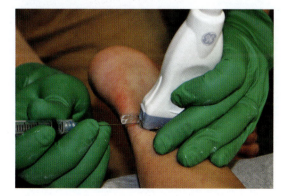

FIGURE 101-5 ■ Sural nerve injection approach: from posterior medial approach (lateral to the AT) with the needle directed laterally toward the nerve.

e. Target

  i. Perineural soft tissues, to create halo about the nerve (Figure 101-6)

f. Pearls and Pitfalls

  i. Avoid intraneural injection and inadvertent saphenous vein injection.

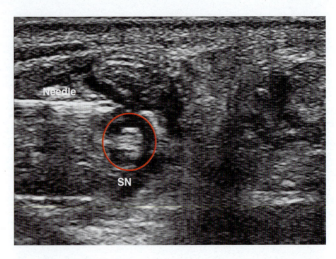

FIGURE 101-6 ▪ Needle with injectate creating halo around the sural nerve (SN).

References

1. Waldman SD. Atlas of Interventional Pain Management. 2nd ed. Philadelphia, PA: Saunders, 2004;512.
2. Fabre T, Monero C, Gaujard E, Gervais-Dellion F, Durandeau A. Chronic calf pain in athletes due to sural nerve entrapment. *Am J Sports Med* 2000;28(5):679–682.
3. Schon LC. Nerve entrapment, neuropathy, and nerve dysfunction in athletes. *Orthop Clin North Am* 1994;25(1):47–59.
4. McCrory P, Bell S, Bradshaw C. Nerve entrapments of the lower leg, ankle and foot in sport. *Sports Med* 2002;32(6):371–391.
5. Lee TH, Wapner KL, Hecht PJ, Hunt PJ. Regional anesthesia in foot and ankle surgery. *Orthopedics* 1996;19:577–580.
6. Redborg KE, Sites BD, Chinn CD, et al. Ultrasound improves the success rate of a sural nerve block at the ankle. *Reg Anesth Pain Med* 2009;34:24–28.
7. Martinoli C, Court-Payen M, Michaud J, et al. Imaging of neuropathies about the ankle and foot. *Semin Musculoskelet Radiol* 2010;14(3):344–356.

Michael Goldin, MD / Brian J. Shiple, DO

KEY POINTS

- Use a 27–25-gauge, 1.25–1.5-inch needle.
- Use a medium-frequency linear array transducer.
- Morton's neuroma is a symptomatic fibrous nodule that classically develops between the third and fourth metatarsophalangeals (MTPs) at the confluence of the medial and lateral plantar nerves.
- The continuity of the neuroma with the interdigital nerve may be seen ultrasonographically somewhat oblique to the nearby metatarsal bone.
- The dorsal approach is preferred.

Pertinent Anatomy

The far lateral branch of the medial calcaneal nerve and the medial branch of the lateral calcaneal nerve combine into one interdigital nerve between the third and fourth metatarsophalangeals (MTPs), which develops a symptomatic fibrous nodule. Less commonly, this can occur in the interdigital nerve right before it sends its terminal branches to the digits between the second and third MTPs (Figure 102-1).

Common Pathology

Plantar interdigital neuroma, also known as *Morton's neuroma*, is a fibrotic lesion of the perineural tissues of the confluence of the medial and lateral plantar digital nerves of the forefoot.

It affects patients young and old, with patients presenting with symptoms at a mean age of 45–53 years of age. Women are more commonly affected (78%). Symptoms include forefoot pain and paraesthesias. The diagnosis can be made clinically through appropriate history and physical examination. Ultrasound or magnetic resonance imaging may be used to confirm the diagnosis.[1]

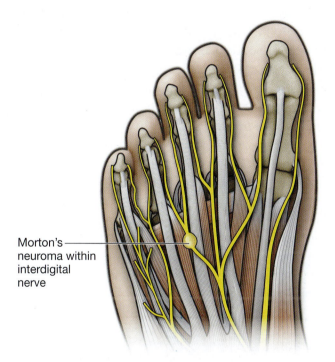

Morton's neuroma within interdigital nerve

FIGURE 102-1 ■ Location of the Morton's neuroma: the interdigital nerve between the third and fourth metatarsal phalangeal joints, which comes from the lateral branch of the medial calcaneal nerve and the medial branch of the lateral calcaneal nerve.

Ultrasound Imaging Findings

Morton's neuroma is best visualized using a medium-frequency linear array transducer at a depth setting at 3 cm or slightly less. A hypoechoic mass greater than 5 mm measured in short axis is usually found in symptomatic Morton's neuroma (Figures 102-2 and 102-3). When viewed longitudinally the neuroma has a more fusiform appearance. If lined up properly, the operator will see the continuity of the neuroma with the interdigital nerve somewhat oblique to the nearby metatarsal bone. The sonographic Tinel's sign refers to squeezing the neuroma between the transducer and the operator's opposite thumb. This may reproduce pain and/or paresthesias. Mulder's sign refers to compressing the metatarsal together with one hand while holding the transducer with the other hand. This can result in the displacement of the neuroma often resulting in an audible click and allow for improved ultrasound visualization the neuroma.

Turn the probe longitudinal over the nodule to visualize the Morton's neuroma as part of the interdigital nerve in long axis. The hyperechoic nature of the nodule may blend in with the surrounding soft tissue. Using color Doppler will help identify the nodule because of the interdigital artery that runs with it. Additionally, using the Mulder maneuver will help differentiate the nodule from the rest of the soft tissue. Some articles state the nodule should appear anechoic. Intermetatarsal bursitis can also be a source of pain in this area and, therefore, knowledge of the anatomy of these structures and their relationship to the interdigital nerves is important (Figures 102-3 and 102-4).

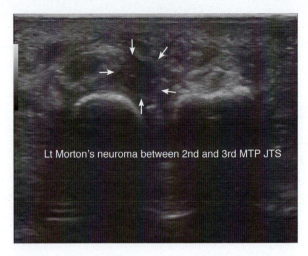

FIGURE 102-2 ■ Long-axis view of intermetatarsal neuroma. *Arrows* are self explanatory.

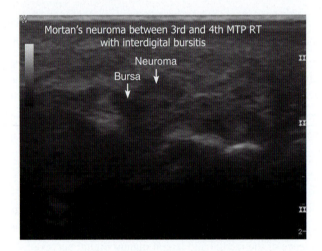

FIGURE 102-3 ■ Short-axis view of intermetatarsal neuroma with intermetatarsal bursa. *Arrows* are self explanatory.

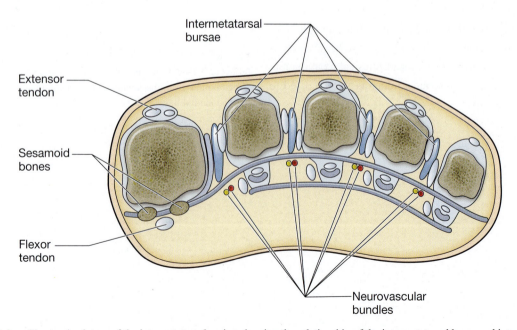

FIGURE 102-4 ■ Short-axis picture of the intermetatarsal region showing the relationship of the intermetatarsal bursa and interdigital nerves.

Indications for Injection of Morton's Neuroma

Injection of Morton's neuroma can be performed for patients with pain that is recalcitrant to conservative treatment with metatarsal pad off-loading, nonsteroidal antiinflammatory drugs (NSAIDs), adjustment of tight-fitting shoes and physical therapy modalities. It is usually symptomatic when Morton's neuroma is >5 mm when measured in the short-axis plane.[2]

In a retrospective study with 27 patients receiving a palpation-guided, single corticosteroid injection, 11% (3/27) people were completely satisfied after the injection.[2] Ultrasound-guided injection has been described by Markovic et al. in a prospective cohort trial.[1] Before injection, the Johnson scale showed 26 patients (67%) dissatisfied, and 13 patients (33%) satisfied with major reservations. At 1 month post injection, 16/39 (41%) subjects were completely satisfied, and at 9 months, 15/39 (38%) were completely satisfied. Clinical outcomes of palpation-guided versus image-guided injection have not been described at the time of this publication.

Equipment

- Needle: 27–25-gauge, 1.25–1.5-inch
- Injectate
  - 0.5 mL of an injectable corticosteroid
  - 0.5 mL of an anesthetic
- Medium-frequency linear array transducer

Author's Preferred Technique

Plantar Approach

a. Patient position
    i. Prone for distal needle entry
    ii. Foot at position that is at comfortable height for practitioner performing injection
b. Transducer position
    i. With skin entry, position the transducer in short axis over the plantar aspect of the metatarsal heads (Figure 102-5).
    ii. When needle is in the neuroma, turn the probe long axis along the interdigital nerve (Figure 102-6).
c. Needle orientation relative to the transducer (see Figures 102-5 and 102-6)
    i. Start in short axis.
    ii. At the middle of the neuroma, turn long axis.

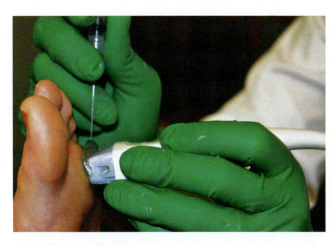

FIGURE 102-5 ■ Ultrasound probe position in the short-axis plane over the plantar aspect of the short-axis metatarsal arch at the level of the metatarsophalangeal joint with the needle directed out of plane in the plantar approach.

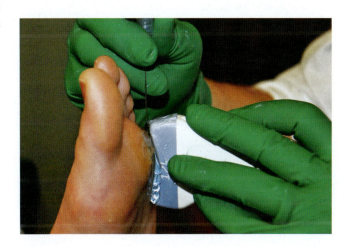

FIGURE 102-6 ■ Ultrasound probe position in the long axis over the plantar aspect of the metatarsal arch at the level of the metatarsophalangeal joint with needle directed in plane in the plantar approach.

d. Needle approach (see Figures 102-5 and 102-6)
   i. Distal to proximal
e. Target
   i. Hyper- to hypoechoic to anechoic nodule at the level of the intermetatarsal space
f. Pearls and Pitfalls
   i. There are three differential diagnoses: (1) inter-metatarsal bursitis with anechoic fluid that is usu-ally compressible; the Doppler effect of fluid flow inside the bursa with injection during color or power Doppler setting would be visible. (2) Metatarsalgia with laxity in the short-axis intermetatarsal ligament system is painful to direct palpation of the metatarsal joint. (3) During history, physical examination, and ultrasound scanning, a mixture of these conditions is seen in the same patient; therefore, more than one treatment approach may be necessary to cure the pa-tient's conditions.

Alternate Technique

Dorsal Approach

a. Patient position
   i. Supine with knee flexed and forefoot hanging off end of examination table for dorsal needle entry
b. Transducer position
   i. Short axis over plantar aspect of metatarsal heads
c. Needle orientation relative to transducer
   i. Start short axis and place needle in middle of neu-roma (Figure 102-7)
d. Needle approach
   i. Start dorsally, distal to proximal, directly perpen-dicular to the probe from the intermetatarsal space.
   ii. Advance until the needle is seen approaching the neuroma.
   iii. Change the probe to long axis (Figure 102-8).
   iv. Adjust the needle medially or laterally as necessary to get the needle into the middle of the neuroma (Figure 102-9).
e. Target
   i. Hyper- to hypoechoic nodule at the level of the inter-metatarsal space

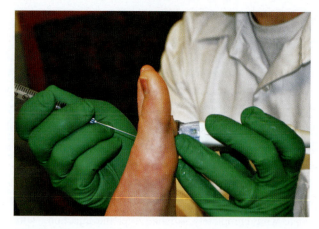

FIGURE 102-7 ■ Ultrasound probe position in the short-axis plane over the plantar aspect of the transverse metatarsal arch, with a dorsal out-of-plane approach.

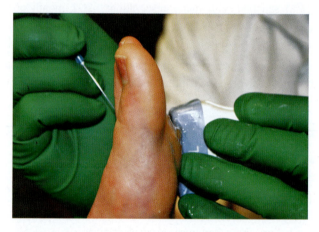

FIGURE 102-8 ■ Ultrasound probe position in long axis over the plantar aspect of the metatarsal arch at the level of the metatarsopha-langeal joint with a dorsal, in-plane approach.

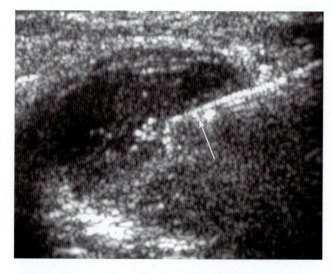

FIGURE 102-9 ■ A 46-year-old woman with Morton's neuroma. Sonogram shows that needle tip is within hypoechoic mass of neu-roma (*arrow*).

f. Pearls and Pitfalls
    i. An alternative to corticosteroid injection is chemical neurolysis. If the symptoms persist despite corticosteroid injection, 4–6% phenol can be used to destroy the nerve. Alcohol requires up to six treatment sessions to effectively destroy the nerve and phenol may take up to three injections. Very small amounts of the solution should be accurately injected into the nodule, because too much solution injected into the surrounding soft tissue may lead to a complication of soft tissue necrosis including slow healing superficial wounds.

References

1. Markovic M, Crichton K, Read JW, Lam P, Slater HK. Effectiveness of ultrasound-guided corticosteroid injection in the treatment of Morton's neuroma. *Foot Ankle Int* 2008;29(5):483–487.
2. Rasmussen M, Kitaoka HB, Patzer GL. Nonoperative treatment of plantar interdigital neuroma with a single corticosteroid injection. *Clin Orthop Relat Res* 1996;326(11):188–193.

Special Procedures

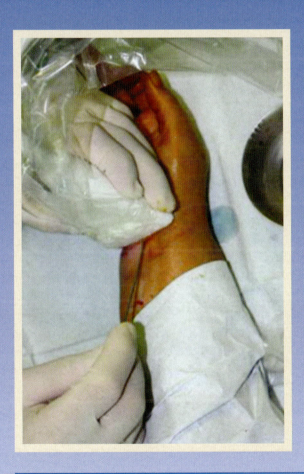

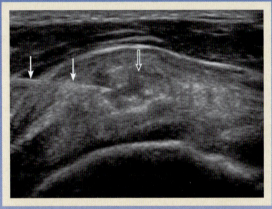

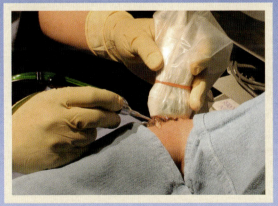

Gregory R. Saboeiro, MD

Pertinent Anatomy

Rotator cuff calcific tendinosis, by definition, involves deposition of calcific material within one of the four rotator cuff tendons of the shoulder. The most commonly involved tendon is the supraspinatus, followed by the infraspinatus and subscapularis tendons. Involvement of the teres minor tendon is rare.

Common Pathology

The calcific material that is deposited within the rotator cuff tendons is in the form of calcium hydroxyapatite, which is a crystalline calcium phosphate. The calcification most commonly lies within the distal tendons near their attachment to the greater or lesser tuberosities and is less likely present more proximally at the muscle-tendon junctions. Calcification may also lie within the adjacent subacromial bursa, and is most likely secondary to decompression of rotator cuff calcification into the bursa and less likely primary bursal calcification.

The diagnosis of calcific tendinosis may be made clinically, but imaging is also necessary in confirmation of this condition. The patient will usually present with limited range of motion and shoulder pain that is greatest with elevation of the arm. Symptoms may vary depending on the location of the calcification within the rotator cuff. The pain is generally greatest at night. Differential possibilities include rotator cuff tears or tendonopathy, subacromial-subdeltoid bursitis, glenohumeral joint arthrosis, and adhesive capsulitis.

Ultrasound Imaging Findings

Imaging of this condition involves visualization and localization of the calcific focus. In most symptomatic cases, the calcification will be large enough to see radiographically and depending on its position on the various shoulder views obtained (anterior vs. posterior), the precise tendon involved can often be determined (Figure 103-1).

Ultrasound and magnetic resonance imaging (MRI) may both allow a more precise localization of the calcification. If the calcification is visualized radiographically and the patient's symptoms are concordant with the diagnosis, an MRI is usually not necessary. In addition, smaller foci of calcification may not be readily visualized on MRI but are easily seen with ultrasound.

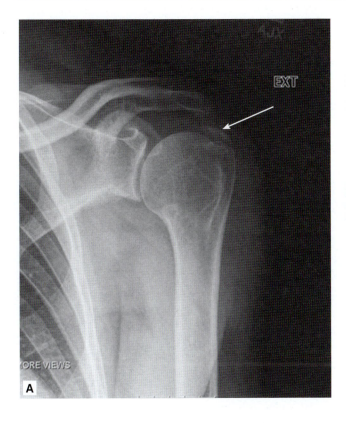

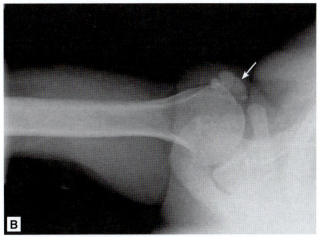

FIGURE 103-1 ■ **A.** Large focus of calcification (*arrow*) at the level of the greater trochanter and confirmed to be within the insertional supraspinatus tendon. **B.** Calcific focus (*arrow*) anterior in position and confirmed to be within the subscapularis tendon insertion.

Ultrasound provides an excellent means of identifying and quantifying the amount of calcification present. The calcification appears as a hyperechoic focus within the tendon, with varying amounts of posterior acoustic shadowing depending on the size and composition of the calcification (Figure 103-2). The calcification may be seen as a single large focus or as multiple small foci. Ultrasound also allows evaluation of the adjacent bursa for evidence of coexisting subacromial bursitis, a common occurrence. The feasibility of performing percutaneous treatment of the calcific tendinosis is also determined at that time.

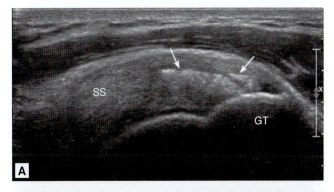

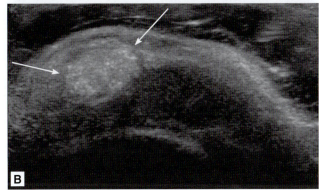

FIGURE 103-2 ■ **A** and **B**. Two large foci of hyperechoic calcification within the rotator cuff tendons (*arrows*). SS, Supraspinatus; GT, Greater tuberosity.

Indications for Calcific Tendinosis Lavage and Aspiration

If the patient's clinical presentation is concordant with calcific tendinosis and ultrasound confirms the diagnosis, there are several treatment options. Physical therapy and antiinflammatory medication are usually of limited value in obtaining long-term pain relief and patient improvement. Extracorporeal shock wave therapy has some proponents but is not widely accepted. Although injection of anesthetic and corticosteroids into the glenohumeral joint or subacromial-subdeltoid bursa may provide some symptomatic relief, this does not address the underlying problem of calcium deposition within the rotator cuff. Surgery for this condition is difficult, often requiring significant tendon resection and subsequent repair, and is generally the therapy of last resort.

Ultrasound-guided percutaneous lavage aspiration of rotator cuff calcific tendinosis was first reported in 1995[1] and was performed with fluoroscopic guidance as early as 1978. Over the intervening years, the procedure has been modified and the outcome improved such that today it is the primary means of treating this disorder. Multiple studies have demonstrated a high rate of success with this therapy. Although the criteria for a positive outcome varies throughout the literature, a good or excellent result has been generally reported in 70–90% of patients.[2-5]

Equipment

■ Needle
  • 25-gauge needle for anesthesia administration
  • 16–18-gauge needle for calcium lavage and aspiration
■ Injectate
  • 2–4 mL local anesthetic
  • 1–2 mL corticosteroid
■ Lavage syringes (3–10 depending on the amount of calcification)
  • Mixture of 7 mL saline and 3 mL of anesthetic in each 10 mL syringe
■ High-frequency linear array transducer

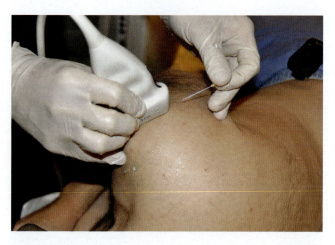

FIGURE 103-3 ■ Long-axis approach to a focus of calcification within the supraspinatus with the patient in the lateral decubitus position.

Author's Preferred Technique

a. Patient position
  i. The patient is positioned such that the calcification to be treated is well-visualized and amenable to needle placement and both the patient and physician will be comfortable throughout the procedure. Depending on calcification location, particularly within the supraspinatus tendon and deep to the overlying acromion process of the scapula, it may be necessary to experiment with various arm positions of the patient to achieve this goal. Generally, the procedure is performed with the patient in the lateral decubitus position for supraspinatus and infraspinatus calcifications and in the supine position if the subscapularis tendon is the target.
b. Transducer position (Figure 103-3)
  i. Transducer position is variable and dependent on the location and orientation of the focus of calcium hydroxyapatite. The best position is generally one that visualizes the calcium in its longest orientation and allows needle placement into the epicenter of the lesion with a single puncture.
c. Needle orientation relative to the transducer
  i. The needle is seen in long-axis to the transducer, and should be as parallel as possible to the transducer position for optimal visualization.

d. Needle approach
   i. Variable depending on the location of the calcific body(ies)
e. Target
   i. The epicenter of each individual focus of hydroxy-apatite.
f. Technique
   i. A liberal amount of anesthetic is administered, being sure that no air is introduced into the soft tissues or adjacent subacromial bursa, extending from the skin entry site to the margin of the calcification along the expected path of lavage needle placement. If air is injected and is superficial to the target calcification, particularly within the subacromial-subdeltoid bursa, the calcification may be entirely obscured and the procedure may need to be postponed until the air is resorbed. With continuous ultrasound visualization, the needle is advanced into the epicenter of the calcific focus with a single puncture (Figure 103-4). Using the syringes filled with anesthetic and saline mixture noted above, intermittent plunger pressure and release is performed until a cavity forms within the focus of calcification (Figure 103-5). At this point, swirling of echogenic material (calcium) will be seen within the cavity and with plunger release, this calcific material will be expelled into the syringe. If more than a single puncture is made into the lesion, the lavage material may decompress and the yield of calcium removed will generally be significantly diminished.

   As large amounts of calcium fill the syringe, exchange is made for new syringes until no further calcification may be removed and the fluid expelled is clear. Ideally, a large amount of layering calcium will be present within the syringes used (Figure 103-6). At this point, any remaining calcification along the wall of the original focus is fenestrated using the needle. If additional foci of calcification are present, these are treated in the same manner. At the conclusion of this process, any remaining calcium fragments too small for lavage are also fenestrated with the needle. Finally, the mixture of anesthetic and corticosteroid described above is injected into the adjacent subacromial bursa. This will provide significant pain relief over the next several weeks to months as additional calcific material decompresses into the bursa from the involved rotator cuff tendon.

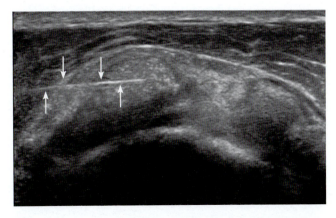

FIGURE 103-4 ■ Sonographic image demonstrating needle placement (*arrows*) within the center of the focus of calcium hydroxyapatite, using a single puncture.

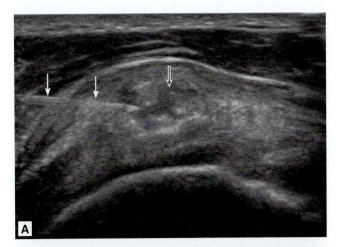

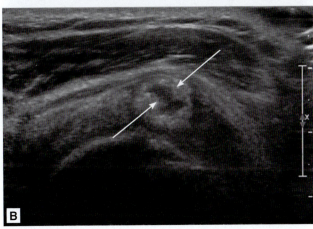

FIGURE 103-5 ■ **A.** Needle (*arrows*) within the focus of calcification with development of a central cavity (*open arrow*) within the calcification during the lavage procedure. **B.** Second patient, demonstrating cavity formation (*arrows*) within a calcific focus during lavage and aspiration.

g. Pearls and Pitfalls

i. A single puncture into the epicenter of the calcific focus is necessary.

ii. No air should be administered into the regional soft tissues.

iii. Linear calcifications with strong acoustic shadowing, which may represent enthesopathic change and not calcium hydroxyapatite deposition, generally do not respond well to lavage and often no calcium may be removed, although they may be fragmented with the needle.

iv. Some authors advocate a two-needle technique in which the lavage solution is injected through one needle and the calcific material is removed through the second needle.[4,6] In the author's experience, this does not improve the yield of calcium removal and unnecessarily complicates the procedure.

v. Some authors advocate the use of smaller (22–25 gauge) needles for the procedure.[7] In the author's experience, this results in a longer procedure time and a lower yield of particulate calcium.

vi. Some clinicians actually perform only needling the calcifications without aspiration of the particulate calcium at all with similar success in outcome.

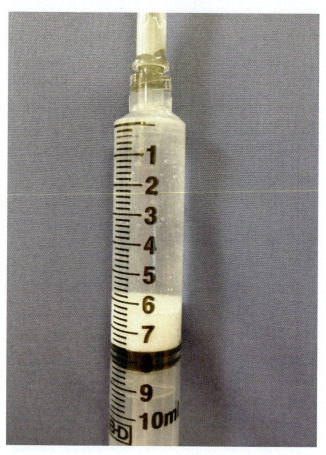

FIGURE 103-6 ■ At the conclusion of the procedure, a large amount of calcium is seen within the dependent portion of the aspiration syringe.

References

1. Farin PU, Räsänen H, Jaroma H, Harju A. Rotator cuff calcifications: treatment with ultrasound-guided percutaneous needle aspiration and lavage. *Skeletal Radiol* 1996(6):551–554.

2. Del Cura JL, Torre I, Zabala R, Legorburu A. Sonographically guided percutaneous needle lavage in calcific tendinitis of the shoulder: short- and long-term results. *AJR Am J Roentgenol* 2007;189(3):W128–W134.

3. Lin JT, Adler RS, Bracilovic A, et al. Clinical outcomes of ultrasound-guided aspiration and lavage in calcific tendinosis of the shoulder. *HSS* 2007;3(1):99–105.

4. Serafini G, Sconfienza LM, Lacelli F, et al. Rotator cuff calcific tendonitis: short-term and 10-year outcomes after two- needle us-guided percutaneous treatment—nonrandomized controlled trail. *Radiology* 2009;252(1):157–164.

5. Yoo JC, Koh KH, Park WH, et al. The outcome of ultrasound-guided needle decompression and steroid injection in calcific tendonitis. *J Shoulder Elbow Surg* 2010;19(4):596–600.

6. Farin PU, Jaroma H, Soimakallio S. Rotator cuff calcifications: treatment with US-guided technique. *Radiology* 1995;195(3):841–843.

7. Aina R, Cardinal E, Bureau N, Aubin B, Brassard P. Calcific shoulder tendinosis: treatment with modified US-guided fine-needle technique. *Radiology* 2001;221:455–461.

Jose Manuel Rojo Manaute, MD, PhD / Guillermo Emilio Rodríguez-Maruri, MD / Alberto Capa-Grasa, MD, PhD

KEY POINTS

- A high-frequency linear array transducer (depth <3 cm) is placed longitudinally over the anterior aspect of the metacarpophalangeal (MCP) and checked transversely for a correct radial and ulnar position (centered over the tendon).
- The release requires a 3-mm hook knife (eg, Orthomed® or Acufex®) introduced 1 cm distal to the MCP crease of the thumb and at the proximal phalangeal crease of the rest of the fingers, at the finger's mid-longitudinal axis.
- Major pitfalls: Instruments must be located precisely at proximal cutting point (PCP) to avoid the risk of transecting any proximal neurovascular crossing structures (especially at the thumb). Keep the release specifically restricted to the synovial sheath without intruding into the more superficial anatomy.
- Major pearls: Extending or hyperextending the MCP joint allows for an easier reach of the proximal edge of the first annular (A1) pulley. If there is a severe stricture and/or the relative size of A1 is too small, we recommend splitting the release of A1 into two or more segments.

Introduction

The trigger digit (TD) is one of the most frequent pathological conditions in hand surgery, with a 2.2% incidence throughout life in the nondiabetic population older than 30 years in age and 10% in those patients with diabetes mellitus.[1]

Anatomy

The fibrous retinacular synovial sheath consists of a pulley mechanism of the digital flexor tendons that starts at the neck of the metacarpal and ends at the distal phalanx. Condensations of the sheath form the flexor pulleys. The first anular (A1) digital pulley is at the level of the metacarpophalangeal (MCP) joint.[2]

Common Pathology

TD is caused by tendon entrapment secondary to mechanical impingement of the digital flexor tendons as they pass through a narrowed A1. Pathologic changes at the A1 pulley include gross hypertrophy, degeneration, cyst formation, fiber splitting, lymphocytic or plasma cell infiltration, and chondrocyte proliferation (fibrocartilaginous metaplasia).[2]

Diagnosis and Ultrasound Imaging Findings

The diagnosis can normally be made based on clinical findings and, for severe catching, it can be confirmed with a simple lidocaine injection into the flexor sheath to unlock the digit. Differential diagnoses include dislocation, Dupuytren disease, severe de Quervain disease, hysteria, focal dystonia, localized enlargement of the flexor digitorum profundus at a stenotic A3 pulley, and profundus entrapment by synovitis at the superficialis decussation.[2] Thickening of the A1 pulley can also be identified on sonography using a linear array transducer (8–12 Hz, depth <3 cm) as a general and focal thickening, with impingement of flexor tendon movement identified dynamically during active and passive movement.[3]

Treatment Indications

Corticosteroid injections are widely accepted as the first choice for treating TD and, at present, we recommend one injection prior to proceeding with surgery if there is no demonstrable catching requiring passive extension or inability to actively flex (clinical grade III of Froimson). However, we proceed directly with surgery in grades III and IV (flexion contracture) because we believe that the symptoms are annoying and the success rate is low enough for the patient as to avoid more delay.[4] We do not use splints for treating TD at our practice.

The success rates for releasing the A1 pulley are relatively similar for classic open surgery (COS) (60–100%) and palpation-guided percutaneous release (73–100%).[5] Although COS is a simple procedure, dissatisfaction rates can be as high as 17–26%.[6] Very few complications have been reported for palpation-guided percutaneous release but, in agreement with other authors,[7] we believe that the potential complications of the different palpation-guided percutaneous release techniques exceed their possible benefits.

As an alternative to palpation-guided percutaneous release, different percutaneous ultrasound-guided A1 release (USGAR) has been recently described by either pulling (retrograde)[7,8] or pushing (anterograde),[3] from an extra-[7] or an intrasheath[8] position, a surgical instrument (ie, needle[3] or hook knife[7,8]). Experimental[9] and clinical[7,10] data have shown a higher complete pulley release rate when using a hook knife instead of a needle. Moreover, accidental intrusions into the neurovascular compartment and moderate injuries to flexor tendons have been described with extrasheath USGAR techniques.[9] For overcoming these difficulties, we recently described, first,[8] a safe volar area in volunteers for aiming a surgical instrument (Figure 104-1) and a procedure in cadavers for performing safely and effectively a retrograde intrasheath USGAR with a hook knife; second,[10] we assessed clinically that the procedure was safe and successful. Favorable results in 48 patients, followed up for 11.3 months on average (83.3% excellent, 14.6% good and 2.1% acceptable), using this technique remains on theoretical grounds because extrasheath retrograde USGAR using a hook knife[7] has yielded similar clinical results. Thus, the hypothetical clinical advantage of the retrograde intrasheath USGAR is based on the potential prevention of accidentally aiming instruments toward a neurovascular structure. The USGAR procedure is performed as an office-based ambulatory procedure and, in a randomized comparative study of the economic impact of three surgical models, we recently described that our USGAR procedure offered the shortest turnover time and the best economical results with a quick recoup of the fixed costs of ultrasound-assisted surgery.[4] In fact, based on our true net income, a recoup of the fixed costs (ultrasound equipment) is achieved after 19.78 procedures.

Equipment

- Needle: 25-gauge × 5/8" needle
- Injectate
  - 2.7 mL injectable anesthetic, without epinephrine
  - 0.3 mL sodium bicarbonate
- 1.5 mm Kirschner wire (KW)
- 16-gauge Abbocath®
- 3 mm retrograde reusable hook knife
- 2% chlorhexidine aqueous solution (instead of ultrasound gel)
- High-frequency linear array transducer

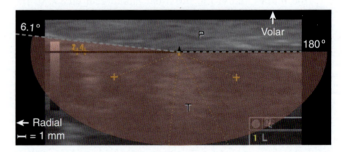

FIGURE 104-1 ▪ Safe axial area for a percutaneous release. Our previous anatomic results,[8] using ultrasounds in volunteers, showed that there was risk of damaging the flexor tendons and neurovascular structures in a semicircular-like area (*red zone*) dorsal to the point from which the first annular (A1) pulley is released (*black triangle*). Therefore, we believe that a surgical instrument should be directed volarly (which required an intrasheath positioning). P, A1 pulley (sheath); T, tendon.

Author's Preferred Technique

a. Patient position

i. With the patient either seated or in supine position, our nurse performs a preoperative cleansing with 2% chlorhexidine solution for 5 minutes, protects the affected hand in a surgical drape, and leaves it resting supinated on an auxiliary table (covered by another surgical drape) at the patient's side (Figure 104-2).

b. Transducer position, approach, orientation, and target

i. After injecting local anesthesia at our skin approach (1 cm distal to the MCP crease of the thumb and at the proximal phalangeal crease of the rest of the fingers, at the finger's mid-longitudinal axis), we perform a two-step release of A1 guided by ultrasound. Every step is initiated with the transducer placed longitudinally over the volar aspect of the MCP and checked transversely for a correct radial and ulnar position (centered over the tendon):

- Step 1 (dilatation): We introduce an ultrasound-guided 16-gauge Abbocath for piercing a point of entry (PEN) on the volar tendon sheath 3 mm distally from the base-shaft junction of the proximal phalanx. We then push the blunt tip of a 1.5-mm KW through the PEN and inside the synovial space to our proximal cutting point (PCP), at 3 mm proximal to the junction of the head and neck of the metacarpal for the thumb and at 5 mm proximal for the rest of the fingers. This step creates an adequate space for introducing next a cutting device.

- Step 2 (release): We introduce the hook knife inside the tendon sheath and push it to the PCP, releasing A1 by turning the edge toward the palm, pressing it volarly, and pulling it to exit through the PEN (Figure 104-3). Adequate release is shown by the disappearance of triggering on active movement of the digit by the patient.

ii. The final skin wound is approximately 1 mm wide, and it is covered with an adhesive dressing that is removed in 2 days. No suturing is necessary. Patients are encouraged to restart their normal life from the same day of surgery and are given instructions for performing constant active and passive full range of motion during daytime.

c. Pearls and Pitfalls

i Once the instrument is inside the synovial sheath (checked longitudinally and transversely), extending or hyperextending the MCP joint allows for an easier reach of the proximal edge of A1.

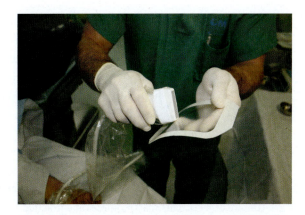

FIGURE 104-2 ■ Patient position and field sterility. In this example, the patient is in supine position, our nurse had already performed a preoperative cleansing, and the hand was left supinated and protected on an auxiliary table at the patient's side.

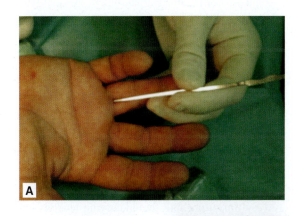

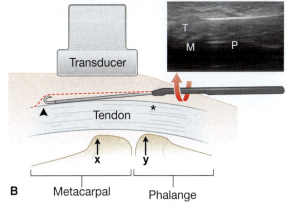

FIGURE 104-3 ■ Release. **A.** The hook knife is introduced inside the tendon sheath at point of entry (PEN). **B.** Diagram shows how the Acufex hook knife is positioned for the release. The device is introduced flat on its widest side, checking its position on long- and short-axis transducer positions until we reach our proximal cutting point (*arrowhead*). We then turn our device toward the palm, press the hook volarly, and pull to exit through PEN (*asterisk*) for releasing first annular (A1) pulley. M, metacarpal; P, phalanx; PEN, point of entry; T, tendon; x, metacarpal head-neck junction; y, proximal phalangeal base-shaft junction.

ii. For hyperextending the MCP in TD located at a second to fifth finger, we normally use the surgical table's edge that is closer to the operator (Figure 104-4). This maneuver requires a conscious effort to keep field sterility for that edge throughout the procedure because we do not use surgical gowns.

iii. For TD of the thumb, the operator will need to hold the patient's finger on a vertical position for extending and hyperextending the MCP while using a surgical instrument, all with the same hand (Figure 104-5). This may require some practice.

iv. Instruments must be located precisely at the PCP to avoid the risk of transecting any proximal neurovascular crossing structures (especially at the thumb). PCP location requires careful monitoring of the distance from the tip of our instrument to the head-neck junction of the metacarpal (unless the quality of our ultrasound equipment allows for a good visualization of A1's proximal edge).

v. If the instrument goes too far proximal, it can be pulled back distally, without damaging the surrounding anatomy, by oscillating the tip in an ulnar and radial direction and pulling gently. The idea is to "unhook" the tip if it is trapped.

vi. Keep the release specifically restricted to the synovial sheath for avoiding complications, without intruding into the more superficial anatomy (longer recovery times) nor into the underlying tendons (risk of rupture). This can be done by checking that the blade of the instrument is precisely located at the sheath before starting the release, on longitudinal and axial views, and as it is pulled (longitudinally).

vii. If there is a severe stricture and/or the relative size of A1 is too small (eg, in some women's thumbs), our instruments may encounter difficulties for reaching the PCP. Moreover, a stricture can force our instruments into an intratendinous position, which will probably damage the flexor tendons. In our experience, the Orthomed hook knife can overcome more easily these strictures than the Acufex because its stem is a bit smaller. When the stricture is too severe, we recommend splitting the release of A1 into two or more segments (Figure 104-6).

viii. We advise training the use of both hands for manipulating the instruments with similar dexterity.

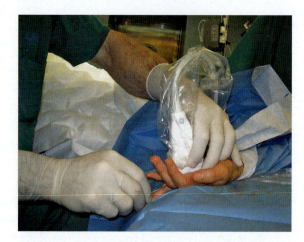

FIGURE 104-4 ■ Extending or hyperextending the metacarpophalangeal (MCP) joint allows for an easier reach of the proximal edge of the first annular (A1) pulley. Keep the field sterile for that edge throughout the procedure if you do not use a surgical gown.

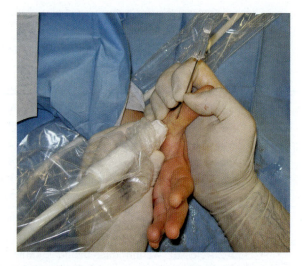

FIGURE 104-5 ■ For the thumb, the operator will need to hold the patient's finger on a vertical position for extending and hyperextending the metacarpophalangeal (MCP) while using a surgical instrument.

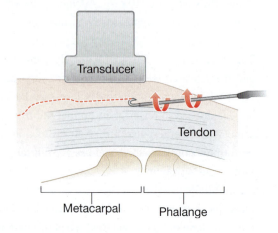

FIGURE 104-6 ■ When the stricture is too severe, we recommend splitting the release of the first annular (A1) pulley into two or more segments.

References

1. Saldana MJ. Trigger digits: diagnosis and treatment. *J Am Acad Orthop Surg* 2001;9:246–252.

2. Wolfe SW. Tenosynovitis. In: Green DP, Hotchkiss RN, Pederson WC, Wolfe SW, eds. *Green's Operative Hand Surgery*. 5th ed. Philadelphia, PA: Churchill Livingstone; 2005: 2137–2154.

3. Rajeswaran G, Lee JC, Eckersley R, Katsarma E, Healy JC. Ultrasound-guided percutaneous release of the annular pulley in trigger digit. *Eur Radiol* 2009;19:2232–2237.

4. Rojo-Manaute JM, Capa-Grasa A, Cerro-Gutierrez MD, et al. Sonographically guided intrasheath percutaneous release of the first annular pulley for trigger digits, part 2: randomized comparative study of the economic impact of three surgical models. *J Ultrasound Med*;31:427–438.

5. Gilberts EC, Beekman WH, Stevens HJ, Wereldsma JC. Prospective randomized trial of open versus percutaneous surgery for trigger digits. *J Hand Surg Am* 2001;26:497–500.

6. Thorpe AP. Results of surgery for trigger finger. *J Hand Surg Br* 1988;13:199–201.

7. Jou IM, Chern TC. Sonographically assisted percutaneous release of the A1 pulley: a new surgical technique for treating trigger digit. *J Hand Surg Br* 2006;31:191–199.

8. Rojo-Manaute JM L-SV, De las Heras Sanchez-Heredero J, Del Valle Soto, Del Cerro-Gutierrez, Vaquero Marín J. Percutaneous intrasheath ultrasonographically guided first annular pulley release. *J Ultrasound Med* 2010;29:1517–1529.

9. Smith J, Rizzo M, Lai JK. Sonographically guided percutaneous first annular pulley release: cadaveric safety study of needle and knife techniques. *J Ultrasound Med* 2010;29:1531–1542.

10. Rojo Manaute JM, Rodríguez Maruri G, Capa Grasa A, Chana Rodríguez F, Del Valle Soto M, J. VM. Ultrasound guided intrasheath percutaneous release of the A1 pulley for trigger digits. Part I: Clinical efficacy and safety. *J Ultrasound Med* (in press).

Jose Manuel Rojo Manaute, MD, PhD / Alberto Capa-Grasa, MD, PhD /
Guillermo Emilio Rodríguez-Maruri, MD / Jay Smith, MD / Javier Vaquero Martín, MD, PhD

KEY POINTS

- For performing an ultrasound-guided carpal tunnel release (USG CTR), a linear array transducer (8–12 Hz, depth <3 cm) is placed over the anterior aspect of the distal forearm and proximal wrist.

- A 3-mm hook knife (eg, Orthomed® or Acufex®) is introduced at the most proximal antebrachial skin crease (approximately ≥2 cm proximal to the pisiform) thru a 16-gauge Abbocath® skin incision.

Introduction

Carpal tunnel syndrome (CTS) results from median nerve dysfunction at the wrist and is the most commonly diagnosed entrapment neuropathy, with a prevalence of 50 cases/1000 person-years. More than 400,000 operations each year are performed for CTS in the United States at an average cost of approximately $30,000 per case.[1,2] Clinicians have continued to explore carpal tunnel release (CTR) techniques to reduce cost, operative complications, or postoperative recovery. In recent years, ultrasound-guided carpal tunnel release (USG CTR) techniques have been developed with these goals in mind.[3-6]

Anatomy and Pathology

CTS has been attributed to high carpal tunnel pressure, which may impair median nerve microcirculation and result in demyelization and axonal loss.[1] Three volar fibrous layers have been described at the hand and forearm: a superficial (superficial fascia[7]), an intermediate (antebrachial fascia and palmar aponeurosis) and a deep fibrous layer.[7,8] Histological and immunohistochemical cadaveric studies suggest[7,8] a mechanical function for the deepest layer, whereas the intermediate layer could play a more proprioceptive role. The deepest fibrous layer has been subdivided[8] into proximal (deep investing fascia), central (transverse carpal ligament [TCL]), and distal portions. CTR safety is theoretically maximized by maintaining a release path that bisects the space between the most ulnar point of the median nerve and the most radial point of the closest ulnar vascular structure.[4,9] Incomplete release is the most common cause of CTR failure,[10] and previous studies have indicated that clinical improvement is contingent on jointly releasing the distal and central portions of the deep fibrous layer.[11,12] Recent studies[7] have also hypothesized that postoperative pain may result from surgical damage to local nerve structures lying within the more highly innervated superficial and intermediate layers. Furthermore, both clinical[4] and anatomic[7] findings suggest a denser innervation in the palm when compared to the forearm. These data suggest that a limited release through a forearm approach targeting the deepest fibrous layer may not only be effective, but may also reduce morbidity.[5,10]

Diagnosis and Treatment Indications

A diagnosis of CTS can be made on the basis of signs, symptoms, and electrodiagnostic tests, as recommended by the clinical guidelines of the American Academy of Orthopaedic Surgeons.[1] Although nonsurgical treatment is an option in many cases, surgical intervention is considered following failure of nonoperative management or in the setting of median nerve denervation.[1,2]

Multiple CTR options have been developed primarily to reduce the surgical morbidity associated with larger incisions.[1,4,9] Improved results have been reported with smaller incisions and reduced dissection. CTR incisions have been described as classic (>4 cm),[2] limited (2–4 cm),[10] mini (1–2 cm),[4,9] or percutaneous (0.4–0.6 cm).[3,4,6] Although some studies have demonstrated better outcomes with endoscopic versus classic CTR (1–2 cm),[11,12] concerns persist regarding the inability of the endoscopic techniques to identify the ulnar neurovascular bundle and the rate of incomplete releases.[1,2,9] Mini-open CTR has closely matched endoscopic surgery in its reduced morbidity, but the procedure is performed non-ultrasound-guided (palpation-guided mini-open CTR).[4]

Percutaneous approaches have only been described under real-time ultrasound visualized surgery[3,4,6] as either ultrasound guided[3,4,6,10] (continued ultrasound visualization) or ultrasound assisted[9] (alternating ultrasounds and direct

TABLE 105-1 ■ DIFFERENCES AMONG REPORTED STUDIES IN LITERATURE FOR CARPAL TUNNEL RELEASE UNDER REAL-TIME ULTRASOUND VISUALIZED SURGERY

	Procedure		Approach Location and Size (mm)		Cutting Direction		Released Portions of the Deep Layer		
	USG	USA	Distal	Proximal	Retro	Antero	Proximal	Central	Distal
Nakamichi[9]		+	10–15			+	+	+	
Nakamichi[4]	+		4			+			
Lecoq[3]	+			5	+			+	
Rowe[6]	+			6	+			+	
Rojo[5]	+			1	+		+	+	+

USA, ultrasound assisted; USG, ultrasound guided.

The method described by Rojo-Manaute et al.[5] has the smallest incision (≤1 mm) for releasing all portions of the deepest fibrous layer through a forearm approach and without intrusion into superficial tissues (less theoretical collateral damage). The distal and central portions must be released for achieving a complete clinical decompression.

vision), from either a distal (palmar)[4,9] or a proximal (antebrachial)[3,6,10] approach, by either pulling (retrograde)[3,6,10] or pushing (anterograde)[4,9] the cutting instrument and by releasing the central,[3,6] central plus proximal, or all portions of the deepest layer[4,10] (Table 105-1). Nakamichi et al. clinically compared an ultrasound-assisted mini-CTR against a classic CTR[9] and, in a later study,[4] a USG percutaneous CTR against an ultrasound-assisted mini-CTR. The results of both studies,[4,9] favored the less-invasive approach in terms of grip strength, pain, and scar tenderness (until the sixth week) and scar sensitivity (until the thirteenth week). Prior research has also demonstrated the feasibility and safety of percutaneous USG CTR in cadaveric models.[3,6] However, some technical aspects of these ultrasound-guided procedures have raised concerns about their generalizability, including: (1) a large list of contraindications[4,9]; (2) the extent of the release at the deepest layer[3,4,6]; (3) the lack of formal anatomic safety studies on retrograde techniques; (4) the best location for the approach[4]; and (5) the best advancing direction of the instrument.[10]

In an effort to overcome these perceived limitations of the prior techniques, we recently performed an anatomic study in volunteers and cadavers for describing a retrograde USG CTR thru a 1-mm (ultra-minimally invasive surgery [*Ultra-MIS*]) distal antebrachial approach.[10] We defined Ultra-MIS as the incision size left by a 16-gauge Abbocath® (1.7-mm diameter), approximately 1 mm because of the skin's elasticity. Our results identified a safe release path following a coronal direction almost parallel to the longitudinal axis of the forearm and directing the cutting edge of the knife toward a volar-radial safe sector of at least 80.4 degrees on an axial plane (Figure 105-1). We recently clinically compared Ultra-MIS CTR versus mini-CTR (unpublished data) in a pilot study (40 randomized patients) to assess the safety and efficacy and subsequently in a randomized controlled trial of 92 patients with 1 year follow-up. Relative to mini-CTR, patients treated with Ultra-MIS were three to five times faster to return to work and daily activities (including work), to restore range of motion, and to stop the use of postoperative analgesics. Grip strength was improved in Ultra-MIS patients only during the first postoperative week, and there were no differences in the time course of paresthesia reduction between groups. Neither group developed relapses or neurovascular complications. An additional potential advantage of Ultra-MIS is that it is performed as an office-based ambulatory procedure, with potential cost savings as previously demonstrated for office-based ultrasound-guided trigger finger release.[13] At present, we hypothesize that similar findings could be expected for CTR, and an economic study is underway.

Thus, the clinical proposed advantages of an Ultra-MIS are (1) increased safety of the technique based on our formal anatomic studies; (2) decreased list of contraindications (none at present); (3) release of the etiological portions of the deepest fibrous layer; (4) decreased collateral damage to nonetiological structures (smaller skin approach and reduced damage to superficial anatomy to the deepest fibrous layer); (5) shorter recovery times; (6) better cosmesis; and (7) potentially more efficient outcomes.

FIGURE 105-1 ■ Position of the "safe zones" for aiming our instruments on an axial plane. The positions of the ulnar artery (a), ulnar vein (v), and median nerve (m) were measured from the safest theoretical point for releasing the deepest fibrous layer (1/2 h, midpoint between the ulnar artery and the median nerve) at three locations: the distal edge of the distal portion (CP_{dis}), the proximal edge (CP_{prox}) of the transverse carpal ligament (TCL), and at the "conflict zone" (CP_{cz}). The axial safe zone was the sector that excluded all these structures. Diagram **A** shows how we made our measurements,[5] and diagram **B** represents the position of the structures at risk and of the safe zones (which had at least 80.4 degrees and were located volar and radially from our origin). The conflict zone (CZ) was the section with the narrowest distance between the ulnar bundle and the median nerve and/or the most "out of line" release origin.[5] (Reproduced with permission from Rojo Manaute JM, Capa Grasa A, Rodríguez Maruri G, et al. Ultra minimally invasive ultrasound guided carpal tunnel release. Anatomic study of a new technique. *J Ultrasound Med.* 2013.)

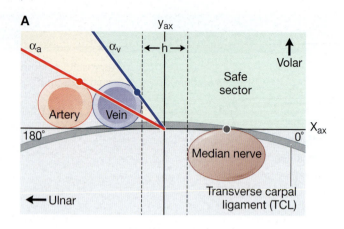

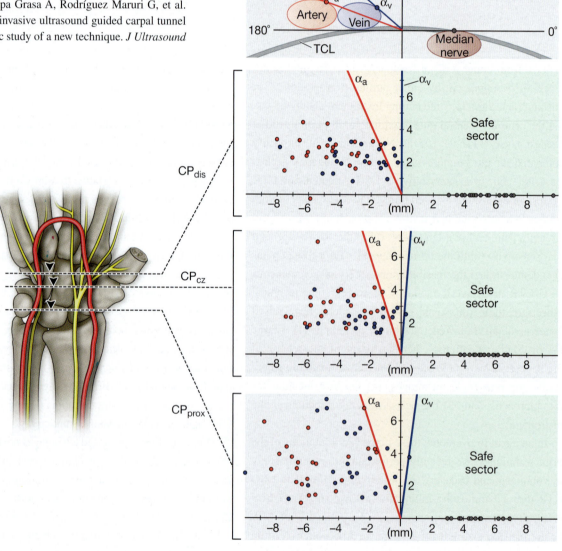

Equipment

- Needle: 25-gauge × 5/8" needle
- Injectate
  - 2.7 mL injectable anesthetic, without epinephrine
  - 0.3 mL sodium bicarbonate
- 1.5 mm Kirschner wire (KW)
- 16-gauge Abbocath
- 3-mm retrograde reusable hook knife
- 2% chlorhexidine aqueous solution (instead of ultrasound gel)
- High-frequency linear array transducer

Author's Preferred Technique

a. Patient position
   i. With the patient either seated or in supine position, our nurse performs a preoperative cleansing with 2% chlorhexidine solution for 5 minutes, protects the affected hand in a surgical drape, and leaves it resting supinated on an auxiliary table (covered by another surgical drape) at the patient's side.

b. Transducer position, approach, orientation, and target
   i. After injecting local anesthesia (Figure 105-2), we perform a three-step release of the deepest fibrous layer. Every step is double checked under long- and short-axis views.

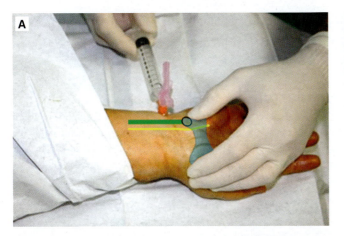
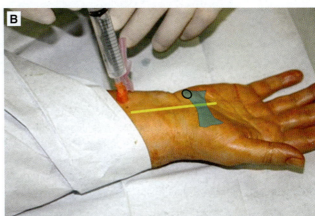
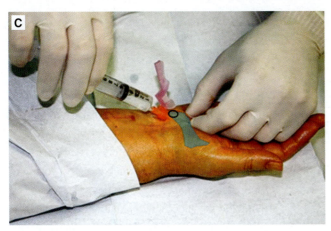
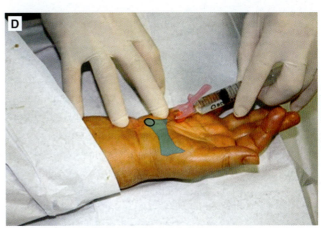

FIGURE 105-2 ■ Classic sequence followed for injecting local anesthesia. The ulnar nerve is anesthetized at the level of the desired skin crease and care is taken for adding a subcutaneous block at the level of the technique (**A**) followed by injecting anesthetic medially to the median nerve (**B**) and to its palmar cutaneous branch (**C**). Infiltration of tunnel's distal edge (**D**) allows for proceeding with the release seconds after, however, it is relatively more painful than the other punctures and it should be done lastly if elected. Note: at present, we prefer to inject 2 cc of local anesthesia using just step C under ultrasound guidance, keeping a 21G (11/2") needle between the intermediate and deep fibrous layers, from our entry point to the distal position where we will start the release.

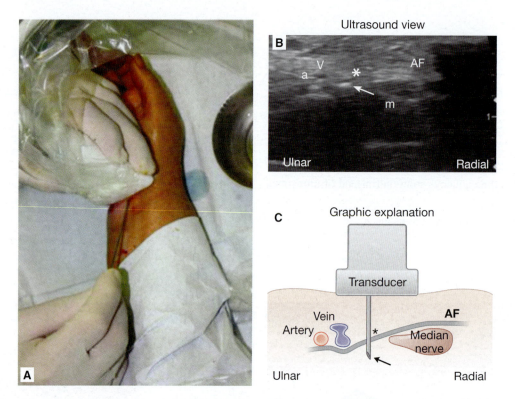

FIGURE 105-3 ■ Distal antebrachial technique. **A.** With the transducer applied transversely, we puncture the first available antebrachial skin crease ≥2 cm proximal to the pisiform. This technique maximizes esthetics, allows for comfortably maneuvering the instruments under the deep fibrous layer and for releasing 1 cm of the proximal fibrous portion before exiting. **B.** The ultrasound view. **C.** Graphical explanation of ultrasound view. *Arrow,* Abbocath's tip; a, ulnar artery; AF, antebrachial fascia; m, median nerve; v, ulnar vein. (Reproduced with permission from Rojo Manaute JM, Capa Grasa A, Rodríguez Maruri G, et al. Ultra minimally invasive ultrasound guided carpal tunnel release. Anatomic study of a new technique. *J Ultrasound Med.* 2013.)

ii. Step 1 (the approach): With the transducer placed transversely across the forearm, the skin is punctured with the Abbocath at the first available antebrachial skin crease approximately ≥2 cm proximal to the pisiform over the midpoint between the median nerve and the closest ulnar vascular structure. All fibrous layers are pierced to create a point of entry to the anatomic plane of the flexor tendons (Figure 105-3).

iii. Step 2 (intratunnel check): For assessing an intratunnel position, a blunt 1.5-mm Kirschner wire is advanced under ultrasound guidance from the entry point to the distal portion of deepest fibrous layer, while remaining in contact with its dorsal surface. The Kirchner wire is generally advanced using an in-plane approach (parallel to the long axis of the transducer), but its position is checked using orthogonal out-of-plane imaging (perpendicular to the short axis of the transducer), to monitor its proximity to the median nerve (located radially) and the ulnar neurovascular bundle (located ulnarly), as well as ensure that the wire remains in the same plane as the flexor tendons.

iv. Step 3 (the release): The cutting blade is advanced via the same approach with the blade facing ulnarly. The blade is advanced similarly to the Kirschner wire, using direct ultrasound guidance. To release the deep fibrous layer, the knife is advanced distal to a sudden narrowing of the deepest fibrous layer (which we have named the "duck's beak" because of its similar appearance), where it lies at least 2–3 mm proximal to the superficial palmar arch. The blade is then visualized out of plane (anatomic axial) to orient the tip of the knife such that is bisects the "safe zone" between the radially located median nerve and ulnarly located ulnar neurovascular bundle. After confirming placement in this out-of-plane view, the knife is revisualized using the in-plane view, and the tip is pressed volarly to position it ≤0.5 mm volar to the deepest fibrous layer. Once this position is confirmed, the knife is pulled retrograde in a controlled

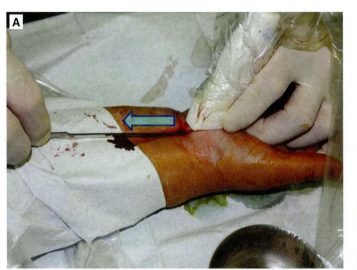

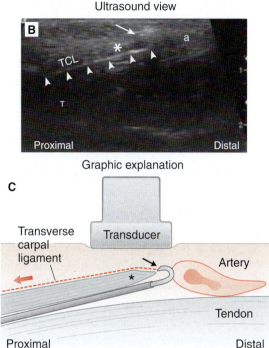

Ultrasound view

Graphic explanation

FIGURE 105-4 ■ Release. **A–C.** Under long-axis guidance, we introduce the hook knife to our distal cutting point, which is set distal to the "duck's beak" (*asterisk*). We check axially that the tip of the instrument is centered between the median nerve and the ulnar bundle for then turning the edge of our instrument toward our axial safe zone. The hook knife is then pulled retrogradely to exit through our skin approach, keeping the path of its tip ≤0.5 mm volar to the deepest fibrous layer (*grey dotted arrow*) while bisecting the axial safe zone. *Arrow,* hook knife's tip; a, ulnar artery; T, flexor tendons; TCL, transverse carpal ligament (central portion of the deepest fibrous layer). (Reproduced with permission from Rojo Manaute JM, Capa Grasa A, Rodríguez Maruri G, et al. Ultra minimally invasive ultrasound guided carpal tunnel release. Anatomic study of a new technique. *J Ultrasound Med.* 2013.)

manner to release the deep fibrous layer. The proximal fibrous layer portion is released for 1 cm proximal to the pisiform before exiting through our skin approach (Figure 105-4). The final skin wound is covered with an adhesive dressing that is removed in 2 days (Figure 105-5). Patients are encouraged to restart their normal lives from the same day of surgery and are given instructions for performing constant active and passive full range of motion during daytime.

c. Pearls

   i. The ulnar vessels and superficial vascular arch are the primary landmarks for the extent of the distal release and the major vasculature at risk.

   ii. If the distal extent of the flexor retinaculum (deepest fibrous layer) is not clearly distinguishable, the release should be started 2–3 mm proximal to the vascular bundle (superficial arch) bundle to ensure a complete distal release.

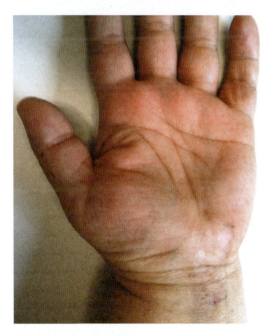

FIGURE 105-5 ■ Photograph of the wound 4 days after ultra-minimally invasive ultrasound-guided carpal tunnel release. (Note: the marks of the adhesive tape are still visible.)

iii. Axially, the blade must be directed toward the "safe zone" located radially and volarly from our release path.

iv. During the initial technique, the Abbocath should pierce all the fibrous layers four or five times to allow an easier introduction of the Kirschner wire and hook knife.

v. When introducing the 3-mm blade hook knife through the Abbocath skin incision, introduce the tip first for pushing, then gently the curved shape of the blade, and twist the instrument. At the same time, stretch the skin gently with the fingertips of the free hand.

vi. Once at the "right floor" (plane of the flexor tendons), the ulnar side of the tunnel will be the safe side: The ulnar bundle will now be in "another floor," and there will be a safe osseous wall ulnarly. However, the instrument should be kept against "the roof" (deepest fibrous layer), otherwise the hook could get tangled within the flexor tendons (if this happens, oscillating the instrument will free up the hook).

vii. The ulnar vessels should be the "lighthouse" throughout the process. Real time visualization will allow accurate CTR within less than 1 mm from the vascular bundle, however, be aware that the vessels may be collapsed by exerting too much pressure on the transducer with a loss of this reference. Thus, it is best to exert pressure on the transducer intermittently to check the location. The primary landmark for longitudinally positioning the distal cutting point should be the ulnar artery and superficial arch because the exact point at which the deepest fibrous layer ends distally ("duck's beak") may not always be clearly distinguishable. In this case, start the re-lease 2–3 mm proximally from the ulnar artery and superficial arch to avoid an incomplete release.

viii. When performing the release, the deepest fibrous layer may become undistinguishable from the intermediate fibrous layer if excessive transducer force is exerted. Use intermittent transducer pressure to facilitate distinguishing between the two layers. With practice, one may also feel a change in resistance at the tip of the instrument when the correct plane is identified.

ix. The proximal portion of the deepest fibrous layer is much thinner. As the cut is extended proximally, care should be taken to keep the blade tip at the correct plane to avoid unwanted intrusion of the more superficial tissues.

x. It is highly recommended to gain experience using both hands for manipulating the instruments.

d. Pitfalls

i. Failure to place the Abbocath at the most proximal antebrachial skin crease will result in a steep insertion angle and compromise the ability to keep the Abbocath and knife superficial within the carpal tunnel

ii. The hook knife should be introduced along the same path as the Abbocath in order to avoid placing the knife in a more superficial plane (eg, Guyon's canal).

iii. The most frequent error after reaching with the hook knife the subcutaneous plane is to push the instrument in a different direction than the one used during the technique with the Abbocath and Kirschner wire. This will usually position the instrument "at the wrong floor" (either in the Guyon's canal or directly over TCL). If this happened, oscillate the instrument in an ulnar-radial direction and pull back gently while keeping the blade away from the ulnar bundle (toward the safe zone).

References

1. Keith MW, Masear V, Amadio PC, et al. Treatment of carpal tunnel syndrome. *J Am Acad Orthop Surg* 2009;17:397–405.
2. Ono S, Clapham PJ, Chung KC. Optimal management of carpal tunnel syndrome. *Int J Gen Med* 2010;3:255–261.
3. Lecoq B, Hanouz N, Vielpeau C, Marcelli C. Ultrasound-guided percutaneous surgery for carpal tunnel syndrome: a cadaver study. *Joint Bone Spine* 2011;78:516–518.
4. Nakamichi K, Tachibana S, Yamamoto S, Ida M. Percutaneous carpal tunnel release compared with mini-open release using ultrasonographic guidance for both techniques. *J Hand Surg Am* 2010;35:437–445.
5. Rojo Manaute JM, Capa Grasa A, Rodríguez Maruri G, Moran LM, Villanueva Martínez M, J VM. Ultra minimally invasive ultrasound guided carpal tunnel release. Anatomic study of a new technique. *J Ultrasound Med.* 2013 Jan;32(1):131–142.
6. Rowe NM, Michaels Jt, Soltanian H, et al. Sonographically guided percutaneous carpal tunnel release: an anatomic and cadaveric study. *Ann Plast Surg* 2005;55:52–56; discussion 6.
7. Stecco C, Macchi V, Lancerotto L, et al. Comparison of transverse carpal ligament and flexor retinaculum terminology for the wrist. *J Hand Surg Am* 2010;35:746–753.

8. Cobb TK, Dalley BK, Posteraro RH, Lewis RC. Anatomy of the flexor retinaculum. *J Hand Surg Am* 1993;18:91–99.

9. Nakamichi K, Tachibana S. Ultrasonographically assisted carpal tunnel release. *J Hand Surg Am* 1997;22:853–862.

10. Rojo Manaute JM CGA, Rodríguez Maruri G, Moran LM, Villanueva Martínez M, J VM. Ultra minimally invasive ultrasound guided carpal tunnel release. Anatomic study of a new technique. *J Ultrasound Med* 2012 (in press).

11. Okutsu I, Hamanaka I, Tanabe T, Takatori Y, Ninomiya S. Complete endoscopic carpal canal decompression. *Am J Orthop (Belle Mead NJ)* 1996;25:365–368.

12. Yoshida A, Okutsu I, Hamanaka I. Is complete release of all volar carpal canal structures necessary for complete decompression in endoscopic carpal tunnel release? *J Hand Surg Eur Vol* 2007;32:537–542.

13. Rojo-Manaute JM, Capa-Grasa A, Cerro-Gutierrez MD, et al. Sonographically guided intrasheath percutaneous release of the first annular pulley for trigger digits, part 2: randomized comparative study of the economic impact of 3 surgical models. *J Ultrasound Med* 2012;31:427–438.

Darryl Eugene Barnes, MD

KEY POINTS

- The common extensor tendon of the elbow is a flat, conjoined tendon consisting of the four superficial extensor muscles originating from the anterolateral surface of the lateral epicondyle.
- The extensor carpi radialis brevis tendon forms most of the deep fibers that are often affected by tendinosis.

- The Tenex procedure is an ultrasound-guided minimally invasive percutaneous procedure that employs ultrasonographic real-time visualization and instrumentation to ultrasonically debride and aspirate tendinopathic tissue (tenotomy).
- The ultrasound-guided Tenex procedure for the lateral elbow approach is in plane and distal to proximal.

Pertinent Anatomy

The common extensor tendon of the elbow is a flat, conjoined tendon consisting of the four superficial extensor muscles: extensor carpi radialis brevis, extensor digitorum communis, extensor digiti minimi, and extensor carpi ulnaris origination from the anterolateral surface of the lateral epicondyle. The extensor carpi radialis brevis forms most of the deep fibers (most commonly affected by tendinosis), whereas a majority of the superficial common extensor tendon is comprised of the extensor digitorum communis. The remaining two tendons contribute minimally to the common extensor tendon. These muscles contribute to wrist extension and radial and ulnar deviation. The radial collateral ligament lies deep to the common extensor tendon and superficial to the radiocapitellar joint. Moreover, anterior and medial to the origin of the common extensor tendon lies the main trunk of radial nerve.

The normal common extensor tendon is characterized ultrasonographically by a dense hyperechoic fibrillar echotextured structure (long axis), located superficial to the dense hyperechoic bone of the lateral epicondyle (Figure 106-1).

Common Pathology

Common extensor tendinosis, commonly referred to as *tennis elbow* or *lateral epicondylitis*, is a common and debilitating cause of elbow pain. It has been confirmed to be a degenerative process and more accurately termed *tendinosis* and has been described histologically as angiofibroblastic hyperplasia of the tendon.[4] It presents clinically with pain located over the lateral elbow that is exacerbated with palpation of the epicondylar area and wrist extension. Most patients (>90%) recover with nonsurgical treatment, such as rest, ice, elbow

straps, physical therapy, nonsteroidal medication, and injection. Patients who fail conservative treatment may be selected for an operative procedure such as an open, arthroscopic tool-guided or percutaneous tenotomy. The purpose of the tenotomy procedure is to incise and partially release the common extensor tendon (all three tenotomy procedures) and visually debride the diseased portion of the tendon (open and arthroscopic-guided tenotomy procedures).[1] Multiple studies have demonstrated 70–95% of patients have "good to excellent" outcomes, with arthroscopic-guided debridement showing the best results.[1] The Tenex procedure uses ultrasound to identify the tendinopathic lesion (tendinosis) and ultrasonographically guide a small tool to debride the lesion in real time through a 4-mm incision. Early data demonstrate similar outcomes found with arthroscopic tool-guided tenotomy procedures.[2]

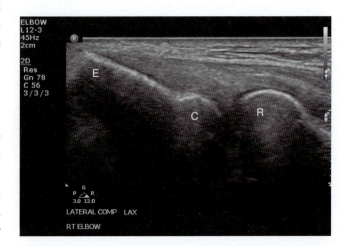

FIGURE 106-1 ■ Normal ultrasonographic appearance of the common extensor tendon in long-axis view. E, lateral epicondyle; C, capitulum; R, radial head.

Ultrasound Imaging Findings

Tendinosis presents ultrasonographically as an inhomogeneous hypoechoic area within a tendon, demonstrating increased intrafibrillar distance or loss of the fibrillar pattern, resulting in thickening of the tendon (Figure 106-2). In some patients, partial tears of the tendon are also found. Cortical irregularities of the lateral epicondyle, which may include an enthesophyte at the apex, are frequently seen. Increased blood flow from neovascularization may also be seen with color or power Doppler function utilization.[3]

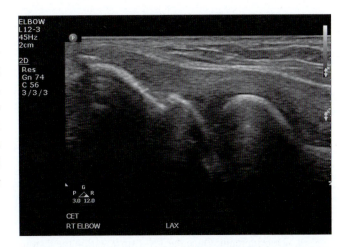

FIGURE 106-2 ■ Ultrasonographic appearance of tendinosis of the common extensor tendon.

Indication for the Tenex Procedure

Patients who fail nonoperative therapy (eg, rest, ice, physical therapy, nonsteroidal medication, and injection) over a period longer than 3 months are candidates for the Tenex procedure.

Equipment

- Needle: 25-gauge, 2-inch needle
- Injectate: 2–4 mL injectable local anesthetic
- TX-1 Tissue Removal System disposable handpiece (Tenex Health, Inc., Lake Forrest, CA) (Figure 106-3)
- No. 11 scalpel
- High-frequency linear array transducer

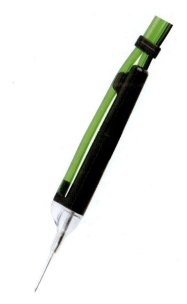

FIGURE 106-3 ■ TX-1 Tissue Removal System disposable handpiece.

Author's Preferred Technique

a. Procedure
   i. Use universal precautions.
   ii. Diagnostic scan: Confirm tendinosis of the common extensor tendon in two orthogonal planes. Confirm the location of the radial nerve near the lateral epicondyle and mark the overlying skin with a surgical marker to prevent any injuries to this nerve during the procedure.
b. Patient position and preparation
   i. Supine with elbow flexed 60–90 degrees resting either on arm board (Figure 106-4) or on abdomen.
   ii. Preparation: Standard surgical scrub and sterile draped applied to elbow (standards may vary by institution or facility).
   iii. Skin marking: Place mark on skin with sterile surgical marker at the distal end of the transducer in long axis (Figure 106-5).

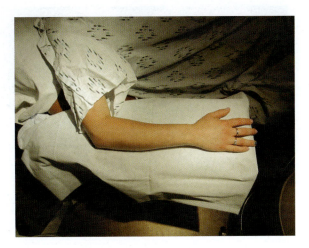

FIGURE 106-4 ■ Patient in supine position with elbow flexed near 90 degrees for the Tenex procedure.

c. Transducer position, anesthesia, and procedure

    i. Position the transducer long axis over the lateral epicondyle (see Figure 106-5).

    ii. Inject 1% local anesthetic into skin, subcutaneous tissue, tendon lesion, and bony area at the origin of the diseased tendon.

    iii. Make a 4-mm long-axis incision (stab wound) distal to transducer (Figure 106-6).

    iv. TX-1 handpiece tip placement: insert distal to proximal into incision under direct visualization and then locate and guide tip to tendinopathic region under ultrasound guidance (Figure 106-7A, B).

    v. Debridement: Once the TX-1 tip is within the lesion, the foot pedal is depressed to activate the ultrasonic tip of the device to start the debridement process (Figure 106-8). Move the tip in a back-and-forth motion along the long axis of the tendon ensuring that the entire lesion has been debrided. This is a process of debriding and scanning in several short sessions lasting approximately 3–5 seconds. Most lesions will require 30–50 seconds of treatment. Microbubbles are produced from the process and are easily seen as a hyperechoic area within the treated lesion, demarcating the area that has been treated. Scan the area to ensure that the entire lesion has been treated and then remove the device and apply pressure to the wound to ensure good hemostasis.

    vi. Dressing the wound: Apply skin closure adhesive tape, occlusive dressing, and compressive bandage or sleeve.

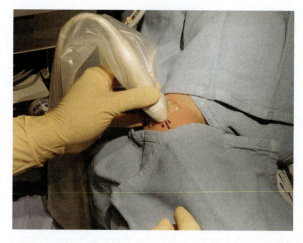

FIGURE 106-5 ■ Skin marking to help position transducer and guide placement of scalpel for the creation of the incision in the long axis of the tendon.

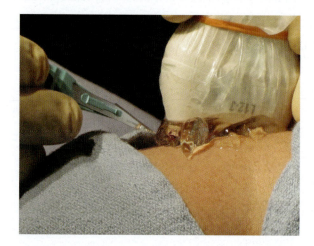

FIGURE 106-6 ■ Scalpel is held in long axis to tendon with sharp edge up to avoid incision into deeper structures.

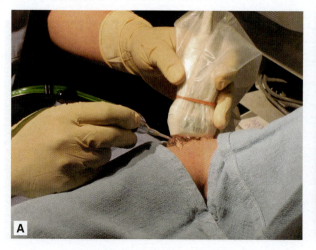 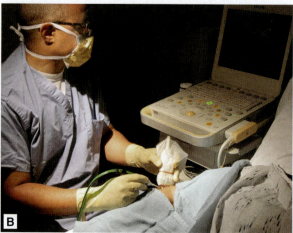

FIGURE 106-7 ■ **A.** Handpiece is inserted into the incision along the long axis of the common extensor tendon. **B.** Demonstrates positioning of patient and equipment.

vii. Post procedure: Encourage shoulder, elbow, and wrist gentle range of motion immediately. Standard wound care protocol (keep area clean, change bandage as needed, use over-the-counter pain relievers as directed when needed and as tolerated and apply ice to area for pain control if needed). Prescribe work and activity restrictions (no lifting, pushing, pulling with upper extremity for 2 weeks and then liberalize over 4 weeks depending on upper extremity activity level). Schedule follow-up appointment (author has patients return in 2 and 6 weeks).

d. Pearls

i. Although this procedure does not take much time to perform, it is a wise to use good ergonomic technique. Make sure that the patient is resting in a comfortable position and that the patients' elbow is just above your waist allowing your shoulder to rest with your elbows at your sides.

ii. It is recommended that you start at either edge of the diseased tendon and work your way to the other edge, ensuring the entire lesion has been treated. As described above, use the microbubbles to help guide you away from the areas that have already been treated.

iii. Communicate clearly to the patient and give written instructions about postprocedural care, including the importance of immediate and continued gentle full range of motion elbow exercises.

e. Pitfalls

i. Ensure that the radial nerve has been scanned during the pre-scan portion of the procedure to avoid damage to this structure. It is good practice to mark the skin overlying the nerve in the procedure area to ensure the patient's safety.

ii. Avoid overtreating an area; it typically only requires 30–50 seconds of energy time (the time the device is activated) to treat an entire elbow tendon lesion.

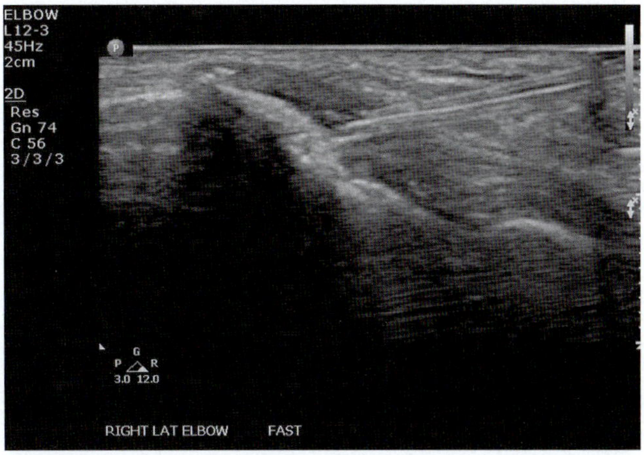

FIGURE 106-8 ■ Showing the tip of the device within the tendinopathic area of the common extensor tendon.

References

1. Szabo SJ, Savoie FH, Field LD, Ramsey JR, Hosemann CD. Tendinosis of the extensor carpi radialis brevis: An evaluation of three methods of operative treatment. *J Shoulder Elbow Surg* 2006;15:721–727.

2. Koh JS, et al. Fasciotomy and surgical tenotomy for recalcitrant lateral elbow tendinopathy: Early clinical experience with a novel device for minimally invasive percutaneous microresection. *Am J Sports Med.* 2013;41:636.

3. Bianchi S, Martinoli C. In: Bianchi S, Martinoli C, Baert AL, Knauth M, Sartor K. *Ultrasound of the Musculoskeletal System.* Berlin, Germany: Springer-Verlag: 2007:378-380.

4. Kraushaar BS, Nirschl RP. Tendinosis of the elbow (tennis elbow), Clinical features and findings of histological, immuno-histochemical, and electron microscopy studies. *J Bone Joint Surg Am* 1999;81:259-278.

Note: Page numbers followed by *f* indicate figures; and page numbers followed by *t* indicate tables.

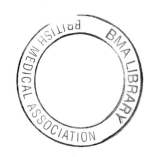